It's Good to Know a Miracle: Dani's Story

It's Good to Know a Miracle: Dani's Story

One family's struggle with leukemia

by

Jay and Sue Shotel

Gordian Knot Books

An Imprint of Richard Altschuler & Associates, Inc.

New York

It's Good To Know A Miracle: Dani's Story: One Family's Struggle with Leukemia. Copyright ©2008 by Jay and Sue Shotel.
For information contact the publisher, Richard Altschuler & Associates, Inc., at 100 West 57th Street, New York, NY 10019, RAltschuler@rcn.com or
(212) 397-7233.

Library of Congress Control Number: 2007943119
CIP data for this book are available from the Library of Congress

ISBN-13: 978-1-884092-74-9

ISBN-10: 1-884092-74-8

Gordian Knot Books is an imprint of
Richard Altschuler & Associates, Inc.

Cover Art: Dani Shotel

Design and Layout: Josh Garfield

Printed in the United States of America

Distributed by University of Nebraska Press

Acknowledgements

We are a blessed family. Blessed with family, friends, professional colleagues, the very finest medical support, caring public school systems (despite their enormity), and great medical insurance. We came to learn that it didn't just "take a village"…it actually took the entire world to help us get through what would be the greatest challenge of all of our collective lives.

From Dr. Schreiner's initial insistence to draw blood, the superb medical practice of Arlington Fairfax Hematology Oncology, specifically, Drs. Robert Christie, John Feigert, Thomas Butler, and Robert Meister; the caring staff of the oncology wing at the Virginia Hospital Center, Arlington, particularly the nursing staff and Dr. William Furlong, an infectious diseases specialist at VHC, to the incredible specialists at the Fred Hutchinson Cancer Research Center (including Drs. Rainier Storb, Mark Stewart, Paul Martin, Mary Flowers, Fred Applebaum and staff, including Betty Stewart P. A., Diane Stayboldt (head nurse, Blue Team), Kerry McMillen (Nutritionist), Andréa Leiserowitz (Physical Therapist), Corrine, Dani's primary nurse at University of Washington Hospital, and the incredibly positive team that drew Dani's blood daily at "the Hutch," our family is forever grateful. Your focus, commitment, expertise and smiles made even the most painful experiences bearable. Several professionals deserve special mention. Robert Christie became Dani's primary doctor the moment she was diagnosed on September 11th. Despite being the bearer of pretty horrific news, he quickly became a favorite. His honesty, no-nonsense approach, helpfulness, and sense of humor were a great asset to Dani, from her initial diagnosis and hospitalization to her post-transplant care. Thanks also to Fred Applebaum, a giant in the field, who took the time to respond directly, within hours, to our request for a consultation and a meeting in Seattle at the Hutch. With great confidence he told us, "they would find a donor" (and they did!). Dani was also fortunate enough to have him as her attending physician for a month, after the transplant occurred. Rainier Storb, internationally recognized as a leader in this field as well, met with our family in October 2002 for our initial consult at the Hutch. He took his turn, as all the doctors do at the Hutch, to interview prospective transplant patients. He also spent a great deal of time educating our family about the transplant process, even detailing ways that their team responded to any problem that might arise, and to assure us that if something didn't work there was always a "Plan B" to make it right. (Boy…did that come in handy!) Finally, Herman Manganzini, our longtime family physician who, when we were being bombarded by advice from all well-meaning people, told us that the initial treatment plan was the right way to go, and there was no need to move Dani after the initial diagnosis, as the treatment protocol was standard and the staff at Virginia Hospital Center was more than up to the task. (Right again!)

Our family and family-to-be (the Greenes) were ever-present. Scott Greene, Dani's boyfriend at the time, managed miracles of all kinds. Not only did he dedicate his life and love to Dani from the onset of her diagnosis, he also organized and implemented our most successful fundraising events — 2 Washington Wizards games. He never missed a day visiting Dani in the hospital in Arlington, and even tele-commuted frequently to his job in D.C. from Seattle in 2003. How he managed to do all of this and continue working was amazing to all of us — especially in light of the fact that Dani and Scott had just started dating in May of 2002. His unquestioning faith in Dani's ability to beat leukemia was a critical factor in her convalescence. Additionally, our son Micah, a brother extraordinaire, researched leukemia and the best medical facilities to treat and cure his sister. His unquestioning willingness to provide his bone marrow for his beloved Dani, his disappointment when he was not a match, and his no-nonsense normalcy became a comfort for us all. Then, there was Dani's Aunt Carol and Uncle Bruce. They joined us in our medical consultations, often asking questions that we didn't think to ask. Dani's cousins Ari, Heather, and Jason all came through, were devoted to Dani, and were quite active in the bone marrow drives.

Like family, our various workplaces provided much needed support. The colleagues who worked with Jay at George Washington University in the Graduate School of Education and Human Development offered hope, best wishes, and hot meals for us in those first weeks when one of us was always at Dani's side. The Montgomery County Public Schools expedited Sue's emergency leave quite painlessly…the Employee Assistance Program helped both of us, as parents, come to terms with our daughter's illness, and helped in the promotion of the county's bone marrow drive. Don Kress, a friend, professional colleague, and the Associate Superintendent, deserves special recognition, along with Dave Brubaker, the now-retired principal of Earle B. Wood Middle School, for their unwavering support in our time of need. Dave not only took the leadership with Susan Hoopes, a Wood Middle School parent, to organize an MCPS and community bone marrow drive in November of 2002 at Wood, but also led "Team Wood" in a 50 mile run in November of 2002, raising over $13,000 to support cancer treatment-related expenses. Arlington County Public Schools, the teachers Dani worked with, as well as the teachers she didn't know, and their special education administrative staff, were equally supportive with their total commitment to Dani in her time of need. Within two months of Dani's diagnosis, 120 days of sick leave had been donated by the teachers of Arlington County — and it was only Dani's second year in the system. Additionally, where other districts chose not to rehire untenured staff in similar situations, Arlington County provided Dani with a non-teaching, supervisory position in the fall following her transplant, to ensure that her immune system had additional time to rebuild. Special mention must be given to Laurie Alderman, her immediate supervisor, who made sure that Dani had every piece of information and document necessary to ensure that the benefits accrued by an employee would seamlessly flow. Within 24 hours of Dani's initial hospitalization, all necessary paperwork, including insurance and disability information, was in our hands. It should be noted that the personal support was just as strong as the professional support, as she was one of many who traveled to Seattle to support us during the transplant and recovery process. She made sure that Dani's students had the best of care as well, and took major responsibility for organizing the Arlington County Bone Marrow Drive, where people had to be turned away.

We never realized how many true friends Dani had. They were amazing. They surrounded her constantly in the hospital, and provided her with support, humor, love, and lots of cards, stuffed animals, and best wishes whenever they couldn't be present. They formed a network to communicate Dani's progress, until her brother established a website, in October, and organized and attended fundraisers for Dani and for the Leukemia and Lymphoma Society, as well as for other cancer research and support organizations. Liz Lichtman, Ally Frank, Yvonne Townesly, roommate Matt Levine, Marisa Tjerandsen, school colleagues Laurie Alderman and Sarah Scorza, and college buddies Topher Patterson and Kat Palotta Fitzgerald rarely missed a day of either visits or calls to keep Dani's spirits up. A special acknowledgement to Liz Lichtman, former college schoolmate of Dani's, and Jay's administrative assistant when Dani was diagnosed. It was Liz's organization, chutzpah, and positive attitude that kept all of us going, particularly her boss, Jay. She led in the organization of all bone marrow drives, was our contact person with all of the various agencies involved in these plans, was instrumental in fund-raising activities, and also prioritized the tasks that needed to be done at Jay's office. She did everything in her power to help her dear friend and her family, as did every member of Dani's "fan club."

Our friends were incredible as well. Sandy Davis and Bonnie and Steve Spivack organized a bone marrow drive at our temple, Beth Ami, and also visited with us in Seattle. In addition, Steve, an attorney, did some investigative work for us about setting up our own charity in Dani's name, and recommended our utilization of the National Transplant Assistance Fund (NTAF) as a vehicle to support our fund-raising activities (more about NTAF later). Burton and Wendy Katzen ran a bone marrow drive

at their temple, Washington Hebrew Congregation, as well. We recall
Burton's genuine sadness at not having a huge turnout because of an
untimely snowstorm. The efforts of Burton and Wendy, Sandy, Bonnie
and Steve, Laurie, Liz, and Susan produced over 1,000 new potential
donors for the National Marrow Donor Programs. To date, at least eight
potential matches for other transplant-eligible patients have been found
from the series of bone marrow drives sponsored by our support system.
These friends and others too numerous to mention, including some we
didn't even know, took us into their lives as they embraced our cause as
their own.

On the other coast, Micah's friends, especially Cameron, Kat, and
Beth, became Dani's friends. From their visits to the U.W. hospital as
well as to our Seattle-based apartment at the Marriott Residence Inn,
they managed to bring laughter and smiles to Dani. Together, we voted
for Clay and Reuben on "American Idol," and sat on the edge of our
chairs for the first season of "24." These West Coast friends made it
bearable to ease the loneliness caused by the distance separating Dani
from her East Coast support system.

It was a group decision (Dani, Micah, Scott, and the two of us)
to welcome all offered encouragement. Scott's parents, Gayle and
John Greene, formed a prayer circle at their church, as did our friends
and colleagues at both of our places of employment. Our rabbi, Jack
Luxemburg, mentioned Dani frequently at services and offered prayers
for her healing. The sisterhood at Beth Ami contacted a temple in Seattle
whose sisterhood in Seattle frequently called with offers of support. Sue's
manicurist, Mindy, even gave her a Buddha to display in our apartment.

We can't imagine a more positive environment than the one we
experienced in Seattle. From the caring personnel at the Fred Hutchinson
Cancer Research Center in Seattle, the staff of the transplant wing at the
University of Washington Medical Center, the overwhelming kindness
shown by the residents of Seattle, to the special treatment we received
at the Marriott's Residence Inn on Lake Union (especially the shuttle
driver, Lewis, who made sure that Dani always had a ride to the Hutch

when she needed one), there was never a doubt in our minds that Dani's comfort was their priority. The Residence Inn has created a normalized environment for the transplant patients who reside there during treatment, and trying to feel normal is critically important for the transplant patient. To this day we believe that the residents of Seattle promote the rumor of rain and gloom to keep the city to themselves. We may have had some rain in Seattle, but for our family, the sun was always shining.

The related organizations were tremendously helpful as well. Special thanks to Sharon Gallop at the Red Cross, Denise Lim at the National Marrow Donor Program, Sarah Singer at the Leukemia and Lymphoma Society, Rochelle Sislen at the Gift of Life Foundation, and the parents of Allison Atlas, who brought the Atlas Foundation assistance to our Bone Marrow Drive efforts. These wonderful representatives of the various support organizations provided kind words, critical information, manpower, and guidance.

And finally there's Tom Heimhuber, Dani's donor, for without him there is no story. By his single act of kindness, he has given us more joy than could ever be imagined.

Contents

Preface

We have several reasons for writing this book. The first is to give cancer patients and their families hope. The second is to stress to the reader that self-advocacy and involvement must be the watchwords for patients and their families. Take nothing for granted, ask questions, take good notes, and take control of the battle against the disease. Perhaps it is the educator in us that has compelled us to tell this powerful story because of its lessons. It is our hope that we can share some of those lessons with the reader to make their lives a bit easier during this struggle. As a family our experience reinforced for us the importance of positive thinking; that love and friendship can be valuable antidotes to illness; that action assisted by knowledge is critical; and that education, advocacy, and self-determination are key factors in this process.

In the words of Laura Landro, assistant managing editor of the *Wall Street Journal* and a leukemia survivor, whose book *Survivor* was of significant help to us when our daughter went through a similar struggle:

...all patients can — and must — arm themselves with the facts, learn to understand medical jargon, get doctors to answer all their questions in layman's terms, weigh conflicting medical opinions, and make the difficult choice among the options open to them.

It is our hope that this book will help in reinforcing that notion, as Ms. Landro's book did for us.

Because of the technical nature of the content and the sheer number of persons who played significant roles, we have provided several resources for the reader in the last two sections of the appendix: the first is a *glossary of terms* that we have attempted to define in non-medical language wherever possible; and the second is a *list of characters* as there are a great many significant people in Dani's battle with the disease. If a person was mentioned more than once in the story, then we have identified him or her in the appendix.

The world is winning the battle against this dreaded disease. Our parents' generation knew cancer as a death sentence where today our generation fears the disease but sees the fight as winnable. Let us hope that our children will learn that cancer, like other diseases, is an enemy that we overcame as part of the history of our civilization.

Prologue

It was the perfect summer for 26-year-old Dani Shotel. She was looking forward to beginning her second year at the Walter Reed School in Arlington County, Virginia. Dani taught 2-to-3-year-old children with special needs in the "Integration Station," an inclusive program for both normally developing and developmentally delayed pre-school children. Teaching was her passion, but we always suspected that she was destined to work with children. Her dad, Jay, was a professor of special education, and chair of the department responsible for teacher education at George Washington University; and her mom, Sue, a former special education and social studies teacher, was now an administrator with the Montgomery County, Maryland Public Schools. It appears that our daughter inherited the "teaching gene." Even as a child, Dani was always the one who was seated next to the new student, the student who couldn't speak English, or the student who had difficulty learning. In a school system that emphasized challenging the best and brightest students, we often described Dani as "gifted in being nice."

Dani had spent her first 18 years in Gaithersburg, Maryland, a commuter suburb of Washington, D.C. She and her beloved younger brother, Micah, had attended Dufief Elementary School (which was across the soccer field from our back yard), Robert Frost Intermediate School, and Thomas Wootton High School. By her middle school years, she became interested in playing softball. Encouraged by her dad, Dani began to practice pitching. Dani always displayed tremendous patience, and was a great listener. Though not what one would call a natural athlete, she was incredibly "coachable." With her dad as her catcher, she would practice for hours, and attended many clinics. So it was no surprise that by her freshman year Dani made the junior varsity fast pitch softball squad at her high school. This desire to excel through hard work and her coachable nature proved to be major factors in Dani's triumph over cancer. Tiny for a fast pitch softball pitcher at 5-foot-3¾-inches and 115 pounds, Dani was urged by her coaches to use her entire body while pitching. She even used her voice in a Monica Seles-type grunt when releasing her pitches. Not overpowering as a pitcher, Dani could throw a variety of pitches with incredible accuracy. As her sophomore season approached, Dani found herself in the role of starting pitcher for the varsity team. In the years that followed, Dani was named first team All County and honorable mention All-Met (D.C. metropolitan area) by the *Washington Post.* Her involvement in a very talented summer tournament travel team led to inquiries by college coaches and several scholarship offers. Eventually, Dani decided on Lafayette College, a small liberal arts college in Easton, Pennsylvania with a stellar academic program and an NCAA Division I Athletic Program, where she continued to pitch until her senior year. With her dad as coach, Dani played women's summer league softball for three years after graduation from college while earning a graduate degree and beginning her teaching career. The many attributes of Dani's involvement in sports, like her physical conditioning and the ability to focus, proved to be essential elements of her treatment.

After graduating in 1998 from Lafayette, Dani attended George Washington University and received a masters' degree in Special Education/Early Childhood. She, along with her chocolate Labrador Retriever, Phoebe, left our home in Gaithersburg and began living the independent lifestyle that is common in the Washington, D.C. area among young professionals. Between school and friends, her life was filled with adventures both challenging and joyous.

By the summer of 2002, Dani had found true love in the person of Scott Greene. They had met casually through mutual friends, and continued an e-mail correspondence friendship for almost a year. Scott, a recent graduate of the University of Virginia, personable, tall and handsome, continued to pursue Dani…and by the end of May, in 2002,

Dani and Scott are an "item." It looked like the real thing.

So, as the reader now understands, life was good. Dani and Scott were together constantly, experiencing the joy of young love. By mid-August, Dani and Phoebe (Scott had to work) joined us in the Outer Banks for a few days of relaxation, enjoying a brief respite before the beginning of the school year. It was a wonderful vacation (even though we were minus our son, Micah, who remained in Seattle where he had completed undergraduate school, and was running his own web development and graphic design firm with two of his college buddies). Dani talked about spending the next weekend at the parents of one Scott's friends on the Chesapeake Bay, and the following weekend camping with Scott and several other friends. Life couldn't get much better!

Chapter One
It's Just a Sore Throat

Dani's Memories: 8/30 – 9/10/02

August 30, Friday night: *I work at Oilily (a children's clothing store in a local mall). I am supposed to meet Scott and some friends after work. I tell him that my throat is sore and I want to be in better shape for our camping trip (the following day).*

    August 31, Saturday morning: *I wake up and my throat feels like really bad strep throat. I call Scott and tell him that I'm going to go to the Prime Care Medical Clinic off of Rte. 50 and that our camping trip is more than likely cancelled. I call Liz and tell her that the camping trip is off and she gives me a hard time (wouldn't you know it!). I see Dr. Schreiner. He cultures my throat. He says that it really doesn't look that red, but it sounds like strep and because I've been prone to it she will start me on the antibiotics. I go to the CVS pharmacy on the corner of Lee Highway and Route 7 (little did they know that those pharmacists were soon to become some of my closest friends). I pick up my Z-Pac and head for home. I camp out in front of the TV for the rest of the day.*

    September 1, Sunday morning: *I wake up and start coughing up blood in the sink. I call my parents crying. They instruct me to call back the medical clinic. The doctor instructs me to go to the emergency room...and says, "Coughing up blood does not sound like strep throat... go to the emergency room." My strep culture with her is still pending and we won't be able to know the results of it for a couple more days. I call Scott and he races over. He drives me to Arlington Hospital Center. We wait in the waiting room for what seems like hours. Finally we are seen for all of 5 minutes. A doctor comes in and tells me that my throat doesn't look all that red and if a strep culture is already taken, then* *that is all that could be done. "Rest and drink lots of fluids" is her advice to me. Walking to Scott's car in the parking lot, I call both my mom and dad. I am crying (not only because I feel sick...but, I also feel stupid). I don't want Scott to think I was being a hypochondriac and I don't want to ruin their Labor Day weekend worrying about me.*

September 2, Monday morning: *Labor Day...and I sleep almost the entire day.*

September 3, Tuesday: *I wake up horribly sick (throwing up, coughing up blood and in a lot of pain). I call my principal, Laurie Alderman. I tell her how I feel and she tells me not to come into work. She says, "Worst case scenario some of the other staff will help your two assistants set up your classroom if you're not able to come in for a few days." I try to make an appointment to see Dr. Deluca...but she isn't in. So I see her partner (Dr. Schreiner). He walks in and I burst into tears. He remains very professional and allows me to explain what hurts. I tell him about everything. He looks into my throat and again it does not appear inflamed. He asks me about what I've done the last couple of weeks. I tell him about Scott and my trip to Matt Sutton's parents' river house (by the mouth of the Chesapeake Bay). He thinks that because the trip had been in August and the water temps had been so warm it was possible that I have developed some sort of bacterial infection. Because of this, he puts me on some steroids as well as pain meds...and I think a couple of other drugs. Again...I stop by CVS on my way home.*

September 4, Wednesday: *I wake up that morning not feeling any better and call Laurie. She tells me to go back to the doctor. I go back and see Dr. Deluca. She tells me that I haven't given the medicine a long enough chance to work. I just need to go home and rest and drink lots of fluids. I call dad and cry on my way home from the doctors. Dad then calls the medical clinic and finds out that my strep culture has come back positive for strep. I continue to cough up blood and can't keep anything down. I start drinking PediaSure...but it doesn't stay down either.*

September 5, Thursday: *I wake up and call Laurie. She tells me to go back to the doctor again. I was delirious and don't remember the rest of the* *day. The medication plus whatever illness I have is making me terribly sick.*

September 6, Friday: *I wake up and call Laurie. Laurie tells me my room is all set up and not to worry about a thing. She is going to run my open-house for the children and their parents. I speak to both mom and dad. They decide that it would be best if I stayed with them for a night and got some chicken soup into my system. All I remember is that I can't drive due to all the medication I am on at that point. Dad comes and picks me up after work. I remember sitting in their sun room looking at the new couches and that was it.*

September 7, Saturday: *My parents drive back with me to my place in Falls Church. We start moving stuff from my bedroom (small room) in to the back bedroom with the bathroom. My parents are disgusted with my sloppy ways. I am exhausted. I want to cry.*

September 9, Monday night: *I discover the bruises all over my body. When I tell my mom, she says to go to the doctor again tomorrow and get a blood draw.*

September 10, Tuesday: *I go into work. It feels like the parents will never leave my classroom after dropping off their kids. I have no energy and the pain is excruciating. After the parents finally are ushered out by Laurie, I sneak into the kid's bathroom in my classroom. I splash some cool water on my face. Leaning on the sink, I begin to cry. Marbea (the Occupational Therapist) follows me in and tells me that I need to go back to the doctor. I have an appointment for later that day...but I go over around 9:00 a.m. The receptionist, who by this time is extremely used to seeing me, fits me into the doctor's schedule as soon as she sees me walk in. Five minutes later I am in an examining room. My doctor walks in and I tell her that she has to draw blood because my mom said to. She tells me she would like to consult with her partner. He walks back into the examining room with her. Dr. Schreiner takes one look at me (remembering me from the past Tuesday) and tells his partner "draw her blood." I go home after the blood is drawn.*

Sue's Memories: 8/30 – 9/10/02

I remember the phone calls back and forth to Dani during that Labor Day weekend. Jay and I are visiting our cousins Jeff and Joann in Margate, New Jersey. The first call comes Friday afternoon while we are having lunch at an outdoor cafe. Dani tells me about her sore throat, her visit to the doctor, the medicine prescribed, and her change of plans for the weekend. Fortunately, the outdoor café is tented as it is raining. I am glad to hear that Dani had cancelled her plans to go camping. The second call comes the following morning. I am sitting in the guest room staring out the window at the gloomy weather. Dani tells me about coughing up blood. I remember agreeing that she should go to the emergency room and I anxiously wait to hear from her again with the results.

We keep in touch more frequently than our normal two or three calls a day the next week. Dani continues to complain about her throat – but tells us that her doctor advised her to be patient and let the medications do their job.

Later on in the week once we return from the Jersey Shore, we alter our plans for Erev Rosh Hashanah (the evening before the beginning of the Jewish High Holiday, Rosh Hashanah). Originally, we planned a festive dinner followed by attending a religious service at our synagogue. Because Dani is feeling under the weather, however, we just have a quiet dinner, which includes matzo ball soup, a sure cure-all for Dani's sore throat. Dani spends the night in her old bedroom and Saturday morning we take her back to her house (which she shares with three roommates) in Falls Church, Virginia. Our plan is to help Dani move from a smaller bedroom in the front of the house to a larger bedroom in the back of the house (which has its own bathroom).

I remember being appalled (which is the universal reaction of all parents upon viewing their adult child's bedroom) at the mess in Dani's bedroom. I let her know my feelings. Dani is pretty weepy. I just chalk it up to Dani being Dani and me being my outspoken self. Since Dani's vacuum cleaner was broken, Jay and I leave (which was a good thing since I am still steaming) to purchase a new one. We continue cleaning and then, on Sunday, we move Dani's "This End Up" furniture (by the way, the heaviest furniture in the world) to the larger bedroom. Dani helps out but continues to look under the weather.

Monday evening, as I am driving home from dinner with a professional colleague, Dani calls me on her cell phone. She tells me that she has bruises all over her body. I am shocked, and don't know what to think. At that point, I say the smartest thing I ever said in my life, something that I don't know where the words came from. I say, "When you go to the doctor tomorrow, tell her to draw blood." When I arrive home, I tell Jay of my conversation with Dani. Jay, as always, balances my panic with his studied calm and says in an understated way, "Oh, she's probably bruised from moving all that furniture this past weekend." He may have said that, but then he gets on the phone with our cousin, a medical doctor, David Laskin. You can depend on David to tell it like is…and David is worried.

Chapter Two
The Plan

Dani's Memories

Wednesday, September 11, 2002: *Our family plan: Dad is not going into work today (his office is very close to the Department of State). Instead he comes over to make me breakfast (my favorite, French toast). For some reason, I'm feeling better that morning. Dr. Schreiner calls me at around 6:30 am. He tells me that he came in early this morning to look into my blood work. He then tells me that I have a high* **blast*** *cell count and that he has made an appointment for me at Dr. Butler's Oncology/Hematology office. Dad arrives by 7:00 am. I tell him that we have an 8:00 a.m. appointment over at Dr. Butler's office. I don't know what dad thinks at this point...but, I think that I may be anemic or have some blood illness...but nothing that would be that big a deal.*

Jay's Memories

September 11, 2001 is one of those dates where everyone remembers where they were. I was traveling along Canal Road next to the Potomac River enjoying that beautiful late summer morning, with the average amount of rush hour traffic that I was quite used to. Heading into work, I remember listening to the continuing reports of chaos at the World Trade Center. I remember looking to the south and west and seeing a rising plume of smoke which I found out a few minutes later to be the plane that hit the Pentagon.

So when September 11, 2002, came closer, the three of us spoke about

---

*NOTE: Individual words and phrases that appear in bold are defined in the *Glossary* in the Appendix. A Glossary term is bolded the first time it occurs only. Some terms in the book also are defined in the context of the discussion, usually within "text boxes."

having a contingency plan for what we might do if that date brought the same kind of chaos that came about a year earlier. Our plan was to head north just because we all live north of the Washington Beltway, perhaps meet in Frederick, Maryland and decide where to go from there. Half serious conversations like this often occur among families and ours was no exception. One thing I knew was that on September 11th, 2002, like many other Washingtonians, I would telecommute. With my office being one block from the State Department and five blocks from the White House, why take any chances!

On the morning of September 11th, when Dani still isn't feeling well, I decide to go over and prepare her favorite breakfast of French toast. When I arrive she greets me with a request that we forego breakfast for awhile as her doctor just called, and told her that her blood work gave him some concern and that we should go to the hematologist at Virginia Hospital Center in Arlington, Virginia.

Sue's Memories

When Dani calls me that evening on September 9th, and tells me about her bruises, I remember that I had been listening to Chris Core on WMAL AM. The discussion on this talk radio station is about the upcoming anniversary of 9/11 and what to do just in case there is another terrorist attack. He speaks about how he and his wife, Anne, and their young daughter, Tabitha, have a family plan in case such an event occurred. So when I am speaking with Dani about how she is feeling, we also begin speaking of a contingency evacuation and rendezvous plan for the three of us. Honestly, I think it takes our minds off of her pain for a bit. When I arrive home, I discuss this with Jay, and we later confirm our plans with Dani. Jay lets me know that he was not planning to go to GWU on September 11th. He thought that he would just head over to Dani's and make her favorite breakfast to cheer her up.

Chapter Three
The Parallel Universe and the Teddy Bear

Dani's Memories (later in the morning of 9/11)

We get to the doctors' office and it was crazy. The receptionist won't let me see Dr. Butler without the correct referral form. I keep pleading with her that Dr. Schreiner is the one that had made the appointment...but she isn't having it. I can't get in touch with anyone from Dr. Schreiner's office because they're not open yet...so, we sit and then finally get in touch with someone from his office who faxes over the referral. Finally we are led into the back to meet Dr. Christie in his office. He is enormous (that was my first impression and continues to this day). Dad sits beside me. He introduces himself and then the woman who is sitting next to him. He explains that she was a medical intern. It all goes in one ear and out the other. I was so happy to finally meet with him...that it is the farthest thing from my mind that this man is about to give me the worst news of my life. He does not sugar coat a thing. He looks at both of us and says, "We've reviewed your blood work and there is a 99% chance that you have a form of leukemia." At first I sit motionless. I look at dad and he has this completely blank expression on his face. The next sentence out of Doctor Christie's mouth is something about that what he suspected I had is a very aggressive form of cancer and therefore I will begin chemotherapy treatments today. That's when I heard the word "cancer" for the very first time. Dad and I both began to cry. Dr. Christie excuses himself from the room. Dad calls mom and I call Scott. The next thing I remember is walking down this twisted hallway by myself that leads me to the "torture chamber" (by the way, I have never again seen this hallway, so I'm pretty sure it was a figment of my imagination). Dr. Christie comes in with his intern. He tells me about the procedure he is about to do. I am on my belly (face down). I am about to have my first bone marrow biopsy. I can't imagine anything more painful in my life. I scream...and I believe Dr. Christie screams as well. I think up until that point the most painful thing I have ever endured is a line drive to the shin while playing in an "18 and under" softball tournament. As soon as he hits the bone, it feels like he is trying to suck every last bit of me through a needle. (I find out later that because my blast cell count is so high...it is like the pressure exploded into the syringe.) He leaves the room and I cry (not little tears...but big crocodile tears with lots of huffing and puffing). What seems like 20 to 30 minutes later, a nurse comes into the room and tells me that I can go out to the waiting room. I open the door and walk out.

Immediately, I see my mom and we hug and cry for what seems like forever. I sit down next to her and we speak. It is a few minutes before I look up and see my boyfriend Scott and cousin Ari sitting across from me. Have they been there this whole time? Then as a family...we walk down another long corridor (but this one really is long)...and wait for a short time in the hospital admissions waiting room.

We are then sent to the emergency room. As soon as I am in my hospital-issue night gown, the curtains open and my small party of four turned into what seems like a party of 20. There was Aunt Carol and Uncle Bruce, Scott, my cousin Ari, Laurie Alderman, my boss, my teaching assistant Lena Rainey and I can't remember who else. Laurie climbs onto my bed (I think pushing my mom aside...). Then, a medical resident and two interns pile into the room. John Schnable, Pamela Herbert and Jack come in the room to ask me all sorts of questions. I think they are a little dumbstruck when they see how young I am and how close to their own age.

Shortly after that we are sent to a private room. We meet Katrina. She is super cute. She tells me that she is going to wheel me down to surgery to have an emergency catheter placed in my neck in order to receive chemotherapy. She is really bad at wheeling the bed and we kept bumping into walls. We laugh together and I immediately know that I really like her. I was then in this super scary room and a lady walks in and reassures me that this surgery is done all the time and I had nothing to worry about. I remember feeling the cutting on my neck...and I am not supposed to feel it... I remember trying to tell them...but the words don't come out. Then I remember laying in a hallway waiting to be wheeled back to my room...back to my family. I start crying and yelling (it probably came out like whispers) for someone, anyone to get me back to my room. I started saying that "I was just diagnosed with cancer and then some people cut a hole in my neck and I think I'm bleeding. I need to get to my room." Finally Katrina is called and we are off for another adventure. I don't remember anything more from that day. No, that is not true, I remember that I don't want my parents to tell Micah. If my brother Micah is told about this then, I remember, I felt like whatever I have is very serious. I would just get better and that was it.

Jay's Memories

9/11 (later that morning)

It took us about 15 minutes to get to the doctors' office and another 30 minutes or so to make sure that the correct referral had been received so that the specialist can look at her. Finally, new blood work is done and the first bit of news we received sounds o.k. to me. We have been fortunate in our family to have never had to develop expertise in the areas of hematology or oncology. With my limited knowledge of hematology I always thought that having a high white cell count meant that your body was fighting disease...a good thing. I am quickly informed by the person reading the test that 140,000 is not the kind of blood count that was fighting disease. It is too high...way too high. We find out later that 90% of those white blood cells are nonfunctional immature blast cells. A few minutes later Dr. Christie calls us into his office and says the following to my daughter: "There is a 99% chance you have leukemia." I am no more knowledgeable about leukemia than my daughter. I am sure that neither of us knows what an oncologist or a hematologist does. The only thing I know is that leukemia is a form of cancer. We stare at each other in disbelief. I remember being a bit annoyed at the suddenness of the diagnosis and the lack of bedside manner. In hindsight, I guess that there is no easy way to say it. What we do know is that leukemia is a form of cancer and that cancer was never a good thing. Things like **acute myelogenous leukemia (AML)** *and bone marrow aspirates were nowhere to be found in either of our knowledge bases. Interestingly, Sue and I had been screened back in the early nineties as part of a drive for potential matches for a young lady named Allison Atlas, who needed a bone marrow transplant, but that certainly is not in my thinking that morning. I later think about the fact that Dani was not eligible to be in the registry because she had mononucleosis in 1992.*

Sue's Memories

I go to work (I am an assistant principal at Earle B. Wood Middle School) on September 11th, comforted by the fact that Jay is going to Dani's this morning. Assured that he will call with any news, I go about my usual morning routine of greeting and encouraging our students to get to their first period class on time as I walk through the halls. When first period arrives, I go to the seventh-grade team room where a parent conference is in progress. I remember receiving a call from Jay. He lets me know that Dani's primary care doctor's partner had called to let Dani know that he is referring her to a hematologist and that she was to go there as soon as possible. He tells me to sit tight until he has more information. I believe that I then informed the main office of my location and asked that they contact me immediately when Jay calls again. Of course I am anxious to hear from him, but I return to the parent conference not suspecting what serious news the next phone call will bring. I remain in the seventh-grade team room after the first period to develop a new schedule, behavior plan, and student contract (the results from the previous meeting). The call comes within the next hour from Jay saying that Dani is very ill and is being admitted to the hospital immediately. I am to meet them at the doctor's office, which is adjacent to the hospital.

I remember feeling numb as I walk to my car. To this day, I don't even recall if Jay told me the nature of her illness...leukemia.

Neither Jay nor I are in any kind of shape at that point to have the presence of mind to get directions for my drive to the doctor's office. Although we live within ten miles of the state of Virginia, we Marylanders often view Virginia as a foreign territory. I keep calling Jay for directions. Scott, a Virginian, who was with Jay at the time, can't really help as he has a similar problem in reverse — viewing Maryland as some distant land. Still the three of us, in our frenzied state, somehow get me to my destination in one piece. I do recall a police car passing me as I make one of several U-turns on Virginia's Route 50! After what seems like hours (when it was actually only about 45 minutes), I arrive at the doctor's office off of George Mason Drive. Jay is standing in the parking lot. I'm not sure who parks the car. Jay and I embrace, say nothing to each other, and together with Scott we walk back into the doctor's office. After that embrace, I believe we both go into a crisis mode of operation. The reality is that our daughter is critically ill. The task before us is to make Dani better...whatever way we can. I mentioned to Dani recently that the only people that I remember who were in the waiting room at that time were Jay, myself, Scott, and our nephew Ari (news traveled quickly in our family and Ari worked nearby in Arlington). I realize now that this was virtually impossible as the medical office of Butler, Meister, Feigert, Christie, and Rodriguez is a very large, successful, and therefore extremely busy practice. I guess at this very point in time my focus has changed from the role of an assistant principal (and having the ability to take in a myriad of events all occurring at the same time) to just that of a mom, and therefore only singularly directed on my child's welfare.

I am sitting next to Jay and across from Ari and Scott. Within a short time (maybe 5 minutes), our Dani enters the room. She sits next to me...we hug and we cry. I don't remember speaking. Eventually we are directed to go to the hospital's admissions office. We walk and walk and walk some more until we arrive at our destination. Surprisingly, Dani is put in a wheelchair and we are escorted to the emergency room to wait until a bed in the oncology wing is made available. Dani is then wheeled into a curtained-off room and given a hospital-issued gown to change into. Things are really moving fast. While Dani is changing (I believe I am in there assisting), my sister Carol, her husband Bruce, Dani's principal, Laurie Alderman, and her classroom assistant Lena join the five of us. I sit next to Dani...holding her hand...never wanting to let go. Laurie enters the very small area where we have all congregated and sits on the bed as well. Somehow, all of a sudden, it is Laurie sitting on the bed, holding Dani's hand. Later on, we would all laugh about this while at the same time being grateful for her streak of chutzpah! So now, by my count, there are nine of us in this extremely small cubby, when three more people enter. They introduce themselves as Dani's personal medical team: John Schnable (resident), Pamela Herbert (fourth-year medical student), and Jack (a third-year medical student). Arlington Hospital Center, a teaching hospital affiliated with Georgetown Medical School, is a part of their rotation. All three are in their 20's like Dani. They are now suddenly and luckily a vital part of our world. They ask us to step outside for a moment as they examine Dani and take her vital statistics. We are then informed that Dani would be taken to a room on the fourth floor of the hospital where the oncology unit is located. We all jam into the elevator.

You hear a lot today about hospital delays in responding to medical emergencies. I can only attest that the time that elapsed from our leaving Dr. Christie's office to our arrival to what was to become Dani's home for the next month was less than one hour. We are eternally grateful to the staff at Arlington hospital for their efficiency and care, as we are told later that week that we were less than 24 hours away from losing our beautiful Dani.

I believe the room number was 424. Within seconds after Dani is placed on her bed, an incredibly petite, adorable, and young nurse (she looks about 15 years old!) enters the room. She writes her name on the white board at the far end of the room, Katrina. (Did she actually make a smiley face dotting the letter "i" in her name?) She appears so sweet, full of life, and genuinely glad to meet Dani and the rest of her entourage. She tells us that Dani, later on in the evening, will be placed on a leukemia

> **Neutropenic** is a condition where a person has an abnormally low number of white blood cells, making it difficult to fight disease that can be caused by chemotherapy.

*medication called **Hydrea**, which will suppress her elevated white blood cell count. She then proceeds to present us with a few house rules. No one will be allowed to visit Dani if they have a cold, and fresh flowers or fresh fruit are prohibited. We learn that these rules are **Neutropenic** precautions taken as Dani's immune system was compromised by leukemia and we cannot risk any chance of outside infections. She presents us with several pamphlets. One, entitled Acute Myelogenous Leukemia, published by the Leukemia and Lymphoma Society and Wyeth, is designed for parents and families, and its focus is educational. The other was comic-book like in appearance and becomes our go to guide over the next several weeks. This pamphlet (i.e., Neutrophil…Your One-in-a-Million Bodyguard) is written in simple language so that people like us with no medical knowledge of leukemia, the treatment, and its side effects, could have some sense of the*

> A **peripherally inserted central catheter (PICC or PIC line)** is a form of intravenous access that can be used for a prolonged period of time, e.g., for long chemotherapy regimens, extended antibiotic therapy or total nutrition. (It is an alternative to subclavian lines, internal jugular lines, or femoral lines, which have higher rates of infection.)

*nature of this devastating illness. She then takes Dani to surgery so that she can have a temporary catheter placed in her neck in preparation for the second pre-chemotherapy treatment, which will occur the next day. An **IV catheter** or **PICC line** is also placed in her arm to allow her to receive both the medication and nutrition needed to begin the fight. We are told that when the doctors feel that the time is right, the PICC line will be replaced by a central venous catheter.*

Jay uses the time, during Dani's absence, to go to the Nurses' Station to ask some procedural questions. A nurse sitting behind the desk is receptive to his somewhat rambling set of questions. Although he doesn't believe he ever saw this person again, she is attentive to his inquiries and commiserated with Jay, saying at the conclusion of their conversation, "Your daughter is one sick puppy."

When Dani (and Katrina) return to the room, she is given the first of what seems to be hundreds of medications, including an antibiotic to stop any infection and some Ambien for relaxation and eventual sleep. Dani, at the time, is grumbling about "that stupid thing in my neck." Soon the Ambien takes effect and she rests, surrounded by her ever-growing posse.

Sometime during that first evening Dr. Christie arrives to check on Dani. Our brother-in-law Bruce asks to speak with him in the hallway. Jay and I follow. Bruce asks Dr. Christie about harvesting Dani's eggs for the future. Dr. Christie, with his no holds barred tell-it-like-it-is style that we come to appreciate, replies that he is more concerned about saving Dani's life, as she could possibly die within 24 hours if they don't begin

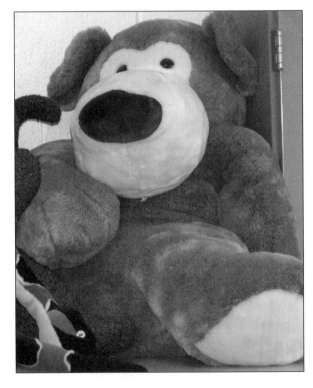

the chemotherapy process immediately. His stunning statement not only silences us all...it underscores the urgency of proceeding with the treatments.

There are a few memories that remain extremely clear about our first few hours in the hospital room. None would be as vivid as the one involving my sister and her husband. We

Dani's new friend, Oaf

remember them leaving for dinner, and surprisingly returning after they have eaten. At around 9 p.m. they say goodbye again...for home we thought. Within an hour they return, but this time they carry the largest stuffed teddy bear imaginable...he has to weigh at least 15 pounds and is over 4 feet tall and quite plump! (I believe Dani retained his FAO Schwartz "given" name of "Oaf.") Oaf and countless other stuffed animals of all sizes and shapes sit vigil over Dani for that first month, filling the window ledges and furniture tops. After that month, most of the stuffed animals are donated to charities, including the pediatric unit of Arlington Hospital and the Walter Reed School in Arlington where Dani teaches. To this day, however, Oaf sits in Dani's classroom as the most special spot for her kids to cuddle when they read.

After Carol and Bruce finally depart for the night for good, Dani is given Hydrea. It is only 11 hours after her diagnosis...and her fight to combat leukemia begins. The next day we find out that this one treatment had reduced the number of immature white blood cells (called "blasts") from 140,000 to 107,000. (The number of white blood cells that is considered normal, by the way, is from 10,000 to 14,000.)

We decide that I will spend the night. Before he leaves for the night, Jay helps me schlep the most uncomfortable chair/bed into the room. This contraption is to be my bed (or whoever relieves me) for the next month or so. Jay leaves for home around 11:30 that evening to feed our dog, Patti, get some sleep, and make plans for the changes in our lives. This night understandably is a sleepless one. Dani's temperature spikes at around 2:30 in the morning. (I don't believe that she remembers any of this.) The nurse and I pack Dani in ice to bring her body temperature down. This seems to have the desired effect; her temperature lowers and stabilizes, and Dani soon returns to sleep. However, this would be the first of many sleepless nights for many of us.

Chapter Four
Advice from Everywhere

I (Sue) begin keeping notes in earnest on that Wednesday (9/11/02). Interspersed between the hourly listing of medication given to Dani and her vital signs (temperature and blood pressure), the notes also include questions to ask the team of doctors and nurses, people to contact, requests to make, as well as any detail or event that transpired. The notebook is a constant companion, and when I'm not present, Jay, Scott, Micah or assorted friends of Dani's are charged with keeping accurate records. (I remember Scott and Kat, Dani's college roommate, being the first to tackle this task outside of the immediate family.) It is no surprise that one of the first pages includes the list of friends and family that we need to contact. This rather large group comes to support Dani immediately. So great is their reaction, that Dani's room immediately fills with those that love her! Honestly…it is standing room only…! The head nurse, Joanne comes into the room and announces to Dani that there are too many people present and that they have to leave. Dani immediately reacts by bursting into tears…and as if by magic… Joanne relents. For the next month and for the next two **consolidation chemotherapy** visits, there are no limits placed on visitors as long as they either follow the guidelines already set by Katrina or if Dani requests quiet time. Joanne and her nurses soon became members of Dani's fan club as well. They not only provide the necessary medical care for Dani, they make sure that her other needs are met. We come to understand how very special the nurses are; we value them greatly and are gratified by their friendship.

A pattern develops immediately where Jay and I spend quiet mornings with Dani, Scott arrives late afternoon after work, and then the visits begin. The room fills with well-wishers. They smile, they laugh, they chat…and they give Dani the strength she needs to fight.

When they can't be in the room, they send their best wishes and prayers on cards and letters and in the form of stuffed animals and photos. Early on, Bruce brings Dani a cherished item, his boxing gloves. They hang by the television, facing Dani 24/7. They serve as a constant reminder to Dani of her personal fight to beat this disease. Another special token for Dani is presented to her by one of her former students, 4-year-old Ben Busey. Her pre-school students from the previous year created life-sized cut out dolls of themselves as superheroes. Ben loved this project and kept his in his bedroom. When he hears that his favorite teacher, Miss Dani is ill, he knows exactly what he can do to make her feel better. He asks his mom to bring Miss Dani, his superhero cut-out, which she does. We hang Ben, the Super Hero cut-out, above Dani's bed. With both the gloves and the superhero prominently displayed the fight begins. Even without the visitors, Dani's hospital room becomes a sight to behold. Gradually, the walls fill with the cards and letters from friends and family and other works of art from former students. Our Dani is surrounded at all hours by love, best wishes, and laughter…a key, we believe, to her recovery.

A problem of a different sort presents itself to us early on during those harrowing first 24 hours…how in the world and what in the world are we going to tell our parents? Jay's mom, Dani and Micah's "Philly Mom-Mom," adores her Princess Dani. We are all pretty sure that she need not know the seriousness of Dani's illness. We all agree to never (never, *never*) use the word **cancer** in her presence. We would just tell her that Dani had a blood disorder and leave it at that. Our plan was to have Dani regularly call her to let her know that she was following the doctors' orders and is feeling much better. My parents, however, are another story. Although my dad is suffering from congestive heart failure, we both know that he and my mother will not hesitate to fly up from Florida to be with Dani. After consulting with several members of the hospital staff, including the social worker, Cathy Dorner, we agree to this scenario. I would call my parents and say the following to them (I actually wrote the speech down word for word in my notebook): "Dani was diagnosed with a blood disorder. There are abnormalities in her blood. We are concerned about her elevated white blood cell count. We didn't want to alarm anyone. So she's in the hospital now and receiving the best of treatments." My dad, being no dummy, first responds with a frantic *"What did you just say*?!" Of course, I then repeat my scripted speech in a stilted monotone only to have my dad, as only my dad could do, raise his voice, his ire, and his concern all at once, so that I immediately drop all pretense and tell them both that their beautiful granddaughter has leukemia. We already know that my parents have scheduled a visit up north in two weeks to attend their great grandson Brandon's Bar Mitzvah in Philadelphia. We agree immediately that they can extend their visit some so that they could come to Arlington Hospital Center as well. Until they arrive on September 25th, my parents call Dani daily with all of their love, best wishes, and important dietary advice!

The question that my dad raised during that tense phone conversation on September 12th was the same one that countless others asked: "How does one get leukemia?" The initial response that Dr. Christie offers us, and the myriad of pamphlets confirmed, was the following: Acute Myelogenous Leukemia has several factors associated with an increased risk of the disease. One factor is the exposure to a very high dose of radiation like that from an atomic bomb explosion. Another cause could be from the exposure to benzene, a toxic chemical once used in cleaning solvents. The third possibility is exposure to chemotherapy used to treat cancers. The last option is just pure bad luck. **AML** is not contagious, and it is not inherited. However, it strikes its victim quickly as the cancer cells reproduce at an incredible rate and block the development of normal marrow cells.

Dani has never been exposed to an atomic bomb detonation. Additionally, her experience with cleaning and cleaning products is quite limited, not only because cleaning was not a big part of her repertoire, but also because the chemical benzene is now a banned substance in cleaning products. Additionally, in her 26 years, Dani never received the treatment of chemotherapy. There is only one explanation. The only answer possible is that our Dani is just the recipient of some very bad luck. Later on in the diagnostic process, we discover that a genetic abnormality had instantaneously transformed a robust, healthy, athletic, energetic, positive thinking 26-year-old into a seriously ill leukemia patient in Room 424 of the Virginia Hospital Center in Arlington, Virginia.

Another interesting problem arises in those first few hours and days. We are blessed with many friends who care about us and about Dani. The problem is that everyone has some advice or has a friend, neighbor or relative that has greater expertise on this topic than we do. As Jay begins to make his series of phone calls to friends and family attempting to tell them what has happened and attempting to keep people informed, these same well-meaning people, trying to help as best they can, make all kinds of suggestions about who to talk to, where to go for help etc. "You need to move her out of the community hospital"…"Get her to Hopkins"…"I know a fabulous oncologist"…etc. An interesting fact about living in the Washington, D.C. metropolitan area is that people who live in Maryland tend to know little about services in Virginia and vice versa. We know nothing about the Virginia Hospital Center in Arlington or the doctors that are affiliated with the hospital. Finally, Jay calls our longtime doctor of almost 25 years and asks him what we should do. As always, he gives us sage advice. "We are fortunate to live in an area where there are many highly qualified physicians. Virginia Hospital Center is no exception." He continues, saying that the treatment that Dani needs for her illness, at this point in time, is a standard protocol. He adds, "I'm sure that the doctors and nurses at Arlington are more than capable of handling this stage of her treatment, and it gives you time to think about the best course of action for the future." With one less thing to worry about, but with our continuing strategy of asking questions about everything that occurs, and keeping a notebook delineating every change, treatment, blood count, temperature and medication, we move forward.

Chapter Five
Overcoming Four Obstacles

Dani's Memory

9/12

Dr. Feigert comes in (he is super cute). He sits on the edge of my bed and starts explaining the plan of treatment for AML. I interrupt him. "Dr. Christie said that there was a 99% chance that I have leukemia...that means there is still a 1% chance I don't have it." I still think sometimes that this was all a really bad dream.

The First Week Continued

9/12

To our Dani, the glass is always half full rather than half empty. She's the one that makes lemonade out of lemons. She always sees the positive. Children with disabilities are children first... with many abilities. All the children in her class are cute and funny and she loves them all. Many things are critical in battling a serious illness but we can never underestimate attitude in this fight. Today is the day Dani will begin her **induction chemotherapy**. The plan is that it will begin

> **Apheresis** means to take away. There are several different types of apheresis but the procedure is essentially the same. It is used to remove specific cells or plasma from your blood. One can be a plasma donor through the Red Cross where they would hook up two lines (one in each arm) and draw blood out of your body with one line, send it through a centrifuge-like machine to separate the blood into its various components (plasma, red blood cells, and white blood cells), and return it through the second line. If one is a plasma donor, then the plasma is retained. This process is then called a **plasmapheresis**.

later this evening. But first Dani will receive a **leukopheresis** (a specific type of **apherisis**) to rid the body of leukemia cells (her second pre-chemotherapy treatment). In Dani's case the target, at this time, is the immature white blood cells or blast cells that are gumming up the works, so to speak. We later learn that this process is called leukopheresis, which is designed to remove as many of the immature white blood cells as possible. About 10 a.m. this lovely lady wheels a huge machine into Dani's room. She attaches some tubes to the new temporary catheter port in Dani's neck and explains the process to us. It is hoped that this apheresis would cause a **leukoreduction** or a reduction of Dani's blast count.

Blasts are bad, immature white blood cells. They are sticky…pus-like, and can clog both arteries and vital organs. She says that her goal is to reduce Dani's white blood cell count from 107,000 (already reduced from 140,000 by the Hydrea) to 75,000. The process lasts at least four hours. As Dani sleeps through most of this process, we sit and watch an IV-type bag fill with the components of her blood separated, because of the different weights, with the white cells as the bottom layer. The technician is able to show us the collection of yellow blast cells that fall to the bottom of the bag. These blast cells will not be returned to Dani's body. It is the goal of this process to remove as many immature white blast cells as possible. At the completion of the apheresis, a nurse completes a blood draw to see how successful the process was. Everyone is pleasantly surprised by the results. Dani's white blood cell count has dropped to 35,000 (which is much better than they had originally anticipated). This is a good start, but a long battle lies ahead. The cavalry of doctors, nurses and technicians win the first skirmish in the fight for Dani's life.

During this day, our first full day in the parallel universe of cancer, our formal education begins. The cavalry speaks a new language here. They use words like **immunocompromised**, induction chemotherapy, **myelogic**, **myeloid**, or myelogenous, blood draws, **mugascan**, blasts, consolidation chemotherapy, etc. Vague memories of biology class return with the discussions of chromosomes, DNA, and liver function. We begin to understand the purpose of distinct drugs…how some are used to ease pain while others are used to cure infections; and we cannot forget the chemical therapy drugs, and the interesting names given to the poisons that were put inside Dani's body to do their discriminate vs. indiscriminate killing. Jay begins adapting and fine tuning his already professional research skills towards Dani's cure. The doctors and nurses are extremely patient with us and answer any questions posed. And it certainly didn't hurt that our brother-in-law, Bruce, a pharmacist by profession, and his wife and my sister Carol are always close by during those first difficult weeks to discuss the purpose of drugs and their effects on the body. We begin to realize that oncology nurses are a breed unto themselves. Their patients are not admitted to the hospital one day and gone the next. These are long-term clients who need continuing and evolving treatment protocols.

We learn that the high fever of Dani's first night in the hospital occurred because Dani was being weaned off of steroids, which masked the symptoms of the infection. Dani is now indeed **immunocompromised** (in layman's terms, she has an infection, and there is little left in her barely functioning immune system to fight it).

Although Dani is advised to sit up, walk around, and eat, she really feels like doing none of that! One nurse even suggests that Dani start drinking Ensure, as it would boost her ever-waning energy.

Dr. Feigert comes in to check on Dani's progress. He patiently explains the induction chemotherapy process to us. He tells us that Dani's form of leukemia, acute myelogenous, comes on suddenly. An analysis of Dani's chromosomes will further define the risk of the disease and the best treatments to use. The chemotherapy protocol that will be followed is, we found out later, quite standard for AML treatment

As of 2001, **Idarubicin** is approved to treat only one single cancer, acute myelocytic leukemia (AML) in adults. Recent research suggests that using Idarubicin results in higher rates of complete remission (CR) and longer survival for patients. CR is the total elimination of all diseased cells detectable following therapy.

Ara-C (Cytarabine) is one of the older chemotherapy drugs, which has been in use for many years. Ara-C is a clear, colorless liquid given by intravenous route. It is most commonly used in treatment of several forms of leukemia and lymphoma. Ara-C is normally given on a daily basis for five to seven days.

and included two chemicals: doses of **Idarubicin** for the first three days as well as seven days of **ARA-C**. These two lethal drugs are used to kill the fast growing disease (the blast cells) in Dani's body. Unfortunately these chemical therapies also kill other fast growing cells (hence the loss of hair). He tells us that in 10 to 14 days Dani's diseased white blood cell count will drop to zero but then the good cells will come back. He further says that Dani will need red blood cell and platelet transfusions. After the drop in blood cell counts, the body will take about three weeks to recover. In the meantime there will be some pretty unpleasant side effects (nausea, vomiting, temporary hair loss, cold sores, diarrhea, and a variety of other pleasantries). He mentions that they will be introducing some other medications to ease some of the side-effects.

Dani sits and listens to Dr. Feigert. The realization of the battle ahead has to be shocking. She knows that this will be the toughest contest she has ever been a part of. No NCAA Division I softball game could ever have been this tough, and yet she displays a quiet determination that she can do this. She already has confidence in the doctors and nurses that are supporting her and is gaining strength from the army of friends that are cheering her on. She often says that this was her body and her personal disease. It doesn't matter what other people have done in their fight. She didn't want to talk to other survivors. It is Dani versus the disease and she will win! She will fight leukemia every way she can. No one can share their experience; no book can tell her the risks. Dani believes that she will win this battle with the same techniques she learned from athletics. She will be disciplined, focused, follow the coaches' suggestions and use her entire mental and physical persona to defeat the opposition.

The fans (visitors) begin to stream in that evening, and it is a sell-out every evening for those first four weeks of Dani's hospitalization. People sit on the floor, wait in the hallway, camp out at the nurses' station, and even send Jay and I to dinner so there could be more room in room 424. Dani, already heavily medicated, welcomes them all. When the guests leave that second evening, Dani asks that my sister and I give her a sponge bath. We shove everyone else out of the room and bathe her. She is shivering so…and she is so weak. We dress Dani in soft warm Karen Neuberger flannel pajamas with a little improvisational tailoring so that the PICC line in her arm for blood draws and chemotherapy and the catheter in her neck aren't disturbed. The reader may be wondering why I'm so detailed about the pajamas. It may seem silly, but fashion becomes another weapon in Dani's arsenal. She will keep up appearances. She vows to keep up her image and she does this throughout the battle. Kids learn things from all who surround them. She may have learned this one from Jay's mom, "Philly Mom-Mom," whom both kids treasure. "The show must go on," was one of her favorite lines…and the kids believe that as well. This second evening remains with me as if it were yesterday, and my heart aches as it did that evening.

After Carol and Bruce leave, the three of us anxiously wait for the chemotherapy to begin. Dot, our nurse for that evening, administers some **Zofran** (anti-nausea medication) to Dani, informing us that it was an excellent drug. (It should be noted that the nursing staff also told us when a medication was not one of their favorites.) Soon after that, she adds ten milligrams of **Decadron** to the IV cocktail. One dose of Decadron, a steroid, is used prior to chemotherapy, normally along with Zofran, and is given intravenously as an additional anti-nausea medication. Around 11 p.m. the chemo begins. If you remember the movie "ET" where the government scientists are in white space suits when they enter Elliot's house, then you will have a picture of what high dose chemotherapy treatment is all about. The nurse enters the room masked and totally encased in protective clothing. She is protecting herself against the poisons (excuse me…chemical therapy medications) that are about to enter and circulate through our daughter's body. Fortunately Dani is basically asleep by then. Needless to say, with that image, neither Jay nor I sleep much that evening.

9/13

As Dani continues to sleep this morning, I leave for home for a quick shower and change. Jay and I then return to the hospital together in one car. On our way, we decide to continue making phone calls to friends and family to inform them about Dani's illness and subsequent hospitalization. The first phone call we make is to one of my childhood buddies, Betsy. I don't think I get through the "hello" part of the conversation before I burst into tears. My guess is that at that moment…it hits me…it is not just words…but our daughter…our beautiful Dani…is critically ill with leukemia. I quickly hand the phone to Jay and compose myself. Jay says "hello" to Betsy and begins to explain my tears. Unfortunately, the tears are catching, and soon he too is unable to speak. Thinking that I've regained my composure, I take the phone from him and continue the conversation until my tears begin to flow again and Jay once more speaks with Betsy. We seem to be passing the phone back and forth across the front seat more than we are talking to Betsy. The conversation is a short one as neither of us can compose ourselves long enough to give Betsy any details of Dani's illness. With a promise to call her later on in the day, we end the call. Emotionally drained, Jay and I agree not to make any more calls at that time. We arrive at Arlington Hospital Center shortly after the call ends, park the car, and head for Dani's room. As we walk, our focus returns. There is no time for public sadness. We both know what we have to do. Focus…Focus…Focus! We must deal with the reality, use our collective problem-solving skills, work with the experts, maintain a positive outlook, and focus only on Dani getting better.

Dani actually sleeps for eleven hours and awakes in a great mood. For the first time in days, she has good color. She uses the commode for the first time and even eats her meals. Her temperature is normal. Scott's parents, Gayle and John Greene, visit Dani that evening after meeting Scott for dinner. We suspect the dinner conversation is quite serious. Gayle and John have already (in the brief three months of Dani and Scott's relationship) fallen in love with Dani. Even though we are just introduced to Gayle and John that evening, Jay and I feel an immediate bond. Carol and Bruce, of course, are among the throng of visitors. After they leave for the evening, Bruce calls us. Bruce is never shy about expressing his opinion and this evening was no exception. He is alarmed about the number of friends, hugs, kisses, and germs being dispensed. We accept a part of his opinion and, as a result, using Purell and antiseptic wipes, will now become the basic rule for visitor entry. But, as stated earlier, Dani's human network of support is critical to her in this time and she will have it no other way. We become adamant at following the rules of the house in terms of cleanliness. (Sometimes we even have to remind the doctors!)

Dani has a good day. Right now, that's all that matters. At about 9:30 p.m. the pre-chemo regimen begins again. Dani is given her anti-nausea medication, which she promptly throws up. Dani's good friend and former college roommate, Kat Palotta Fitzgerald, and our Scott are there for the big event, and quickly demonstrate their devotion by cleaning up the gross mess. They stay by Dani's bedside until about 11:30 that evening after which Dani and I snuggle together for a special mom and daughter time. We settle into a routine that goes something like this: I spend the night, and Jay goes home to feed and walk the dog and sleep. He comes back about 6:30 a.m. I go home and shower and return for the day. Jay tries to hang in until the doctor visits, and then heads into work for a few hours. We figure out dinner when he gets back and between 9 and 10 he heads home. Tonight, however, Jay will head to Baltimore Washington Airport to pick up our son, Micah, who is flying in from Seattle.

Chemo begins a bit later than planned that evening as Dani has some time off of her IV drip when she is unplugged and transported to get a mugascan (a test designed to measure how efficiently your heart is pumping blood).

Dina is our evening nurse and she begins the chemo at 1:30 a.m. after Dani gets her anti-nausea and pain meds. As Dina goes about her tasks, she lets us know that Dani's daily regimen needs to change some. She can't use a razor or tampons; she can only use a soft bristle tooth brush, and may not use a harsh mouth wash. As Dina finishes her task Dani sleeps. She wakes up about 2 a.m. complaining about neck and back pain. She is given some pain meds, but there is a "cougher" on the oncology wing, so neither of us sleeps very well.

9/14

Dani wakes up feeling dizzy. It appears that the anti-nausea medication is having that effect! The nurse delivers Dani's very own stethoscope and thermometer so that nobody else's germs can be transmitted. She reports that Dani's white blood cell count is down to 8,000. The chemo sure works fast! Dr. Christie arrives and we find out that before he was an oncologist he was a veterinarian. Dani, a lover of all things animal, is instantly taken by that piece of information.

The day is uneventful except for her brother Micah's arrival from Seattle. He's tired but relieved to finally be with his big sister. Later on that evening, Dani is administered the last dose of the Idarubicin.

9/15

New meds are introduced today. **Alpurinol** is administered to prevent gout. Dani is also given a stool softener, as she hasn't pooped since Tuesday, September 10th. Dr. Christie visits in the morning with Dani and tells her that her blast count is down to 25% of her white blood cells, which is far less than the 90% on 9/11. He also reports that her white cell count is down to 1,900, she has no fever, she doesn't appear to need blood or **platelets** (a transfusion), and at the moment she's finished with Idarubicin.

> **Platelets** are one of the main components of the blood that forms clots, sealing up injured areas and preventing hemorrhage.

He tells us about consolidation chemotherapy, which is a protocol used to keep Dani's leukemia in remission. He tells us that it will begin about four weeks after the induction chemo ends. He predicts that this protocol of straight chemo treatment will go on for about five months. A chromosome analysis will be completed in the meantime to tell us whether chemotherapy alone, or radiation, or a bone marrow transplant will be necessary to permanently rid her body of leukemia. He asks that we have Micah get a blood test to see if his marrow matches Dani if the need for transplant were to arise. He also mentions that another possible treatment would be to have Dani donate her own bone marrow cells.

Dr. Christie also informs Jay about the National Headquarters for the Leukemia and Lymphoma Society of America, where doctors are working on "cutting edge stuff" and also provide some financial support.

When Dr. Christie leaves, Dani is given the drug **Phenergan** for her nausea. We learn that her other anti-nausea medication has been changed to **Ativan**, as the Zofran makes her dizzy and, as Dani says, "loopy!." Dani immediately falls asleep despite the onslaught of visitors. Dani's high school softball coach Matt Boratenski and his wife Estelene arrive. Estelene, the former "Wootton softball team mom," brings Dani's favorite white chocolate macadamia nut cookies. Dani sleeps through their visit. Food seems to be the gift of the day. Today is Yom Kippur, the Jewish Day of Atonement. During this day, Jews all over the world fast. As is tradition, the fast ends at sunset with a feast. Our good friends, Bonnie and Steve and Carol and Bruce, bring enough delights to feed the entire oncology wing.

Dani spends most of the day sleeping. At night, the stool softener has the desired results. The hospital decides to reduce Dani's Ativan dosage by half, but they agree to give her Phenergan first for nausea. Additional medications are now starting. Dani is given 25 milligrams of **Benedryl** for the "gunk" in her throat.

I get to go home to sleep and Jay spends his first overnight with Dani. It's a bad night for Dani. At midnight, she's given **morphine** and Zofran after she vomited. At 4 a.m. these medications are repeated. Dani tells me later in the day that this was the worst night yet. She and Jay cry together that night as they struggle through the experience and the side effects Dani was feeling from the illness and the chemo. Neither of them go back to sleep until 6:30 a.m. when Dani's IV bag is changed. Dani is promised another dose of morphine by 7:45 a.m. Dani wakes at 7:15 a.m. She tells Jay that her neck hurts where her catheter is. Finally at 7:45 a.m. she's given another dose of morphine and some Phenergan.

Dani tells the nurse that her pain level is a twelve on a scale of 1-10.

At 8:45 a.m., Dr. Christie drops by. Despite Dani's pain, she chats with him about their respective weekends. He pokes her in places that hurt and lets her know that his partner, Dr. Rodriguez, will also drop by. By 9 a.m., Dani's favorite nurse, Katrina, arrives. Dani cheers. Dr. Rodriguez comes into the room, checks Dani's neck and suspects that she may have developed an infection near her catheter. She tells us that someone from the Infectious Disease Department will stop by to culture her.

What a busy morning this turns out to be. The dietician stops by and recommends Carnation Instant Breakfast or Slimfast for Dani. Katrina brings Dani **Tylenol**, **Pericolace**, and **Alpurinol**. Dani's team of residents arrives at 9:30 a.m. They chat for awhile and decide to add an additional antibiotic to the medication cocktail.

By 10 a.m. Katrina has drawn blood from both the PICC line and the peripheral line. Dani's red blood cell count is down from 30 to 25 (normal is 36–46), and her **hematocrit** (is the percent of whole blood that is composed of red blood cells) is down as well. Later on today, Dani will receive two units of blood. Katrina places a hot compress on Dani's neck and administers a stronger antibiotic. She says that it might take three to four days to get the results of the culture. On the positive side, she tells Dani that her temperature is down from 101 to 99.5.

The drug regimen continues, first with Zofran at 11:45 a.m. A few minutes later she is given an antibiotic called **Fortaz**. At 2 p.m. she receives morphine and Phenergan.

Today we meet Dr. Furlong, an Infectious Disease Specialist. Our first encounter is not so pleasant, as he tells Scott and Micah to leave the room while he performs his exam of Dani. The two young men stand their ground and introduce themselves as Dani's boyfriend and brother. The crisis is quickly averted as Dr. Furlong accepts their reasoning. After his initial exam, he comments that sometimes a vein becomes irritated by drugs, but that a PICC line should not become infected. We're not really sure what this means at the time. At 3 p.m. the nurse begins preparation for the blood transfusion. She also believes the PICC line is infected. Dani's mood continues to be gray. Jay calls Dr. Christie with our concerns.

In the midst of all this, the social worker arrives and suggests that Dani speak with a 26-year-old survivor of leukemia. She also suggests counseling. Dani is polite but declines her offers at the moment. She is determined to fight this thing her way.

At 4 p.m. the blood transfusion finally begins. By 4:30 p.m. Dani's temperature has risen to 101.9, and she is given Tylenol and morphine. By 5 p.m. Dani's temperature is 103.1. Katrina stops the transfusion and calls Dr. Rodriguez with her concerns. Dr. Rodriguez says this sometimes happens during a blood transfusion. So after another dose of Zofran, the transfusion is restarted at 5:30 p.m. By 9 p.m. the blood transfusion has ended, Dani's PICC line has been flushed and she begins to receive a platelet transfusion.

In the midst of the platelet transfusion, at 10:15 p.m., Dr. Furlong returns. He suggests **Betadine** and covers the wound where the catheter is. As Dr. Rodriquez predicted, Dani's temperature drops, to 99.5, by 11 p.m. She is able to go to the bathroom with my assistance. She prepares for bed by having a "cocktail' of Zofran, morphine, Ativan, and Tylenol. We talk a bit before she finally falls into a fitful rest at 11:30 p.m.

9/17

Dani sleeps until 4:27 a.m., a great night for her. Erica, Dani's nurse for the evening, gives Dani her pain and anti-nausea medication and she falls back to sleep. At 6:30 a.m. Dani awakes and uses the bathroom. She asks for more pain and anti-nausea meds. She comments that she feels like she just exercised without first stretching. She attempts to drink a can of Carnation Milk Chocolate Breakfast Drink before receiving doses of morphine and Zofran. By 7 a.m., her temperature is rising again. Erica gives Dani Tylenol. Erica and I agree that prior to blood transfusion, Dani should be given Tylenol. Jack the resident stops by and Dani tells him about this "muscular pain." Jack thinks that it is probably a slight infection and that the antibiotic they are using will help. As Erica finishes up, Katrina enters the room. She is able to draw blood from the PICC line without incident. She takes Dani's vital signs, and gives Dani her anti-gout and stool softener meds. With Katrina back on call Dani seems to rest more comfortably.

Later that morning Dr. Feigert arrives with what appears to be good news. He tells Dani that she has sensitive veins (of course!) and that the team is considering the placement of a more permanent catheter (Groshong) in her upper chest. Additionally, he reviews her progress. Her white blood cell count has dropped to 1,500. He predicts that by the end of the day, the count will be at zero and free of all blasts — an excellent sign. He also tells us that her LDH enzyme level was at 5,000 with 500 being normal (LDH is most often measured to evaluate the presence of tissue damage. The enzyme LDH is in many body tissues, especially the heart, liver, kidney, skeletal muscle, brain, blood cells, and lungs). This level was now down to 1,500. These numbers show us that the leukemic activity in Dani's body is way down. He believes that Dani's chromosome report is normal, although he had not yet seen the written report, but that her risks of relapse are still somewhere in the middle because of her extremely high white blood cell count upon admission.

> **HLA typing**: The human leukocyte antigen (HLA) test, also known as tissue typing, identifies antigens on the white blood cells that determine tissue compatibility for organ transplantation.

He thinks that she'll be discharged in about two more weeks and have three courses of consolidation chemotherapy. He still recommends **HLA typing** for Micah. Once more he tells her that the practice believes that the leukemia was brought on by a very bad case of bad luck.

Dani and the rest of us pass the day as relieved as we can be after getting through the first week.

The Second Week

9/18

A week has passed since Dani's diagnosis. We're awakened at 1:20 a.m.

by the continuous beeping of the IV monitor. It beeps for one of two reasons: the medication has been completed or the monitor just decides to beep for no apparent reason. It will take awhile before we figure out the cause of the beeping (and discover the mute button!). For the next four hours, Dani is given a boat-load of drugs (antibiotics to fight infection, serious pain medication and anti-nausea medication, primarily to deal with the side effects of the chemo). It seems as if the monitor never stops beeping. By 7 a.m., after what is obviously not a very restful evening, blood is drawn and our beloved Katrina arrives with the Phenergan and morphine, and teaches us how to work the monitor. With the arrival of a new day, we continue to hope to hear some good news.

When Dr. Christie arrives, Dani tells him that she only takes the anti-nausea meds with morphine. She reports that she's not experiencing any mouth soreness or neck pain. Dr. Christie seems pleased with that report. He seems concerned about Dani's spirits and suggests that Dani speak with a survivor of AML. He says that most patients feel that it's helpful. Dani only nods. He then reports some pretty good news. With the blast count now at zero, he reports that she has dodged two major bullets, that is, the worry of an extremely high white blood cell count and the fear of tumor lysis occurring. **Tumor lysis syndrome** is caused by the sudden, rapid death of cells, particularly cancer cells in patients with leukemia or lymphoma, in response to cancer therapies. As the patient's cancer is sensitive to the chemotherapy, the leukemic cells break down rather quickly. If we think of the leukemic cells as little balloons containing poison, the chemotherapy drug destroys the balloons and the poison is then released into the patient's blood stream, which then has to be filtered by the kidneys. This syndrome is prevented through additional treatment including intravenous fluids, Allopurinol and, in some patients, aluminum-based antacids. In Dani's case the fluids and Allopurinol, he tells us, have appeared to do the trick.

Then the conversation turns to Dani's cytogenetic studies (**Cytogenetics** is the study of chromosomes and the diseases caused by numerical and structural chromosome abnormalities.). Dr. Christie says that even though the initial report on Dani's chromosomes is relatively normal, it could be better. He continues saying that "the issue is whether a bone marrow or stem cell transplant should be considered so that the leukemia will not return in the future." For that matter, he's hoping that Micah is a match. He then proceeds to give Dani a pep talk. He says that things are going really well even now when her body's white blood cell count will soon be at its **nadir** (or lowest point, as it is called). At this time, Dani will have the greatest risk of infection (primarily from germs that were under control, in her own body). He recommends that she needs to keep fighting by doing what she is doing — keeping up her spirits, eating, hydrating, and walking around. As Dr. Christie is about to leave, his partner, and Dani's second favorite doctor, Dr. Feigert, arrives. It's only later that we realize that he had some news and wanted to share it with Dr. Christie first. As they leave the room, they tell us that Dani will be given two units of blood today to fight the fatigue that accompanies a low blood count even though her hematocrit (the percentage of red blood cells in the blood) is essentially on the borderline for transfusion at 26 (and quite a bit below the normal range of 36-46). Katrina draws blood, doses Dani with Phenergan , Pericolace, and Benedryl , and then, with nothing else to do, Dani showers.

The daily shower becomes a ritual for mother and daughter. Dani's strength had declined greatly by now, and she needs major assistance in showering. We have to seal up the PICC line and the catheter, because of the risk of infection. Dani has requested that I wash her and help her keep her balance as she can barely stand now. The last time, I bathed my daughter was probably when she had the chicken pox at seven years old. Dani is extremely weak. Her beautiful athletic body that had the lowest percentage of fat on the entire Division I Ladies Softball Team at Lafayette College is now limp. I dry her off with big, fluffy sheet towels that we brought from home, and dress her in her soft and comfy pajamas before returning her to bed. This daily shower quickly becomes part of our morning routine. It's my time to spot any new rash, discolorations or bumps that appear on Dani's body.

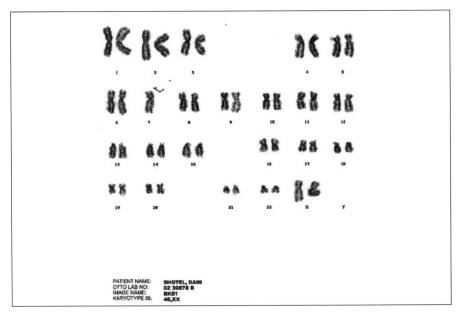

The image above depicts the cytogenetic study showing a missing chromosome #7

Once returned to her bed, Dani is given an antibiotic. She also asks for some morphine (for her just-starting-to-ache throat), anti-nausea meds and some Tylenol as a fever preventative medication for the upcoming blood transfusion. We are pleasantly surprised by a visit from our Rabbi, Jack Luxemburg. Rabbi Jack has known Dani for over 20 years. He has always doted on her and Dani on him, as well. When she was in high school, Rabbi Jack came on several occasions to Wootton's softball games to watch her pitch. Their relationship was, is, and will always be special. For this reason, it is kismet or fate that he is sitting by Dani's side when Dr. Feigert enters the room. The Rabbi asks if he should leave. Dani tells him it's okay, and that she wants him to stay. The doctor's report stuns us. He says that in further analysis of the cytogenetic study there are some abnormal chromosomes. In the 20 tests that underwent analysis, four of them showed abnormal results. In Dani's case it was a partial deletion of the long arm of chromosome 7, which is one of the abnormalities associated with AML in a small but significant number of cases. Because the research suggests that this deletion is of critical importance in a tumor suppressor gene (a so-called "cancer killing gene"), Dani becomes an AML patient with a high risk of relapse and a prime candidate for a bone marrow transplant. It appears that a missing gene in a portion of Dani's DNA had instantaneously transformed a robust, healthy, athletic, energetic, positive thinking 26-year-old into a seriously ill leukemia patient.

He further states that once her bone marrow is clear, she'll be referred for a transplant consultation. He mentions Georgetown Hospital, Johns Hopkins, a place in Seattle, and Sloane Kettering as options. "We'll get there when we have to," he says, and informs us that a referral could happen with one day's notice. He continues informing us that instead of five months of chemotherapy, Dani will now go for a bone marrow transplant, a very intense treatment. "But," he states optimistically, "that would be the end of your chemotherapy treatments. Dr. Christie will tell you all about transplants." He repeats, "It's an intense process, but you're young and healthy." (Little did we know how important that is!) He continued, "Our focus now is to get Dani into remission." Dani, our eternal optimist responds, "It's shorter?" Dr. Feigert says, "Yes, it's shorter, and more intense. The experience will be memorable. The goal is to cure you and there is a good chance of a cure. Our total expectation is that you are going to beat this. Right now you need to have an absolutely positive attitude of 'I can do this!' So...accept it for what it is." Dr. Feigert repeats, "Just focus," and looks at her PICC line, and returns to his normal "doctoring." He reports that her phlebitis (inflammation of the wall of a vein) looks worse today than it did yesterday as it appears extremely tender and, at the same time, hard. He believes her vein is infected, and will request that a Dr. Schwab, a radiologist, check the line later on in the day.

Dr. Feigert then departs. Dani continues her sunny disposition, telling Dr. Feigert to have a great day, and even reassures the Rabbi that she'll be fine. For the first time in our 20 years of knowing Rabbi Jack, he appears to be at a loss for words. Dani's strength is contagious. Her reaction to this "breaking news" finds Jay and me even more confident in her treatment and eventual cure. The Rabbi says goodbye to Dani, and Jay and I walk him to the elevator. We hug him and thank him for being with us. His concern for Dani was so much more than that of the obligatory caring which comes with being the leader of a congregation comprising

> The **Mi Sheberakh** is one of the central Jewish prayers for those who are ill or recovering from illness or accidents, whose name is taken from its first two Hebrew words. With a holistic view of humankind, it prays for physical cure as well as spiritual healing, asking for blessing, compassion, restoration, and strength, within the community of others facing illness, as well as all Jews, all human beings.

1,150 families. Dani touches him, as her spirit touches all of us. He tells us that members of the congregation will be saying the Mi Sheberakh for her recovery, every chance they get.

The day's routine resumes. More Benedryl is ordered for itching. The blood transfusion begins at 5 p.m. Dr. Schwab appears and checks Dani's PICC line. He says that it appears okay for now, but he'll check it again tomorrow. Later on that evening, after Dani's fans depart, Dr. Furlong, the infectious disease doctor, drops by. He checks Dani's arm where the PICC line is. He reports that it doesn't appear infected, but that "since you are neutropenic and you have a fever, we probably need to add more drugs." In some pain, Dani reports to him that she is past due for her Phenergan. As Dani says goodnight to Dr. Furlong, the night nurse, Erica, arrives with drugs aplenty and begins the second transfusion, which lasts until the early hours of the 19th.

9/19

The day begins with news that Katrina is off. Jack, the first-year intern, stops by at 7 a.m. Dani reports a new pain to him — in her eyes. The area around Dani's eyes appears darker than normal. As Jack leaves, Erica takes the empty transfusion bags out of the room. She also cleans up blood droplets on the floor (a result of the evening's transfusions). Dani and I let Erica know that it would be okay for her to turn on the room light at night! An hour later, Dr. Butler arrives. He appears pleased with all the signs so far. He explains that Dani's eye pain is occurring because her sinuses are clogged. He is the most humorous as well as the most senior member of the oncology practice, and he confirms what his colleagues have previously said. Dani's leukemia is very sensitive to chemotherapy and that Dani's body is handling the chemotherapy quite well. Chemotherapy is at its worst the first time around. "Some people," he says, "don't feel 'crappy' (a technical term!) at all when they get subsequent treatments." He is pleased with her blood chemistry, reports to us that Dani's numbers are all on target and that her vital signs (kidney, heart, lungs, liver, etc.) are all good. He predicts that one course of consolidation chemotherapy may be all that will be needed as the search begins for a bone marrow donor match for Dani. He tells Dani that she will most definitely lose her hair, and that any tingling in her scalp will not be a sign of dandruff but that of upcoming baldness. She thinks that this is not a big deal when put in perspective.

Dr. Butler then tells us about a study done at Johns Hopkins about whether patient isolation during chemotherapy treatment benefits the patient. He states that the study found that the patient is more at risk from his or her own body than from catching infections from others. He reiterates that it's okay to have visitors as long as they are not sick. Visitors should not touch Dani, and they should wash their hands when they enter room.

Around midday John Schnabel enters the room, checks Dani's eyes and orders Sudafed to Dani's ever-growing list of meds to combat the eye pain and quell the sinus infection. Dani begins to develop a rash on her thighs. Dr. Furlong thinks that it is a reaction to the antibiotic used for her sinus infection. He reminds me once more to report any new rashes as well.

The big news of the day for Dani the over-achiever is that she had three poops!

9/20

At exactly 5:58 a.m. Dani's induction chemotherapy is completed! Dani sleeps through this momentous occasion. At 7 a.m., Jack and Pamela begin their rounds by visiting Dani, who is becoming a bit of a team favorite. They think that the rash is dissipating and that Dani's arm looks less swollen. An hour later, Dr. Feigert confirms this and says that Dr. Furlong has recommended a change in the antibiotics to Imipenem (Primaxin), which is used to prevent and treat bacterial infections and has lots of potential side effects (rash, vein irritation, nausea, vomiting), but since Dani has these already it probably doesn't matter much. Dani reports pain in her throat, which Dr. Feigert calls chemo eutrophi (a raw throat). The cells that line the throat are also fast-growing and are therefore affected by the chemo as well. He suggests that Dani begin taking what he calls "magic mouth wash" (this nickname alone intrigues us). He also says that Dani's blast count is finally at zero and that they'll perform another bone marrow aspirate within a week to check that the blast cells have not returned. Dani recalls her introduction to this process and is not looking forward to having it repeated. Dr. Feigert assures her that it will be less painful as, hopefully, there will be no blast cells. If blast cells are found at that time, he says that she'll receive two more days of chemotherapy — "not a big deal." "Dani," he says, "it doesn't really matter how long it takes to get you into remission in terms of prognosis. The only thing that matters is that you get into remission."

Today is the big day for Micah. He will have some blood drawn to see if he is a potential match to be Dani's donor. We are informed that he will have a one-in-four chance of being a match. The results, we are told, won't be known for about one week. He returns from the process, looking a bit green, but he is hopeful that he will be the match that Dani needs.

The morning routine continues with an antibiotic eye drop added to the regimen. Dani's temperature is elevated (102.5). She naps and when she awakens an hour later her temperature has dropped. The nurses are having more difficulty taking a blood draw from Dani's PICC line. They begin to draw blood from Dani's other arm, using a **butterfly** (children's size needle), as it appears that our Dani has rather small and delicate veins.

When Pamela, John and Jack come in later that day, the discussion focuses on the rancidness of magic mouthwash. Dani had envisioned it as a wonder drug…what with the name magical mouthwash…tasting sweet and having an instant soothing effect on her sore throat. Once gargled, she swears that it is has the most vile after-taste of anything that has ever entered her throat! Dani says she would rather have the PICC line pulled without any numbing medications than ingest that stuff again. The three of them attempt to reassure Dani that it can't really be that bad…and it will eventually take care of the chemo eutrophi. At this point, Scott throws down the gauntlet. He tells them that his Dani will only take it again if John takes it as well. John says he will, but that this will have to wait until he's back on call, Monday morning. Some excuse! They quickly exit, only to return to say that they'll now give her a pill for the **thrush**. This also gives Jack the opportunity to tell Dani that he will try the magic mouthwash…as he will eat anything! That's just Jack for you!

Later that day, Dr. Rodriquez, the fifth member of the oncology/hematology practice, stops by and tells Dani that she looks terrific. Dani does not feel terrific. She

> **Thrush** is an infection of yeast fungus, Candida Albicans, in the mucous membranes of the mouth. Candida is present in the oral cavity of almost half of the population. These changes can occur as a side effect of taking antibiotics or drug treatment such as chemotherapy.

has pain, fever, the eye meds make her eyes sting, the magic mouth wash is disgusting, she is not sleeping well, and the rashes are popping up in various places on Dani's body. Our guess is that Dani looking terrific is relative to the other oncology patients on the wing. A new anti-fungal medication, **Diflucan**, is introduced. Dani and I begin to notice that as her ailments and rashes increase, Dr. Furlong's visits occur even later at night. It is not unusual for him to visit post-midnight. He stands at the entrance to Dani's room and shines a flashlight on Dani's face, arms and the rest of her torso. Our guess is that infectious disease specialists take no chances regarding germs. Despite this, Dani and I look forward to Dr. Furlong's somewhat quirky late night visits.

9/21

A new day dawns with a new drug being introduced. The Diflucan is being replaced with **Intraconazole**, another anti-fungal medication that promises broader coverage. Dani reports that her throat is a little sore and her eye pain is a bit less with the edema (swelling) around her eyes lessened. Despite her report of less pain, the nursing staff, already sensitive to her pain, begins to use a small blood pressure cup on Dani's arm (usually used with children). Dani appears to be having an allergic reaction to the **Cephalosporin**, which is used in the treatment of infections caused by bacteria, as she vomits. When Dr. Rodriguez arrives an hour later, Dani has showered, put on new pajamas, received her dose of Phenergren and has requested some Demerol. Dr. Rodriguez is upbeat saying that Dani's eyes look better, and her lungs sound good. She tells us that Dani will get a blood transfusion today, but until that happens she recommends that Dani get up and out of bed and walk around. A new anti-fungal drug is introduced into Dani's IV catheter, Sporanox (also known as Intraconazole).

The "chemo" is having its effect on Dani's eating habits. She reports that all foods are beginning to have a metallic taste. Dani is also disgusted by the awful smells of most foods. She does try some of my special homemade apple sauce, and drinks some water. Later on in the day, she directs my sister and me to buy some white bread. When we return with her favorite, Martin's Potato Bread, she is at once nauseated by its yellow color. Carol, Jay, and I start searching for information about food and food preparation for people undergoing chemotherapy. We find that Dani's reaction is normal and that a way to reduce the metallic taste is to prepare food using wooden, plastic, or glass kitchen products and utensils. For the limited time when we're not by Dani's bedside, our new goal is to locate our discarded Corning Ware products and prepare food that Dani will find acceptable.

That afternoon Dani is visited by Dr. Furlong's associate (Dr. Furlong has a well- deserved weekend off). The doctor squeezes Dani's arm and asks her if it hurts. She says that it does. He leaves the room for some reason. During this time, Dani quickly turns to me, grabs and squeezes my arm real hard several times, and asks me if that hurts.

I scream and we both laugh. She has caught me by surprise but her message is loud and clear. It amazes us that through all of this pain, my daughter is able to maintain a sense of humor. We are no less amazed by how disciplined Dani is. She follows the doctors' orders perfectly. She ingests drug after drug (Demerol, Zophran, Benedryl, Promaxin, Phenergren, Vancomyacin, eye drops, etc., etc.) without blinking an eye. The parade of medications even made Uncle Bruce's head spin (and he's the pharmacist of the family)! When the doctor returns, he has the nurse change the bandages surrounding the PICC line. She winces a bit when this dressing is changed. "Whoa!" she says, "My arm feels like it just got waxed."

Today is Saturday, and Dani has lots and lots of visitors. When your child goes off to college, you tend to lose touch with the friendships they develop. We are amazed by the quality and quantity of friends that Dani has amassed over the eight years since she has been out of our home. One special visitor stops in today, one of Dani's first pitching coaches, Don Dillingham. Dani attended a clinic led by Don early on in her softball career. During her high school career, Don was actually the varsity coach at a rival high school. Although Don knew how to coach the mechanics of pitching, his greatest strength was the building of mental toughness and motivation. Throughout her high school years, Dani kept one of his motivating poems right on her mirror…so that she began each day from a position of strength. This poem became the home page for the website Micah created as well:

> *If you think you are beaten, you are.*
> *If you think you dare not, you don't.*
> *If you like to win, but think you can't,*
> *It's almost certain you won't.*
> *If you think you'll lose, you're lost.*
> *For out of the world, we find*
> *Success begins with a person's will.*
> *It's all in your state of mind.*

If you think you are out classed, you are;
You've got to think high to rise
You've got to be sure of yourself,
Before you can win a prize.
Life's battles don't always go
To the stronger or faster person;
But sooner or later the one who wins…
Is the one who thinks "I can!" Anon

He sits himself next to Dani, and holds her hand. He speaks "fighting words" to her. He speaks about winning this game, believing in herself and her teammates. His inspiring words come from the heart. A small portion of his words include the following: "Don't let the cancer own you, and you should not own the cancer! When I walked into the room, you said, "I have cancer." You don't have cancer! You are a survivor and a fighter! You are not and never will be a person with cancer. People with cancer die…and that is not you!" When he finishes speaking, there was an awed silence in the room. Each of us is touched by the strength of his caring words. Dani seems to gain strength, sitting up straighter, smiling more broadly. If she needed any additional strength, these past few mnutes with her former coach stiffens her resolve to beat this thing.

Today is a special day because tonight Dani and Scott will have a date. Their plan is to watch the Miss America Pageant on TV. Scott is charged with keeping the notebook going. Jay, Micah and I leave Dani and Scott around 10 p.m. only to return twelve hours later. It is the first night that Jay and I are at home at the same time since the diagnosis.

9/22

During the early morning hours, according to Scott's very precise notes, Dani is given two blood transfusions. The nurse has to put an IV line into Dani's right arm as the PICC line isn't working fast enough to get the new blood flowing. Scott spends the entire night watching that blood flow ever so slowly into Dani's body. The second transfusion is completed by 7:10 a.m. Nick, the resident stopped by at 8 a.m. Now adding insult to injury, Dani has developed, as she says, "zits on my face." Scott leaves Dani's bedside to go home and rest a bit. He leaves Dani in good hands, as Katrina is back.

Later on that morning the doctors complete their rounds. The infectious disease doctor checks out Dani's arm. He says that if the hardness continues they will have to insert a new PICC line. When Dr. Rodriguez arrives, she is puzzled by the fact that Dani's counts are lower. She asks that another blood draw be done to verify the numbers. In the meantime, she advises Dani to keep exercising…that exercise will make her feel better. When the blood count is redone, it shows the white blood cell count recovering to 1.6. Dr. Rodriguez thinks it's a bit too soon (but then again, she doesn't know the power of the Dani)! Elizabeth, the technician who performs the second blood draw, is an eight-year survivor of **ALL** (acute lymphocytic leukemia). We continue to marvel at the quality of Dani's caregivers. The inhabitants of this parallel universe are truly awe-inspiring.

Later on that day, we all settle in and begin to watch the Redskins game. Dani tries Bruce's special compounded anti-nausea cream and it works! Even though the Redskins continue to suck, we are all delighted with Dani's upbeat mood. She eats five peanut butter crackers and has a great shower despite the fact that she now has a rash all over her body. Katrina goes out in quest of the infectious disease guy. A fourth-year resident shows up and checks out the rash that has now spread to Dani's posterior. He decides to leave it alone. After he leaves, the fan club reassembles and has a good laugh at the resident's expense. Dani remarks that she is beginning to believe that "this is really just a bad dream with really nice people in it." The Redskins lose…the company departs. Jay spends the night, which is, for the most part, uneventful.

9/23

At 2 a.m., Dani wakes up freezing. The evening nurse brings in more blankets and the heat is turned up. She falls back to sleep until Pamela and Jack stop in around 7 a.m. Jack downplays the rash by saying that it really doesn't look like a big deal! Pamela helps Dani out by changing her Phenergren dosage orders to "as needed." We're also told that we can use Bruce's anti-nausea cream without calling a nurse. Dani's blood is drawn and we find out that the counts are essentially the same. The staff notes that Dani's liver function is a bit off at this time.

Dani has a huge lunch today — some peanut butter crackers and three cups of juice. The decision is finally made to pull the PICC line. One of the nurses jokes that maybe they should have given Dani platelets first. The joke is lost on us. Later on in the afternoon, we all meet Dr. Leonardo Mendez, a **gastroenterologist**, who has been brought on board to keep an eye on things (such as potential liver damage problems). Right now, there is a borderline diagnosis. He will be checking for damage in how Dani's cells process and how well the liver filters out what he calls "the bad stuff." He says that today's test is down from yesterday's, which is a good thing even though her **bilirubin** (a pigment that is produced from the break down of red blood cells) is up. The liver is an amazing organ. Damage from high dose chemotherapy happens about 50% of the time. But the liver, with some rest, tends to heal itself. Dr. Mendez is optimistic but will remain connected to Dani's case and let us know if any problems develop. The day passes relatively quietly. Two-thirds of Dani's medical team, John and Pamela, stop by. Dani was given Diflucan (the latest anti-fungal medication) orally because her blood counts were low. Later on it seems that Dr. Furlong stopped the Diflucan, as her blood work confirmed that Dani never had a fungal infection. He also thought, according to John and Pamela, that it might be adding additional stress to her liver. Dani tells John and Pamela that she is worried about getting sores in her mouth. She also talks about eating, which is good news for all of us. As they leave, they promise to get her any take-out fast food that she wants!

Later on that evening Dani's nurse takes Dani off of IV fluids for the first time. She is not hooked up to anything for four entire hours. Freedom, however short, was sweet.

9/24

Dani spends a restless night, waking up at 3 a.m. and complaining about how cold she is. We wrap her in blankets, bump up the heat, and by 7 a.m. and Jack's visit she is warm and toasty and ready to face the day. Even though she says that her arm hurts, her throat is dry and she now has one sore in her mouth, she proudly announces that today she is going to make a new commitment to eating. She then proceeds to eat her cereal and drink all of her grape juice. We feel that we have experienced a miracle! On his way out, Jack mentions that they'll be introducing a new anti-fungal drug, **Abelcet** (also known as Amphotericin B) to Dani. We're told that it covers just about everything when a person does not have the **neutrophils** as protection from disease. (If this medication covers everything, we wonder why Dani is on thirty other medications!) Dani's body has overcome the first two crises in her battle with the disease: the extremely high blast count that invaded her body and had begun to clog her organs has been significantly reduced; and the leukemic cells appear to be highly vulnerable to the induction chemotherapy regimen of the first seven days. The immediate crisis is over, but now Dani has to face other risks caused by the treatment as

> **Abelcet** is used to treat a variety of serious fungal infections. It is often used in patients who cannot tolerate or who do not respond to the regular amphotericin treatment. It works by stopping the growth of fungi.

> A **neutrophil** is a particular type of white blood cell that is made in bone marrow, and whose absence would put Dani at continuing risk for disease. Its job is to find and kill any germs (bacteria) in your body. Neutrophils seek and destroy bacteria and keep you healthy.

well as the disease. Her liver now has to work extremely hard to get rid of the waste products caused by the successful first round of induction chemotherapy. In addition, her body is at risk from the various forms of fungi and germs/bacteria etc. that are kept under control by an intact immune system. They are now free to reproduce. For this reason, blood counts will be taken daily to monitor the need for transfusion of blood products, and to keep her as safe as possible during this period when her counts will be extremely low.

My sister arrives at 10 a.m. and comes bearing gifts: Danish pastries. Dani actually eats two pieces. Carol also brings a message from our favorite pharmacist, her husband Bruce. He wants her on **Colace** (a stool softener) and not Pericolace, as our Dani is having the opposite of constipation.

Prior to Dr. Butler's arrival at 11 a.m., Dani amazes us further by consuming eight pieces of matzo with butter and salt and washes it down with cranberry juice. Dr. Butler approves of Dani's commitment and states, "Food is medicine!" He then moves on to some interesting news. Dani's white blood cell count is zero. She has finally reached the nadir. When Dani tells Dr. Butler that she's totally exhausted, he explains that she is exhausted because she has very little blood, she'll be in nadir for about a week, and her exhaustion is par for the course. We come to learn that chemotherapy will affect the ability of Dani's bone marrow to make new blood cells of all kinds (red blood cells that carry oxygen through your body, white blood cells that protect you from illness, and platelets that enable your blood to clot). As a result, her blood counts will be lowest 10-14 days after chemotherapy. Dani is now officially what is medically called, neutropenic (which is a lack of neutrophils necessary to protect the body from disease). He's pleased with her progress and informs us that she won't need any red blood cell or platelet transfusions today. Despite the good news, he tells us that he's still quite apprehensive about this formidable enemy, AML. He compares it to a hand-grenade with a loose pin; it can explode at any time. Then, he adds, today there are many more victories in the battle with new methods of harvesting bone marrow, similar to the apheresis process that Dani went through almost two weeks ago.

Shortly after he departs, Joanne (the head nurse on the wing) confirms the rumor that Dani will be receiving Abelcet soon, along with Tylenol and Benedryl. She says this drug is "big guns" and "shows that we're not messing around." Dr. Furlong has prescribed one dose a day for several days as Dani's liver was not fond of Sporanox (Intraconazole). She tells us that the side effects may be some simultaneous fever and chills or rigors (severe shivering). Dani receives the dose and rests peacefully. Pleased by her positive reaction, Jay and I decide to go out to lunch around noon, leaving Micah with Dani. At 12:26 p.m. the rigors hit Dani, and it isn't a pleasant experience. Micah covers Dani with blankets, pushes the nurse call button, and yells for assistance. She is shivering so severely that the bed is shaking as well and Micah is afraid that Dani will hurt herself. The 4 minutes until Joann arrives, he later tells us, feels more like four days…but she arrives with reinforcements in the form of a Benedryl/Demerol cocktail. The cocktail achieves the desired effect quickly. Our Micah has always been devoted to his big sister, but usually it was Dani that was taking care of Micah's needs. Micah now takes on the role of big brother…the protector. It is much harder work! But throughout her illness, Micah, without being too mushy, demonstrates his love and willingness to do anything that would bring his Dani back to her normal nuttiness. Micah, Dani, and Joanne recount the Abelcet episode to us, when we return. Joanne tells us that Dr. Furlong will slow the infusion of the drug to four hours, but that it will continue through the duration of Dani's **neutropenia**. The remainder of the day and night are peaceful.

Week 3

9/25

Two weeks have passed since Dani's diagnosis and admission to Virginia Hospital Center at Arlington. Jack makes his usual round at 7 a.m. and Dani keeps to her commitment by eating Cinnamon Toast Crunch with some milk. She also announces that her bowel movement is normal. The big news of the morning is that Dani showers unassisted at 8:45 a.m. to be exact. Afterwards, she sips some water and comments that for the first time in two weeks it doesn't have the metallic taste and "doesn't taste bad." She takes Tums to help with her heartburn and tells us that it's working. She then snacks on some popcorn and awaits Dr. Butler's visit.

Upon his arrival, Dr. Butler wisely states that from now on Dani will be pre-medicated for Abelcet. What a concept! This was the drug that Joann told us was not one of her favorites, one of the "big guns," yet no one thought about pre-medication. At this point all we could do was laugh! He goes on to say that we're now at the half-way point of her induction chemotherapy treatment, but that there are still some bumps in the road yet to come. She's sure to have some ups and downs, as the treatment is complicated. He announces that tomorrow, Dani will have a second bone marrow aspirate and adds that we may want to pre-medicate for this. Based on her memories of her first time the aspirate was completed, Dani thinks it is an excellent idea. Dani is feeling so "chipper" after Dr. Butler's departure that she decides to give Philly Mom-Mom (Jay's mom) a call. It is short, upbeat, and sweet. Shortly after she hangs up the phone, John, Pamela, and Jack enter the room to be with their favorite case study. Soon, they get down to business and discuss Dani's reaction to the Abelcet. They agree with Dr. Furlong's changes to the protocol, and tell Dani that the drug will treat her fungal

sores. They also suggest a **Mycelex** troche, a lozenge that may ease the throat pain.

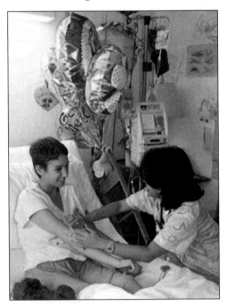

At 11 a.m., Dani and Katrina get all fancied up as they have been chosen to have their picture featured in the hospital's annual report. The fame and glory, however, is short lived, because by 11:10 a.m. Dani gets pre-medicated for round two of Abelcet. The cocktail of Benedryl, Tylenol, and Demerol works well today in reducing the fever, chills and general discomfort caused by

Dani & Katrina in Virginia Hospital Center

this powerful drug. By 3:22 p.m., the Abelcet has been infused into Dani's body without incident... thank goodness. With her temperature at 102 Katrina introduces a new antibiotic, **Aztreonam**, to fight off the bacteria and at the same time puts Dani back on IV fluids.

At 4:45 Dani is visited at long last by her Poppy and Grandmom. Never very fond of hospitals, they find it very difficult to see their beloved granddaughter in a hospital bed attached to a vital signs and IV monitor. I sense that they really feel Dani's pain figuratively and literally. During their visit, Laurie Alderman arrives, as she always does, like a sudden gust of wind! She has great news for Dani. In two weeks Arlington teachers have donated 45 days of their sick leave to Dani. And if that wasn't enough good news, she adds that Dani's insurance covers bone marrow transplants. (It wasn't until later that we find out that the search to find a donor, a critical part of the transplant process, is not covered by her insurance.) My sister Carol, who brought our parents to see Dani, wisely keeps the visit short. My dad, in failing health himself, looks as sad as I have ever seen him as Jay and I walk them all to the elevator.

And so begins another episode of the visitors' parade that crowd into Dani's room every evening. After their departure, Dani awaits the appearance of her favorite infectious disease doc. Dr. Furlong arrives sometime after 11 p.m. and tells us of the new medication regimen. He says that they'll cut back on the Vancomycin and stop the Immipenim. He'll now place Dani on round-the-clock Benedryl. Her rashes and swelling he dismisses as drug reactions. He favors Dani having a more permanent PICC line rather than the temporary butterflies used for infusions and transfusions. He agrees that Dani should be using a heating pad to ease the phlebitis in her right arm. With that advice, he bids us adieu.

Today is Jack's last day of his oncology rotation. He comes by in the early a.m. for his final examination of Dani. He looks at her rash (which is now mostly on her stomach) and the one sore on her tongue. He says, "You're looking great." In appreciation of his care, Dani has gifts for Jack. Since his next rotation will be pediatrics, Dani (an expert in her own right in meeting the needs of young children) gives Jack several childrens books to read to his patients. Jack is so appreciative of her thoughtfulness. He and Dani chat about his next rotation and Dani's job. Then, they discuss the upcoming bone marrow aspirate. Recounting the first one (the scream heard round the world!), Dani is not looking forward to this one. Jack reassures her that it won't be so bad now, as she doesn't have any of the blasts that exploded out of her marrow when the needle first entered, and besides, she will be pre-medicated. Dani nods but I'm sure she's thinking, "That's easy for you to say. You aren't the one being stuck!" She wishes Jack well, and he leaves.

A bit later, Dr. Christie pops in. He tells Dani about Aztreonam (Exactan) a new antibiotic. He inquires about Dani's rash and throat, which she says feels better. He tells her that her puffy stomach is par for the course, and that the rash is probably the result of the Ara-C chemotherapy.

For the past few days, there has been some discussion among the nurses about giving Dani the drug **Neupogen** to help speed the growth of healthy white blood cells. When we ask Dr. Christie about it, he replies, "She's doing so well, she doesn't need Neupogen." He also confirms that all of her reactions to the medications are normal.

> **Neupogen** or **Filgrastim** are man-made versions of substances naturally produced in your body. These substances, called colony-stimulating factors, help the bone marrow to make new white blood cells.

The morning continues with hydration, Tylenol, and Benedryl. There seems to be a problem finding a vein from which to draw blood. The nurses begin to apply heat to Dani's arms before they draw blood. She's taken to X-ray, returned to the room, and then returned for another X-ray due to some snafu. The highlight of the morning is the now infamous "butt check" (for rash and infection). We collectively cheer and laugh (like fifth graders) as we hear that Dani passed the test. As the morning ends, we learn that Dani's platelets are up to 27,000 (normal is about 150,000 to 450,000 platelets per micro-liter of blood), her red blood cell count is up and her hematocrit is a rousing 27.5% (36-45% is normal).

The afternoon begins with some Demerol and Phenergan. They'll serve dual purposes now as Dani first has a bone marrow aspirate, without incident, and then ten minutes later starts on her IV Abelcet. As is expected and despite the drugs, Dani does not have a great afternoon. She's cold once again, so we pile on the blankets, and she actually naps for two hours. She wakes up and feels too warm now. She tells us that she feels awful but will feel much better once the Tylenol kicks in. She readies herself for the evening's visitors with a heating pad on her right arm and an ice pack on her left!

The day is a gloomy one. It begins to rain in earnest in the late afternoon. Micah, Scott, and Matt, Dani's housemate, are none too pleased about this forecast, since tonight is the D.C. Light the Night Walk for the Leukemia and Lymphoma Society on Freedom Plaza in Washington D.C. Two other "F.O.D." ("Friends of Dani") teams have already participated in New York and Philadelphia.

They leave the very warm hospital room in late afternoon to meet up with other "F.O.D.s." They return hours later looking like three drowned rats, each carrying a slightly deflated red "Light the Night" balloon. Their somewhat pitiful appearance brings a smile to Dani's face.

The evening ends with an 11:30 visit by Dr. Furlong. He detects some fluid in her left lung. He suggests cutting back on her fluid intake. He also has some concern about Dani's breathing. The next day a set of pulmonary

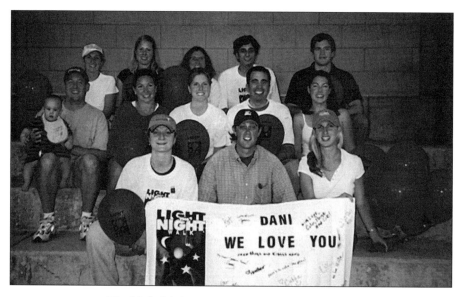

The Philadelphia Light the Night Team for Dani

function tests determine that her oxygen intake is in the high 80s and the normal should be in the high 90s. The tests determine how much air your lungs can hold, how quickly you can move air in and out of your lungs, and how well your lungs add oxygen and remove carbon dioxide from your blood. The tests can diagnose lung diseases and measure the severity of lung problems. He will recommend putting Dani on oxygen to relax her breathing. Dani's will to fight continues to amaze us. What we view as a very rocky road, Dani looks at as just one more bump.

9/27

The day begins with another chest X-ray. Pamela arrives promptly at seven, listens to Dani's lungs and detects a bit of a "crackle." Dani shows Pamela her disappearing rash (from both her arms and her tummy). After Pamela leaves, Dani decides to tackle the oxygen issue her way, and with her IV stand and monitor for support, walks two laps around the fourth floor of the hospital. When she returns her oxygen intake is at 88. Dr. Schnable (John) stops by a bit later and downplays the latest set-back saying, "Your lungs don't sound too bad. But for now, we'll keep the oxygen flowing." As John leaves, Dr. Feigert enters. He tells us that Dani will have a **lung scan** to make sure her lungs are clear. Dani downplays all of this by telling Dr. Feigert that she's always had limited lung capacity, and was even diagnosed with exercise-induced asthma during her years as a college athlete. Dani has now taken the role of reassuring the doctors! Dr. Feigert goes on to say that her bone marrow looks pretty good, but the pathologist will do a double check. He states that her white blood cell count is up to .6, which is "on schedule." On the other hand, he reports that Micah does not look like a potential bone marrow donor for Dani based upon the initial screening. Micah had a one-in-four chance in being a match, a two-in-four chance of being a partial match (three of six factors) and a one-in-four-chance that he will have zero

A **lung scan** is a nuclear scanning test that is most commonly used to detect a blood clot that is preventing normal blood flow to part of a lung. (It should be noted that we didn't know this at the time.)

of six primary factors in common with Dani. In fact, our son had zero out of six factors in common with his sister! We are not really surprised by the news as we joke that our kids are very different in every way. The search for a donor will have to extend outside of the immediate family. He goes on to tell us that he's going to give Dani some **Lasix**, to reduce fluid retention, and will order a **nebulizer** to facilitate her breathing. The Lasix, he warns Dani, will make her pee a lot. He suggests that hydration be cut in half. He asks Dani to

> A **nebulizer** is a machine that changes liquid medicine into fine droplets (in aerosol or mist form) that are inhaled through a mouthpiece or mask inhaler (MDI). It is powered by a compressed air machine and plugs into an electrical outlet.

begin measuring her fluid intake and output. Before he says goodbye, he tells us that Dani's oxygen numbers are no worse than last night, and that he's ordered some platelets for later today.

Just as he said, Dani has the lung scan at 11:20 a.m. We are told that it is done to insure that there is no infection. Even though Dani didn't have a fever, a sure sign of infection, they just want to be sure. A bit after Dani returns to the room, we are visited by Dr. Casolaro, a pulmonary specialist. As a welcome, Dani vomits in his presence! She tells him that earlier in the day she had difficulty breathing. When he asks if she has any chest pain, she tells him, "No." She repeats her tale of exercise-induced asthma, but said that she hasn't used the inhaler for at least a year. Jay's recollection is that she hasn't used the inhaler since she stopped doing "suicides," or running a mile at her college softball practices. She also informs him that she had pneumonia while attending Lafayette College. He checks her arms and legs for swelling. She also lets him know that last night she had trouble lying flat. The doctor explains that her stomach is distended, so it pushes her diaphragm up, which makes it hard to breathe. He states that there is less than a 10% chance that she threw a blood clot. Ah hah…we now know what the doctors were worried about! He suspects that the decreased air flow is caused by Dani's asthma plus some fluid retention. He prefers not to do a definitive test (a CAT scan) because the dye involved could affect her kidney function which already took a beating after the chemo. He decides that a nebulizer is the appropriate course of action. The nebulizer will give her increased oxygen levels and he warns that the oxygen will act as a diuretic (more peeing!). But he says that if this makes her hyperactive, they'll cut the dose down. He informs us, again, that Dani's pulmonary function is at 88% and it's supposed to be between 99% and 100%. He comments that the normal practice to treat patients with breathing problems occurs when pulmonary function is at 87%, but he recommends that Dani receive the treatment now, just to be safe. The nebulizer will be used every four hours for seven minutes. After he leaves, Dani lets us know that as long as the oxygen is going, she experiences no shortness of breath.

Pamela comes into Dani's room with her eventual replacement, Caroline, in tow and introductions are made. She also brings in an incentive spirometer and tells Dani she needs to breathe into it ten times an hour when she's awake. She tells Dani that her goal should be to get the little ball to the number 2,000 on the side of the machine. When Dr. Feigert arrives a few minutes later, he appears very concerned about Dani's swollen arm and the potential that she may have a clot in her troubled veins. He orders an ultrasound for her arm STAT! He wants it completed before the technicians begin their weekend. He's pretty sure that she hasn't thrown a clot, since her platelets are so low, and she's been given Lasix, which acts as an anti-coagulant as well as a diuretic. If we had any concerns about the quality of Dani's care at the beginning of this ordeal, it is now quite clear to us that any symptom or sign would be checked, double checked and followed up on. It seems that Dani's will is matched by the commitment of the staff. The old "ounce of prevention" adage seems to ring true. By 6:30 p.m. the test is completed and initially nothing dangerous shows up in the results.

When Dani returns to the room, her nurse, Lisa, attempts to insert a new IV line. She calls a specialist to get two IV's going, as Dani is behind on her medications with all the special treatments she has received today. Lisa places warm compresses on both arms and is finally successful in inserting the new line. Dani celebrates by having a banana, some Cheerios, and by doing her breathing exercises as directed.

When Dr. Furlong makes his late night call, he tells us that the tests were negative for clots, but Dani is still on fluid overload, and an anesthesiologist will soon stop by to begin the IV. As we are all relieved by the good news after what was a rather anxious day, he bids Dani a good night.

9/28

It is Saturday morning and Dr. Feigert pops in with some good news. The results of the bone marrow aspirate and the **flow cytometry** that analyzes the marrow show Dani's marrow to be totally clear. We all cheer with his great report.

Pamela drops in. Today is her last day in the oncology rotation. We've bought her pearl earrings to show our appreciation for her dedication to Dani. Pearl earrings have become a symbol of our best hopes for Dani's recovery, as those are the only earrings Dani ever wears. So now they have a special meaning. Pamela finds it hard to say goodbye and keeps dropping by all during the day. She promises to stop by on Thursday evenings so that we can continue the routine of watching the TV show "Survivor."

Dani has a pretty exciting day. Not only does she consume an entire peanut butter and jelly sandwich and a bag of potato chips, but she washes it all down with chocolate milk. We all find this to be very good news. The next bit of excitement involves a medical emergency but it is not Dani who has it. About 6 p.m., Dani's room is once again filled with her fans. Her dear camp friend Jason is among the well wishers. He smiles, and partakes in a few minutes of conversation. Then, suddenly, he says goodbye, jumps up, and rushes out of the room. We all hear a loud thump in the hall, and run out to find Jason on his back in the hallway with four nurses by his side. His blood pressure is extremely low at 68/44. He is immediately rushed to the emergency room of the hospital. I follow him down and when I arrive he is resting comfortably, and slightly embarrassed at the excitement he caused. The staff wants to keep him overnight for observation, but he balks at this, and says he is feeling much better. Rumor has it that he escaped, and fled before the ER staff returned to his enclosure. We call his home later in the evening and receive the good news that he made it home just fine. It's only a good memory today because Jason is okay, but this one episode reminds us how both funny and fragile life can be. Jay spends the night with Dani, while Micah and I return home.

9/29

Despite Katrina's positive thoughts that it might be possible that Dani would not lose her hair, Dani begins to suspect that was not going to happen. Dani's hair-endowed pillow case presented the clue that total hair loss was imminent! The head tingling reaches its crescendo this morning. Still, Dani maintains her beauty, as it's not her hair that is her shining glory but her beautiful smile and positive outlook on life. Early this morning, Dani announces that they may as well shave her head. Jay agrees to complete the task.

The following is Dani's account of the event:

My wonderful nurse, Katrina, has tried to assure me that she has known a few chemo patients who did not lose their hair during the course of induction chemotherapy. Unfortunately, I do not turn out to be one of those patients. We are nearing the end of the second week of my stay at Arlington Hospital Center when my hair begins to fall out in clumps and I begin to look like a mini "Cousin Itt" (from the Adams' Family). That night when my dad stays over, we talk about not letting the hair fall out on its own but by us "taking the bull by its' horns" and getting rid of it ourselves. The next morning, our only focus is in finding clippers to shave my head. One would think that with all of the surgeries and procedures that occur in a hospital, a pair of head-shaving clippers would be easy to find. It turns out that this is not the case! Katrina eventually presents us with a "nasty" pair of clippers. In fact, they appear as if they haven't been used since the early seventies! They look rusty and don't appear that they could perform the important task of removing all the hair from my head! We are correct. Undaunted though, my dad assures me that we will rise to the challenge! He asks for a pair of hospital scissors... and my dad begins to tackle my head of hair. The result is uneven and messy...but completely fabulous! I finally felt like we were personally doing something to fight back at the mess we are in. In a celebratory mood, I then shower myself and slip into a comfy pair of blue and white striped flannel pajamas. Feeling victorious, I hop back into bed, feeling quite smug. Soon after, my mom and brother arrive. She pales when she sees me. "Oh no," she said, "This will not do! Let's get you into something pink and girly. You see, my new uneven messy hairdo and blue and white striped pajamas, paired with my significant weight loss, make me appear like a concentration camp survivor...and my mom is not having any of that look. We laugh, I change, and I'm ready to face another day.

We learn later in the morning from Dr. Feigert that Dani's oxygen level has improved to 93%. He reports that her lungs "sound pretty good" with "less crackles." Dani's skin now has some **petechiae**, small red or purple spots on the body, caused by a minor hemorrhage (broken capillary blood vessels). Petechiae are a sign of **thrombocytopenia** (low platelet counts), which Dr. Feigert describes as, "a good thing, an arm band of courage." We can't figure out why. He also informs us that Dr. Furlong has reduced the level of Abelcet, as Dani's kidneys are "getting pretty beat up." Even though Dani's white blood cell count is a bit down today, he expects it to turn around soon. For that reason, he is continuing to keep the neupogin shot on a remote back burner. He tells Dani that all this silliness and pain from the PICC line will soon be a bad memory because tomorrow she'll have a more permanent "port," a **Groshong Catheter** placed in her chest. He says that she'll be sore for a bit, but all the tissues will heal. Dani merely takes it all in, smiles, and nods her head. He suggests that she receive platelets before the procedure. Later on in the afternoon, Dani performs a taste test of the entire dried fruit spectrum (since her chemo diet prevented her from having fresh fruit). She approves of the apple and apricots but offers the dried pineapple to her guests.

In the evening Dani complains that her PICC line is burning. Dot, Dani's night nurse, replies that in 24 hours she won't have that to complain about any more! She also reminds Dani that she can't have any food prior to the Groshong procedure (which we thought would occur by mid-morning the next day). Soon after the nurse leaves Dani's room

> Because of a greater risk of infection with a central catheter, the PICC line was utilized initially, and when the doctors felt the time was right, a **Groshong Catheter** was then inserted in Dani's chest. The Groshong Catheter is a long, thin tube made of flexible silicone rubber. It is surgically inserted into one of the main blood vessels leading to the heart (this is basically done to dilute potentially damaging medications by having them flow into a main artery so they can be diluted quickly inside the body). It can be used for drawing blood samples and for giving intravenous fluids, blood, medication or nutrition. It basically reduces the number of needle sticks you need to have while you are being treated.

Dr. Furlong enters. He looks Dani straight in her eyes and tells her that she appears to be in good shape. Coming from Dr. Furlong, this is good news indeed! He further states that her lungs sound clear, and he's not too worried about her kidneys at this point in time. He asserts that, as her blood counts rise, her fever will go away. He then tells us a bit about the Groshong procedure. Dani will be sedated but she's not to worry about that because "it's not big time surgery." He also mentions that a Dr. Wagner is performing the surgery. Dani says goodnight to Dr. Furlong and has a restful evening.

9/30

The day begins with a blood draw at 7:34 a.m. Dani's temperature is normal as is her blood pressure and pulse. Dani has been told to fast until after the surgical procedure of implanting the Groshong Catheter in her chest is completed. Dani decides that her daily shower will wait as well. When Lisa, Dani's nurse for the day, arrives, she informs Dani that the procedure won't take place until 3 p.m. at the earliest.

Dr. Rodriguez arrives and is pleased with the blood counts even though the white blood cell recovery is a bit slow. Dani complains a bit that her stomach doesn't feel so good. Dr. Rodriguez says, "Dani you're doing well," but that the kidney function is still down a bit. She's further impressed with the increase in Dani's oxygen intake level. The treatments seem to be having a great effect as Dani's oxygen level is now at 96%. The day passes slowly. Finally, at around 6 p.m. the surgeon, Dr. Wagner, drops by to meet Dani. He, too, is a comedian as he tells Dani that he is happy today because, "he always wanted to do one of these surgeries!" Prior to being wheeled down to surgery, Dani places her food order. She's now been without food for about 24 hours. She tells Scott and Micah very specifically that she wants Domino's cheese pizza, breadsticks, plus McDonald's fries, a cheeseburger, and a vanilla shake. When she returns from the procedure, she consumes it all. We are thrilled! At 8:34 p.m., Dot, Dani's evening nurse, arrives and takes out the PICC line. Hooray! She checks Dani's vital signs and doses her with Phenergan , Demerol, Vancomycin, Exactim, and Vicodin. Dani doses off early, so when Dot draws blood from the Groshong Catheter successfully, Dani whispers, "Yay!" with her eyes closed.

10/1

Dani's day begins early and with quite a shock. At 2:15 a.m., Lisa, Dani's night nurse, brings an ice pack for the Groshong site. The ice pack opens up all over Dani! But the day improves as at 7:04 a.m. the nurse is able to perform a blood draw once again with no difficulty. Later that morning, Dr. Meister stops by and begins to speak about transplant centers. He says that if Dani is a good candidate for an **autologous transplant**, it might not be necessary to go to Hopkins. He tells us that the Virginia Hospital Center in Fairfax and Georgetown Hospital both do autologous transplants. (In an autologous transplant the person's own stem cells or bone marrow are collected and stored. The patient then undergoes high dose chemotherapy and/or radiation to destroy the disease, after which the stem cells or marrow are re-infused into the patient.) Whether Dani is a good candidate for an autologous transplant is, to some degree, dictated by her chromosomal difference. Jay's research already suggests that this will not be the way to go for Dani. Dr. Meister then tells us that they will begin to set up consultative appointments for Dani in about 10 days to two weeks from today. He also speaks about the possibility of an allogeneic or matched unrelated donor (MUD) transplant as another option. He says that the chosen center will be making the recommendation as to what protocol to follow. As he leaves, the new team of interns enters Dani's room. It appears that only Caroline is familiar with Dani's case.

Later on that evening, when Dr. Furlong drops in, Dani speaks with him about her continuing period. Dr. Furlong doesn't believe that it is related to her treatment, and suggests that if it doesn't slow down, we may need to consult with a gynecologist. For the record, Dr. Furlong seems quite pleased with Dani's progress, as she is **afebrile** (without a fever) for the first time since she was diagnosed.

Week 4

10/2

The morning proceeds routinely. Caroline, Pamela's replacement, stops by at 7 a.m. and, as the nurse completes the blood draw, reports to Caroline about Dani's never-ending period. A respiratory specialist stops by, listens to Dani's lungs and reports that she sounds good! Today is a special one as, for the first time in a month, Dani feels good enough to pay her bills!

Later on that morning Dr. Meister appears with lots of great news. Dani's kidney function is improving; her marrow is recovering; and there is a good chance that Dani will be out of the hospital by next week. He tells us that Dr. Christie will make appointments for us to consult with various transplant centers prior to selecting the correct one for Dani. In our discussion about bone marrow transplants, Dr. Meister informs us that it is his professional opinion that Seattle has the best facility for unrelated donors, the Fred Hutchinson Cancer Research Center (or "The Hutch," as it is affectionately referred to by many).

Dani, once again, brings up the issue of her period. He too appears unconcerned. He says that her platelets are fine, and he thinks that all the medications have messed up her menstrual cycle. He proceeds to tell Dani what she can and can't do when she goes home once her counts are recovered. He wants her to walk for exercise but not to overdo it. The best news for Dani is that she can be around her chocolate Labrador Retriever, Phoebe. Despite the long difficult days and challenges that lie ahead, Dani is grinning from ear to ear as she tells Dr. Meister to have a great day.

Later that evening, we hear about two murders that occurred in Montgomery County. By 10 a.m. the next morning four more lives are taken. In all ten people are killed and three wounded in the three-week spree that begins on October 2, 2002. The D.C. area is in shock for the next three weeks, and we join people all over the D.C. area in taking extra precautions, everywhere we go.

10/3

Today is a momentous day for several reasons. The first reason is Dr. Christie's visit, of course. He tells us that Dani's platelets are up to 97,000 (good news) with her white blood cell count recovering to 1,000. Additionally her **creatinin level** (a measure of kidney function) continues to drop. It is now at 1.4 with .6 to 1.0 considered normal. He checks Dani's phlebitis and tells her that the bumps are caused by her neutrophils that are fighting infection. He expects that her counts will go up every day. Then Dr. Christie gives us another bit of news. He makes a "WAG" (wild-assed guess) that Dani will be out of the hospital in three or four days. After we cheer, he warns us that what awaits Dani in the future compared to her induction chemotherapy treatments will be "a walk in the park with thunderbolts!" He says that we have at least three options for treatment after induction chemotherapy, remission, and consolidation chemotherapy (chemo that will keep Dani in remission until her bone marrow transplant). The first option is an autologous transplant. The second course of action is an **allogeneic** stem cell transplant from a relative. (Since Micah was not a match, we would now proceed to get as many of our relatives tested as possible.) Finally, he spoke about a MUD transplant (Matched Unrelated Donor) that we would find through the National Marrow Donor Program. He believes that a MUD transplant will probably be the most likely option, and that Hopkins and a place in Seattle called the Hutch are the places to go for that process. He explains the process of consolidation chemotherapy to us. He says that after your marrow recovers from chemo, you can go another 14 to 21 days before you receive another dose of chemo that will keep you in remission. He says that the hospital stay would be much shorter, probably four days, and that Dani would be able to go home to recover until the next treatment. Dr. Christie leaves us with a lot of information to chew on.

Jay now begins to work on the schedule to get as many family members as possible tested, although the chances are slim that one will be a match for Dani. We realize that we will have to schedule a day locally as well as one in the Philadelphia area to make it as convenient as possible for as many relatives as possible to be tested. In addition, Jay contacts members of both sides of the family to ask them to get their blood typed. Within an hour of Dr. Christie's departure, Laurie Alderman, Dani's principal and mentor, tells her that the Arlington County teachers have now donated 80 of the 90 days of sick leave needed to cover her until she becomes eligible for disability insurance. That number will eventually reach 120 days — part of the overwhelming support she receives from her fellow teachers, many of whom do not know her personally. She tells Dani that she'll stop by later to have Dani fill out some paper work regarding the school system and the state's longterm disability coverage.

That afternoon I receive a phone call from Dr. Fred Appelbaum, who we later find out is the Director of the Clinical Research Division at the Fred Hutchinson Cancer Research Center in Seattle. He is absolutely charming on the telephone. He tells me that as a child he grew up three doors away from Dr. Meister, one of the partners in Dani's nearby hematology/oncology practice in Virigina. Obviously Cleveland,

Ohio was the hotbed for preparing oncologists! He appears extremely confident on the telephone, saying that they'll begin a preliminary donor search as soon as possible. He estimates that the search will take approximately three months. During that time Dani can have her consolidation chemotherapy back in Virginia. I hang up the phone feeling quite confident about finding a donor for our Dani, and Jay proceeds to contact the next person on the list of guardian angels.

In the next 30 minutes, Jay is on the phone with Rochelle Sislen. Rochelle is the local representative for the Gift of Life Bone Marrow Foundation, whose name we received from Bruce. Rochelle tells Jay that she wants to do a preliminary search for Dani's blood typing of the National and International Registries that are a part of the World Marrow Donor Association. Over the phone, Jay reads Rochelle Dani's blood typing. Within a few hours Rochelle calls Jay back after reviewing the database available to her, and confirms that the numbers of potential matches for Dani are less than for the general population; but she also expressed some confidence that among the 8,000,000 potential donors

The **Gift of Life Bone Marrow Foundation** was established in 1991 as a donor recruitment organization, to help save the life of New Jersey leukemia patient Jay Feinberg. From 1991 to 1995, the organization launched an ambitious campaign to recruit donors of Eastern-European Jewish ethnicity throughout North America and abroad. Although it started as a grassroots effort to save one life, the campaign facilitated transplants for hundreds of other patients also in need of donors. Jay Feinberg's ethno-geographic background was Eastern-European Jewish, the same as Dani's. Since a patient's best chance of identifying a genetic match lies with those of similar ancestry, donor drives sponsored for Jay focused on Jewish communities worldwide. Over 60,000 donors were typed at more than 225 drives around the world, and dozens of matched donors were identified for other patients as a result of this campaign. Then, in 1995 Jay's miracle happened: a donor drive organized by the Foundation identified a closely matched donor! Jay received his transplant in July 1995 at the Fred Hutchinson Cancer Research Center in Seattle, Washington. Since the campaign for Jay Feinberg, the Foundation formalized its evolving role as a Bone Marrow Registry. In early 1998, the Foundation joined the World Marrow Donor Association and began to participate in bone marrow donor drives worldwide. The Foundation currently maintains a database of over 100,000 bone marrow donors, and focuses on the registration of Jewish volunteers of Ashkenazi (central and northern European) and Sephardic (Spanish/Middle Eastern) ancestry. Both minority groups are underrepresented in the worldwide donor pool. The tragic consequences of the Holocaust have caused additional difficulties for patients of Eastern-European Jewish ancestry, which severed potential bloodlines.

a match will be found. She reiterates that persons of Eastern European Jewish ancestry are underrepresented in the potential donor registry. Our awareness of this under-representation phenomenon makes us a bit more nervous about finding a match for Dani. There are several "general" matches within the pool that were made available for her review, but she advises Jay that testing all available family members was still a wise thing to do, as "general" matches could turn out not to be at the level required for a transplant to move forward. Rochelle is quite helpful in gathering the materials Jay would need to test our willing extended family members, and Jay drives to her house the next day to pick up the materials he will need to do the testing. We decide that on Sunday, October 13th we will test the family members that are available to us in the D.C. metropolitan area as well as some close family friends that wish to be tested; and that on Sunday, October 20th, Jay and I will travel to our home town, Philadelphia, to test the majority of both our families that still reside in that area. Individual family members who live outside of the D.C. and Philadelphia areas or who were not available that weekend will be given information about how to get tested or sent test packages by mail, in what is a very simple procedure of a swab with a Q-tip from the inside of the mouth. The search for a donor to save our daughter's life has begun in earnest! If all of these events weren't reason enough for October 3rd to be a momentous day, Pamela topped it off by reserving the hospital's Community Outreach Room for the evening's viewing of "Survivor" for Dani, Pamela and the visitors that showed up that evening.

10/4

Dr. Butler arrives for his morning rounds. He's quite pleased that Dani's body is showing a substantial recovery of healthy blood-producing bone marrow. He emphasizes that the first remission is the "big bump point." *"Dani," he says, "will be even healthier"* when she undergoes consolidation chemotherapy. He reiterates some of Dr. Christie's words, saying that Dani has successfully dodged four bullets: she survived the first 24 hours with the help of the incoming treatment of the drug

Hydrea and apheresis designed to bring down her white blood count; there did not appear to be organ damage from the blast cells or the initial chemotherapy; her leukemia was highly sensitive to the chemotherapy regimen; and she is currently cancer free and in remission. Dani is quite pleased by his assessment. Despite the positive words of Dr. Butler, Dani is still experiencing considerable pain. Her medication regimen continues to increase. Her doctors have told her that with each day the pain will decrease, but such has not been the case. She tells the nurse on duty, that her arms and hands are bothering her. When she makes a similar statement to Dr. Furlong later in the day, he tells her to keep wiggling her fingers and keep hot packs on her arms. As for the phlebitis, Dr. Furlong tells Dani not to worry about it. Dani feels better mentally, if not physically, after the conversation, and relaxes sufficiently to nap for a few hours.

10/5

Dr. Schreiner, the doctor who urged his primary care physician partner to administer a blood draw on September 10th, drops by to visit Dani. He, as always, brings Dani a vending machine pastry (slightly "squished" from being kept in his jacket pocket), and tells Dani that he's glad to see that she is in remission. He says, "it helps being strong and of good stock." We all laugh because it is what Dani's Grandmom always says.

That evening after Dani's visitors have gone home, an elderly female oncology patient enters her room. She surprises us by embracing Dani and initiates some sort of religious blessing before a nurse arrives to escort the woman back to her own hospital room. Dani and I are pretty sure that this is an omen for Dani to hurry up and get released from the hospital real soon!

At 1:15 a.m. Dani is unplugged from her IV. I'm sure that she is dreaming sweet thoughts of her home in Falls Church, Virginia.

10/6

In preparation for Dani's departure from the hospital, we begin to take the cards, pictures and posters off of the walls in her room. Dani remembers that Dr. Christie had told her that she will probably be leaving the hospital on Monday or Tuesday. Dani is so excited about this possibility that she joins in the room clean-up effort. We put together a list of questions for the doctor as we work.

Dr. Butler finally drops in 2:00 p.m. He tells us that Dani is getting stronger, and if her counts continue to be this good, she can participate in her normal activities when she goes home. As her arms are much better, and her white blood cell, platelet and neutrophils counts are doing well, it should be a very boring day. At this point, boring is a good thing! He patiently answers our questions one by one. Here are a few responses to our multitude of questions: do not worry about getting West Nile Virus; Phoebe, Dani's dog, is not a threat; Ted, her 3-year-old pet red-eared turtle is, however, and a roommate will have to continue to take on the care and feeding; as long as your counts are good, you can eat, drink, and exercise as before; and you can pluck your eyebrows and go food shopping, but not at the same time! "Once released from the hospital," he adds, "Dani needs to drop by the office once a week and to have her blood counts checked." He also gives Dani permission to walk outside the hospital, although he says that she should wear a hospital mask. Delighted with all the good news, Dani says goodbye to Dr. Butler and calls her "partner in crime," risk-taking Liz, to plan a clandestine adventure. As Jay and I figure that Dani's place in Falls Church probably could use some cleaning, prior to her release, we depart for a mission we have come to dread! We leave for her home. Without informing us, Dani prepares for an adventure of her own. Liz's response to Dani's request is, as always, supportive. "Dani, I know your mom is going to kill me, but I'll do it." Within one hour of our departure, dressed in plenty of warm clothing, a wool hat, and a hospital mask, and with her partner in crime, Liz and Dani begin their secret mission. Dani wants to surprise Scott by walking the little over a mile to his house. It takes a while as Dani has lost a great deal of muscle strength (and obviously common sense as well!). When they arrive at Scott's house he is nowhere to be found. Dani leaves a message in Q-Tips, spelling out "I LOVE YOU" on his bed. They then begin the trek back to the hospital with the goal of arriving before Jay and I return to the hospital. When we walk into her room, she proudly boasts of her accomplishments and falls into a deep slumber. Our reaction is surprise over concern. We admonish Liz, a tiny bit, but Liz, as only Liz can do, assures us that she would always take care of Dani.

Dani describes Liz and their clandestine mission as follows:

Liz came to the hospital as often as she could. She came by bike, bus, and/or metro. Her laugh warmed my room and probably kept the nursing staff from trying to pair me up with a roommate (her laugh is kinda loud ☺). Thank God for Liz! Liz was with me on one of my most adventurous days in that hospital. Originally the doctors and nurses told me that I would be in the hospital for 28 days. Well, on my 28th day, I was not well enough to be discharged and was beyond upset. The doctors struck a deal with me. They said that I could go for a walk outside the hospital while wearing my medical mask. Well, that was good enough for me. I called Liz, and told her that she needed to come over. So, we went downstairs, and we walked outside, and we kept walking...not around the hospital as instructed, but towards Scott's house (which was a little less than two miles away). Liz kept saying, "Oh my God, your mom is going to kill me!" But, of course, she kept walking with me. We made it all the way to Scott's house. He was not home.

Liz is an angel throughout this trial. Dani had met Liz eight years ago, when she joined the Lafayette College softball team as a "walk on." Armed with plenty of *chutzpah*, and a *joi-de-vie*, she soon become one of Dani's best buddies, and one that Jay and I came to love and respect. After they both graduated from Lafayette, Liz went into the Peace Corps. Upon her return from Malawi, Jay was in the midst of searching for a new administrative assistant in the university department that he chaired. Liz was interested in the tuition benefits for a master's degree and was more than qualified for the position. When she interviewed and was offered the position, she grabbed it and quickly became a most valued asset. Little did we know just how important she would become to the department and to Jay when Dani became ill. She quickly developed a network of university contacts as only Liz could do, streamlined some of the office operations, creatively redesigned some of the office procedures, and was easily able to sort and order Jay's responsibilities so he could concentrate on the issues of greatest importance while splitting his time between the hospital and the office. These abilities became critically important, especially in

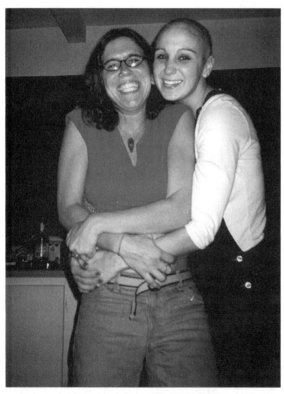

Liz and Dani smiling as usual

the months that would lie ahead, when Dani and I would be in Seattle and Jay would become a commuter to Seattle and a tele-commuter to the office every other week.

Once Dani was diagnosed, Liz essentially increased her sphere of influence at the office, acting as screener, gatekeeper, and organizer, while Jay's energy was divided between our daughter and his responsibilities as a department chair and a faculty member at George Washington University. Liz also was one of the key members of the voluntary group of friends that became the driving force in the various drives and fundraisers that were organized around support for Dani and other leukemia victims. She was the primary contact person for the Red Cross-supported bone marrow drives that were arranged in November, and was key in organizing the "Light the Night Friends of Dani" groups that walked in her honor to raise funds for all people fighting blood related cancers. She also provided much comic relief during Dani's several hospitalizations. One unforgettable memory is her determination to learn how to knit. She had seen me passing the time by knitting, so she asked me to teach her. Even more stubborn than myself, as well as free-spirited, she began to knit (she called it that) a scarf, paying very little attention to my very precise instructions. That "scarf" was proudly given to Dani before her departure to Seattle in January of 2003, and Dani proudly wore it during her stay…provided it matched her outfit of the day!

10/7

We begin to notice that Dani becomes a little less "special" as her counts improve, and her rashes and various aches and pains dissipate. In the morning, Dr. Butler tells us that he is quite pleased with Dani's blood counts, and that her kidneys are functioning normally. Even Caroline, the intern, seems unfazed by the fact that Dani has had her period for seven days. Dr. Rodriquez stops by later in the day, and once more reiterates to Dani that a Neupogen shot is not necessary. She said that this treatment wouldn't do anything at this point, as Dani's counts were rising nicely. She said that Dani's neutrophils were at 300 today, but they should be at a minimum of 500 before Dani would be allowed to go home. She suggests another walk outside, not knowing what Dani had already accomplished. Jay and I bundle Dani up for an unnecessarily protective walk around the neighborhood surrounding the hospital. Later on in the day, we find out that Dr. Christie is setting up our consultation visits to Johns Hopkins on October 14th and Seattle on October 18th. As a further sign of Dani's upcoming departure from the hospital, Dr.Furlong tells us that he is preparing a one page summary of the medications Dani has been on and her reactions to each of them. We laugh as we try to figure out what the impossible-to-read font size would be on a one-page summary of her medications and her reactions.

10/8

In preparation for Dani's release from the hospital the next day, Dr. Christie removes Dani from all antibiotics. He tells us that her counts will probably go down a bit as a result. He is not in a great mood today as he is having some difficulty setting up the consultation with Seattle (at present, both our Seattle consultation and the beginning of Dani's first round of consolidation chemotherapy are slated for the same day, which is obviously problematic). He leaves and returns one hour later, more like himself, and reports that consolidation chemotherapy will probably begin on 10/21 rather than 10/18 as originally scheduled. This will allow us to have our consultation at the Hutch as scheduled. The high point of the day was a call from "Poppy," Dani's grandfather. His sage advice to Dani today was for her to eat eggs, and "not those junky bagels!" In our discussion later that day, we decide that I'll go to work Wednesday morning, 10/9, and Jay will stay with Dani until she is released from the hospital as we're not quite sure what time this highly anticipated event will occur. Jay now begins to plan our strategy for the next few months: getting the relatives tested; making arrangements for consultations; organizing fund-raising activities; and, making sure that Dani's insurance covers what it needs to. Dani has dodged the bullets that came at her so suddenly. Now the work begins for a cure.

10/9

Dani is released from the hospital. It is mid-afternoon by the time I receive this great news. Unfortunately, the call comes after I have served eighth-grade lunch duty, one of my least favorite tasks as a middle school administrator. I rendezvous with Dani and Jay at her home, and together we write up a food list in preparation for the food shopping we will do. We plan a celebratory dinner of lasagna for Dani, Scott, and her housemates, Matt, Lori and Maria.

Some Get Well Notes from the First Month

It is our belief that positive communication can play a huge role in a person's health. Dani received so many visitors and phone calls during that first month wishing her well. She also received hundreds of "get well" cards and notes. A highlight of each day for Dani was mail delivery. Anyone who disputes the influence of love, humor, and positive thoughts on a patient's recuperation, needed to see the impact each note had on her determination to "fight this thing!" Here is a small sampling. You be the judge.

From a student's mom (Dani's student from the previous year who along with this note presented Dani with his prized life-sized cut-out of him as Super Ben): *"Hi! We have been collecting Ben's art for weeks, but Ben keeps pulling it out of the pile and taping it around the house. He loves to admire his own artwork almost as much as he loves his own reflection in the mirror! Ben turned four last week. He celebrated several times, mostly spontaneous. We had a party at the Puffins snack time. My parents were in town so we went out a lot, and Ben managed to tell the wait person at every place that it was his birthday and he expected them to sing to him! They did. He can say that he is four ("dor") and shows four fingers. He knows his colors, except for some red and green confusion. No shapes yet. He can count semi-reliably to four. He counts like this: "One, two, three, four, ninety, twenty".... Ben still listens to your message on our answering machine everyday, often several times a day. It is his never-changing ritual. Heaven help us if the power should ever go off! He asks about you all the time and begs to stop and visit every time we pass Arlington Hospital. He plays with his airplane and pretends he is flying to see you.... We can't wait to see you. Come home!"*

From Dani's attending medical resident: *"I just wanted to let you know what a pleasure it has been to work with you and your family over* *the past few weeks....I hope you realize how much you are touching the lives of everyone who has had the opportunity to get to know you....I had no idea when John gave me your name and told me to get your history and physical done on the day you were admitted how deeply I would grow to care about you....When you're a student struggling every day to learn and remember the immense amount of information that comes your way, it's very easy to lose sight of the human side of medicine. Thank you for not allowing me to do that. Thank you for making getting to work...an absolute joy – and most of all thank you for reminding me why I went into medicine in the first place. Your constant smile, even during the worst of what we put you through, has brightened too many of my days to count....Thanks so much for being you and for being my favorite patient ever...Dani- keep smiling, and know that I'm thinking about you and wishing you all the best, now and always."*

Chapter Six
Extreme Opposites on the Road to a Cure...

Dani's Memory — Coming Home

10/9

Finally the doctors clear me to leave the hospital. It has been so long since I had worn anything besides pajamas. It has been so long since I have played with my crazy dog. It has been so long since I have eaten dinner at a table (rather than a hospital bed). I am so ready to leave. This is not to say that I'm leaving the Oncology Ward without some tears shed. I know that I will be back within a month's time...but, that doesn't matter right now. Saying good-bye to Dot, Katrina, Joann and Lisa is harder than I could have ever imagined.

They have some hospital policy of having to be escorted to the exit of the hospital by wheelchair. This strikes me as pretty weird considering throughout my entire stay I was never wheeled anywhere (except in and out of surgery...but, I think that is pretty standard). Anyhow, I'm wheeled down to the exit of the hospital. Scott and my dad have packed up both cars. My dad is running to Dominoes to pick up some pizza and then planning on meeting us at home. I climb into Scott's car and happily breathe in the smell of unfiltered and untreated air. The car is not sterilized and even has a bit of trash on the floor. I love it. I haven't been allowed to be in an environment like this in what felt like forever. For the entire ride home we speak of all the things we will do, now that we could be a "normal couple" again. We are so happy.

Scott pulls up to my house. I jump out of the car, possibly even before it stops moving. I rush up to the front door and unlock it. I run to my room and immediately tear off my hospital garb. My thought is, "I'm going to be 'normal' and sexy, and I'm going to put on my 'good butt' jeans." I find them neatly folded in a drawer. This was not how I left them. I knew my mom had come by and straightened before I had gotten home. I pull them out and immediately jump into them. Unfortunately, I'm not normal and far from sexy. They fall right off me. These are no longer my "good butt jeans" and things are far from being "normal."

Dani's return to her home is a momentous occasion. Jay and I have stolen away from the hospital in the past week to straighten up her room, do her laundry, change her linens, and to make the rest of the house as sanitary as possible. Dani does have three capable housemates at this time, Matt, Lori, and Maria, but none of them have reached the "fanatic" stage like we have in terms of keeping things clean. Her place not only has to be immaculate (which is nearly impossible for a twenty-something group house), but it also has to be stocked with all of Dani's favorite foods. As both Jay and I are planning to return to some approximation of a normal work schedule, we both want Dani to be as comfortable as possible. We take care of every detail, or so we think.

Dani's first day home is celebratory. Scott brings her home from the hospital in the early afternoon. Jay follows behind with a carload of "stuff from the hospital" plus a special lunch. When I arrive, we do more food shopping in preparation for Dani's homecoming dinner. Her roommates join Scott, Dani, Jay, and me for the feast. We leave shortly after dinner, leaving Dani at peace, finally, but exhausted by all of the activity.

Our plan for the next two days was for Dani to rest in the morning with Scott. Jay and I would be arriving as soon as we could from our respective jobs. We didn't, for a moment, anticipate the anxiety Dani would feel once she returned to her own home. Despite the fact that her roommates are home at night, Dani alone in her bedroom, without the companionship of the nurses (who became her friends) or one of us, begins to process all that she has already been through, and has trepidations about what she will soon face. She has difficulty sleeping with such thoughts, and when she does finally fall asleep, she has nightmares. Even having her beloved Labrador Retriever Phoebe nearby doesn't stop these thoughts. Scott moves in.

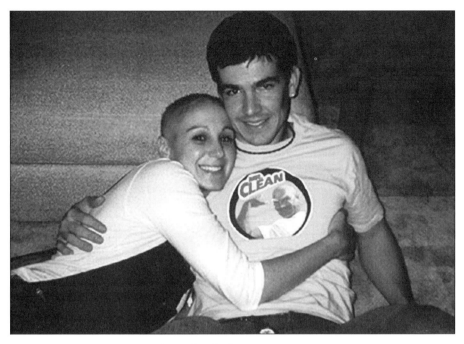

It's good to be home again.

10/10

On her second day at home, she decides to confront the personal demon, leukemia by turning to her creative side. She takes out her paints and creates a self-portrait. The portrait is of a post-chemotherapy Dani. She portrays herself nude, hairless, sad, with tears flowing, yet with a determined expression. A poem written over the self-portrait reads as follows:

> *I remember looking into the mirror that day*
> *And thinking you have Leukemia?*
> *I could stand to be alone in that moment*
> *Lose myself in the reflection*
> *But I wasn't alone*
> *I was thrown into a world of comfort*
> *Filled with friends and family*
> *I could have cried with tears never ending*
> *But instead the worst news of my life*
> *Turned into a time of utter amazement*

Due to the unpredictable amounts of kindness
And compassion shown by many
I will beat this for me and for everyone who loves me.

She shows us the painting when we arrive. We are stunned by the stark beauty and simplicity of the painting and the poem. This painting travels with us throughout Dani's travails. It is hung in her various hospital rooms throughout her treatments. We create hundreds of thank you notes with the image of the painting on the front. People are amazed by her talent and positive spirit. She even amazes those closest to her!

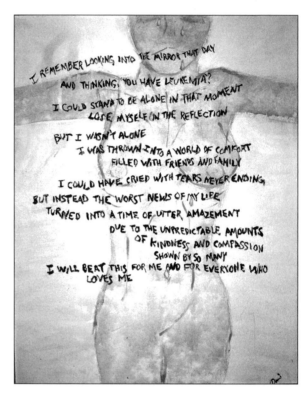

Dani's self-portrait and poem

Several additional paintings are produced during this "in-between" time which are accepted for a gallery show in the area before she leaves for Seattle.

By early October, contact had already been made by Liz with the Red Cross of Washington, which is linked with the National Marrow Donor Program (NMDP) and its local branch office located at the National Institutes of Health in Bethesda. They will provide the materials and the personnel necessary to do the actual testing of people interested in becoming bone marrow donors. The cost of the testing is approximately $50 to $100 per person, but the Red Cross could cover a portion of the cost. In addition the "Fair Lakes League," a community-based organization in Virginia, and the Friends of Allison, a nonprofit corporation providing funding for the recruitment of potential marrow donors, are also contacted by Liz, and both organizations agree to support our efforts. The Foundation was established in honor of Allison Atlas, who was diagnosed in August 1989 at age 20 with a rare form of leukemia. Doctors informed Allison and her family that her only chance for survival was a bone marrow transplant. No one in Allison's family had the perfect tissue type that matched hers, so she was forced to appeal to the community for help. The Atlas family also turned to the NMDP. Family and friends also formed the Friends of Allison in October of 1989. The purpose was to recruit more potential bone marrow donors. A campaign was launched to find a life-saving donor for Allison and the thousands of other patients who needed a matching donor. Unfortunately, a donor was not found in time for Allison. Allison's search sadly failed but thankfully her effort was not to be in vain. The Friends of Allison continues to fund marrow testing for other cancer victims because Allison believed, "No one should die because they do not have a donor." Mr. and Mrs. Atlas both advised us on the bone marrow drives, and members of the family were present at both the Wood and the Beth Ami drives. The Atlas family and the continuing support of other groups and organizations, such as the Gift of Life Foundation and the Red Cross, as well as NIH and the National Marrow Donor Program, have been key to developing a world wide registry that now totals over 13 million potential donors.

10/12

On Saturday we have a meeting of all the people who have volunteered to help in our efforts to test for a possible donor, raise funds for medical expenses for Dani and for leukemia focused charities, and promote the cause generally. About 30 close friends turn up at Dani's house for this organizational meeting. Jay gives a brief introduction, speaking about costs and what insurance will and will not cover. Liz discusses her contacts with the Red Cross, the Gift of Life Foundation, the Allison Atlas Foundation and the Fairfax League, in terms of their support for the bone marrow testing drives we would like to schedule. Laurie Alderman takes over and details the plan for the first drive scheduled for the Walter Reed School in Arlington (where Dani teaches) on November 7th. Laurie's planning becomes the model we'll follow for subsequent drives. By the time the two hours have elapsed, we have planned four drives (Reed School, my school in Montgomery County, our synagogue in Rockville, Maryland, and another synagogue in North West Washington D.C.), who would be the lead person(s) for each drive and who would be responsible for publicity.

In addition we float approximately thirty ideas for fundraising activities with the help of the documentation provided by the National Transplant Assistance Fund. One incredible fundraising event falls into our lap. A colleague of Jay's at Geogre Washington University has a brother who works for the Washington Wizards professional basketball team. Through the kindness of Abe Polin, the owner of the team, and the support of Chip Maust and his brother Brian, tickets for several games are set aside at reduced cost so that we will be able to charge half-price for the tickets, and Dani's fund will receive the differential between the cost of the ticket and the price we paid. Scott will be taking the lead in organizing and marketing the event.

We are astonished at the level of support and commitment shown by Dani's, Jay's and my friends. The feeling of helplessness our friends had felt is now transformed into plans of action. This turns out to be a huge gathering of "Type A" personalities. It is surprising that Dani's house is still standing with all the energy that is concentrated in one space!

Although we know that there would be a slim possibility of Dani finding a match from the local bone marrow drives that are being sponsored on her behalf, we, as a family, become very involved in this activity and several of our friends devote a great deal of their time, effort, and energy to these events. These four drives would not just be supported financially by these organizations but also with voluntary professional personnel.

With Liz, Laurie, Bonnie, Sandy, Wendy, Burton, and Susan ready to set up their respective drives, they had their work cut out for them. In addition we would need both publicity for the drives and volunteers to man the various activities not associated with the actual blood draw necessary for typing (i.e., the welcome station, sign-in and form completion, screeners to review eligibility, the babysitting area, and a station to take voluntary contributions to defray the cost of the testing). We all agree that no monetary donations would be taken for Dani specifically at the bone marrow drives. Contributions would be directed to the groups that made the drives possible. Liz is tasked to work with Laurie Alderman, Dani's principal, on the first drive scheduled for Reed Elementary in Arlington County. A date in early November is targeted.

10/13

This week is another busy one for the Shotel family. Jay has already picked up test kits from the local representative of the Gift of Life Organization, Rochelle Sislen, several days before our mini blood drive at our home. After our Micah proved not to be a match, and even though the chances of finding a match within our extended family are slim, Rochelle suggests that testing family members is still the wise thing to do. The kits do not require a medical person as they are designed to sample DNA by taking a swab of the inside of one's cheek utilizing a long Q-tip. Although the analysis of DNA is a bit more expensive than the traditional drop of blood test that would be utilized in the other drives we were planning, we are pleased to be able to get our family tested in the comfort of our home. So we invite my sister's family to get tested. Close friends of similar Eastern European ancestry, convinced that their bone marrow would be the match that would save Dani's life, decide to come as well. With that element of high expectations present, one would think that the Shotels' were celebrating someone's birthday! The guest of honor, Dani, travels with Scott from Falls Church to visit and thank everyone for their efforts. In total we add twenty more potential bone marrow donors to the national registry on that day and plan another similar activity for our family members based in Philadelphia for the following weekend.

During the last several weeks, Jay utilizes his skills as a researcher to develop a new area of expertise — that of recommending to Dani, Micah, and me the places, based upon the data, which would have the greatest probability of success. The two locations that appeared to have the greatest potential for a MUD (matched unrelated donor) transplant are Johns Hopkins, because of its proximity and general positive reputation, and "The Hutch," because of their significant experience and success rate with Dani's particular form of leukemia. Although the data seemed to suggest that Hopkins has much more limited results with AML patients, proximity convinced us, in the end, that a consultation with them was important.

10/14

We rendezvous with Dani and Scott in the early afternoon and make our way to Johns Hopkins Medical Center, where we are scheduled to meet with an oncologist for a consultation. Because this meeting is so important, we invite Carol and Bruce to join us. Bruce has prepared at least two legal-sized pages of questions for the oncologist.

For the past month Jay, Scott, Micah, Carol, Bruce and I have read every bit of information that has been provided by our doctors and the hospital. Jay went further, accessing various websites, including those designed for George Washington University faculty and linked to the hospital and medical school. One source in particular, *Survivor*, by Laura Landro, is helpful with regard to both treatment options and self-advocacy. It gives Jay, Scott and me a gut-wrenching, first-hand account of what is involved in a bone marrow transplant. The three of us are extremely grateful for that book, as it "pulled no punches" and informed us about the details of the process that no medical journal could ever provide. Dani, as only Dani can, chooses a different path in preparing for the transplant. She refuses to read anything that speaks in statistical terms. Additionally, she is adamant in her refusal to speak with survivors of leukemia. She lets us know that this is her body, her disease, and she will fight it her way. This means doing what her doctors advise, eating well, exercising when she is able, and surrounding herself with her friends and family. She approaches the task as if she is training for the college softball season: focused on the goal, determined to do the right thing, and with the discipline necessary to become ready for the task at hand with her careful preparation. The goal is to destroy the opposition!

By 1:30 p.m., the six of us arrive for our appointment with the Johns Hopkins oncologist. We sit and wait in what appears to us to be a relatively new wing of the building in a football stadium-sized waiting room, with many numbered doors and lots of people waiting for their name to be called. We are joined by Dr. Ryan Katz, an old friend and schoolmate of Dani's, who oftentimes was smarter than the teachers who taught him. Ryan, whose brilliance is only exceeded by his sense of humor, is completing his residency in Reconstructive Surgery. He waits with us, reassuring Dani that she is in great hands at Hopkins. Soon Dani disappears into one of the many doors for a blood draw. When she returns, Dani and her "posse" of five are led to a tiny, windowless, and rather warm office. It is here that Dani, Scott, Bruce, Carol, Jay and I will spend the next two hours and 15 minutes in consultation with the oncologist assigned to Dani's case. Obviously the room that has been selected for this purpose is not designed for the size of our posse. The oncologist is a bit surprised by the number of "family members" accompanying Dani to the consult. He adds three more chairs to the already cramped quarters and begins. He reviews the "givens": she has AML, her chromosome number 7 is a bad marker, and there is little likelihood of a cure with either an autologous transplant (using her own cleansed bone marrow) or with chemotherapy alone. He continues by discussing an allogeneic transplant from an unrelated matched donor, which he states has a 50-50 outcome. In order to have this type of transplant it is imperative that Dani continue in complete remission, as relapse lowers the success rate of the outcome. In addition, he suggests that a donor should be found as quickly as possible to reduce the number of consolidation chemotherapy treatments, as each treatment takes a toll on your body. He then proceeds to detail the matched unrelated bone marrow transplant process with us. He breaks down the process into three phases. The first phase is preparation; Dani will be given high doses of **Busulfan** followed by Cytoxan. He specifically details the toxicity these poisons can have on Dani's organs. Dani listens intently, and tears up a bit. The doctor proceeds to inform us about the second phase, infusion and engraftment of the stem cells. He speaks about the number one problem and reason for "mortality and morbidity" of allogeneic transplants being Graft versus Host Disease (**GvHD**).

Upon hearing these not so pleasant words, Dani tears up a bit more, takes a deep breath, and refocuses on the doctor. He then speaks about the recovery phase. His notes from our October 14th meeting (which we received after the consult) state the following:

> **GvHD** occurs when infection-fighting cells from the donor recognize the patient's body as being different or foreign. These infection-fighting cells then attack tissues in the patient's body just as if they were attacking an infection. Tissues typically involved include the liver, gastrointestinal tract and skin.

It is during this phase...most patients appear to have fairly stable bone marrow function, but the patient remains at increased risk for infections...which can be detrimental.... Matched unrelated donor transplants, even in younger patients, offer an up-front mortality between 30 and 60%, but based on your current excellent health and relatively reasonable tolerance for previous therapy, and provided you are in remission at the time of your potential transplant, and if you find a donor, you are likely to have an up-front mortality between 30-45%.

This notation is quite similar to what he states during the consult.

These words, not unanticipated by Jay, Carol, Scott, Bruce or I, still manage to shock us when stated so nonchalantly. Dani is stunned.

The doctor continues by presenting to us the process of the reconstruction of Dani's immune system and treatments she will receive during her first year post-transplant. He tells us that Hopkins prefers doing a transplant where the donor is a perfect 6/6 match, but mentions other experimental treatments that Hopkins is currently pursuing. He then allows us to ask questions.

We ask questions about the use of cord blood transplants, fertility and egg storage, and the likelihood of finding a related donor. Then Bruce, brazenly asks, "If this were your daughter, where would you want her treated?" The doctor seems somewhat taken back by the question. He agrees that Seattle does more allogeneic transplants per year and with excellent results that have been very difficult for any other center to reproduce. However, he states that Hopkins, being closer to home, will offer Dani her continuing support of friends and family. But he adds, "It will be a relatively short period of time that you would actually be away."

He tells us that he will speak with Dr. Christie after our consult is ended. In closing, he tells Dani, "our goal is to get you as normal as you can be, as soon as you are able." We say goodbye and Jay tells him we will contact him upon our return from Seattle to discuss how we will proceed with the process.

The six of us leave the office, find our way to the parking lot, and decide to meet at Amici Restaurant in Baltimore's "Little Italy" to process what we heard in the meeting. Our Dani is emotionally drained and says little during lunch. None of us appear to have much of an appetite, which is certainly unusual for this family! I check my notes and count the number of times the doctor mentioned the words *morbidity* and *mortality,* which turns out to be four times. After this revelation, Dani asked that we talk about something else. We agree. Our late lunch is eaten in relative silence.

It is not until our ride home from Baltimore that Dani speaks again.

We have just driven through a rain shower. Suddenly, Dani looks out the car window and spots a rainbow. Like our Dani of old she says that the rainbow is meant for her, and that she's pretty sure that the end of the rainbow is on top of her house in Falls Church!

10/15
Dani calls me at work in the afternoon. I am shocked by what she has to say. The oncologist from our consult at Hopkins has just called her. He said that he had already spoken with Dr. Christie and would be consulting with Dr. Rainier Storb from Seattle later in the day. The doctor told Dani that it was a pleasure meeting with her and her family and said that it would also be his pleasure to help her in any way possible. He also expressed regret if his words upset her. We laugh and look forward to our trip to Seattle.

10/17
Several days after our less than comforting consultation at Johns Hopkins, we fly to a consultation at Fred Hutchinson Cancer Research Center (the Hutch) in Seattle. Micah's initial recommendation for the Hutch to be considered for treatment options, with only a slight bias because he lives out there, was now backed by data about the center. The National Marrow Donor Program keeps a database on each of the transplant centers by cancer type as well as a variety of other factors, including success rates broken down by patient age and type of cancer. It turns out that the Fred Hutchinson Cancer Research Center in Seattle is the world leader for the treatment protocol that Dani would need. Under the structure of the Seattle Cancer Care Alliance: the University of Washington Medical Center, Children's Hospital of Seattle, and the Fred Hutchinson Cancer Research Center work together to serve the Northwest and the world.

Micah meets us at Sea Tac Airport. He takes us to the Silver Cloud Inn, a hotel that is a few blocks from the Hutch and right off of Lake Union. Just over four years ago our family began our love affair with the "Emerald

City," when Micah enrolled as a freshman at the University of Puget Sound. We actually stayed on a tugboat, which was converted to a "bunk and breakfast" on Lake Union, so we were somewhat familiar with the area. However, in our many visits to Seattle over the last four years, the Fred Hutchinson Cancer Research Center and its multiple buildings that line the east side of the lake went unnoticed by our family. Now it was possible that it would become the center of our world for the months to come.

That evening, we go to our favorite Italian restaurant in East Lake (obviously East of Lake Union), Serafina. We are introduced to the owner, Susan Kaufman, and we ask for special seating in as secluded a place as possible, since Dani's immune system is not what it should be from the induction chemotherapy. Susan is glad to make our acquaintance, and more than willing to comply with our request. She and Dani form a bond, as Susan is a survivor of breast cancer. She extols the virtues of the Hutch, the University of Washington Medical Center, and Seattle. She then sees that our dining experience is a fabulous one. Serafina becomes another comfortable and special place for our family, and Susan becomes a new friend of Dani's. Her enthusiasm and positive spirit that evening were just what the doctor ordered.

10/18

In the morning, the four Shotels embark from the Silver Cloud Inn to the Hutch. We enter the building's lobby and are immediately struck by the warm atmosphere. In front of us sit two smiling volunteers stationed at the Information Desk. The walls of the lobby contain inspirational artwork and motivational statements. The volunteers direct us to the sixth floor. As we arrive there, we are greeted by the receptionist. The waiting room is incredible, not just because its 80-foot expanse of windows overlook Lake Union and the Olympic Mountains, but also for its child-friendly play area and easy computer access. In the future, we will pass time marveling at the magnificent view and watching the seaplanes take off and land on the lake.

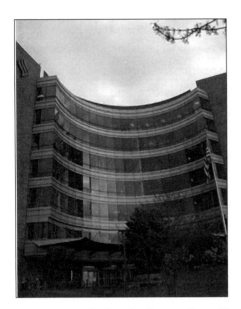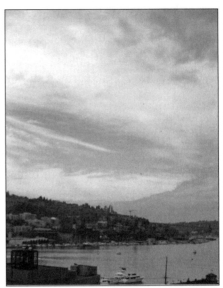

*The Seattle Cancer Care Alliance Building at the Hutch and
the view from the sixth floor*

Soon, we are escorted into an "airy" and windowed conference room, replete with a round table, five chairs, and a white board. Dr. Rainier Storb enters and introductions are made. Dr. Storb, an imposing figure, is casually dressed in khaki slacks and a blue oxford cloth shirt. He is wearing Birkenstocks on his feet. We later learn that he often kayaks to and from work across Lake Union. We meet for over two hours with Dr. Storb, the head of the Transplantation Biology Program, a member of the Clinical Research Division, and a Professor of Medicine at the University of Washington. We later find out he is the originator of the protocol utilized to treat bone marrow transplant patients. He begins the consult on a positive note, saying that the search had already begun for a matched unrelated donor for Dani at the Hutch on October 3rd, and they are optimistic that one will be found. He tells us of three well-matched donors (from the United Kingdom, Italy, and Germany), four broadly-matched possibilities from France and the United States, and sixty-four split mismatched donors. Of course, with this news, we are all smiles. Dr. Storb estimates that the time it will take to find and test the donor and prepare for the transplant to be approximately three months so that he expects Dani to have two additional rounds of "consolidation" chemotherapy before her trip to Seattle around the 15th of January. The time spent in Seattle for preparation, transplantation and recovery is likely to be another four months, with much of the time spent as an out-patient in an apartment a few blocks from the clinic facility.

Then, he begins to educate us. Occasionally using the white board to draw, spell, or define terms, Dr. Storb at once becomes the master teacher and the Shotels his attentive students. The information he imparts is familiar, as we have heard most of it from the oncologist we met with at Johns Hopkins on Monday. The difference, quite frankly, is in his delivery. He is enthusiastic about the work being done in AML research and treatment and optimistic about the potential for a cure. "Matter of factly" he tells us that Dani is at high-risk because of the missing chromosome 7, and because of that a transplant is the correct treatment. Each year, he tells us, they perform from 140 to 160 transplants with a 60% success rate. Each day, with new research findings, these numbers have improved. He then proceeds to explain the three phases of Dani's treatment; pre-transplant preparation, transplant treatment, and out-patient care. Despite the sometimes gruesome details he mentions, he is quick to detail the preventative and on-going treatments put in place to bring the patient some comfort. Dani, he says, will begin her high dose chemotherapy as an out-patient. None of us will have to wear masks during this time. He explains that the process of receiving a new immune system does have the possibility of long-term side effects, like secondary tumors forming in the next 10 to 15 years, sterility, and the possibility of lung disease. This information, at this point, is no longer shocking to us!

He then discusses the treatment phase, saying that Dani will be in a private room on the 55-bed oncology wing of the University of Washington Hospital. "There is 36 hours between the last **Cytoxin** dose and the stem cell infusion." He mentions that she may need a **plasma exchange** at this time to facilitate the change of blood type during the time prior to the actual transplant. After the transplant the donor's bone marrow or peripheral blood stem cells should engraft in 11 to 12 days. Dani will be in the hospital for approximately 28 days and will be released to outpatient care when her blood counts come back.

When he begins to discuss the post-transplant recovery phase of the process, his focus is on Graft vs. Host Disease (GvHD). This affects 75 to 80% of transplant patients. He tells us that it presents as a rash or the stomach just doesn't feel right about three weeks after the transplant. When and if this occurs, it's treated. A separate consultant team is called in and medications are prescribed to prevent possible damage to the liver, kidneys, lungs, and other organs. He mentions that Dani will be placed on **Methatrexate**, as a GvHD prevention, as well as **Cyclosporine** and immunosuppressive drug. These two drugs work together to prevent the donor cells from attacking Dani's organs. But, he adds, we find that a little bit of GvHD is a good thing, as it shows her new blood system is beginning to work. When a person has some GvHD the relapse rate is lower in matched unrelated donor transplants. Dr. Storb, although intent on presenting a realistic picture of the entire transplant process, demonstrates great confidence in the institution's ability to react to "bumps in the road" but says to us, "so as complications arise, and they will, treatments are prescribed."

Dr. Storb tells us that when we choose the Hutch for the transplant, Dani will be assigned to a team that will include a senior attending physician (like Dr. Storb), three primary care professionals (an oncology fellow, a hematology fellow, and a physician's assistant) as well as a Hutch oncology nurse and a University of Washington oncology nurse. Other specialists will be called upon as needed. But for now, he says that the search is underway for her donor. Once a donor is found, his or her blood typing will be completed by the lab, a transplant date will be set, Dani will begin high dose chemotherapy as an outpatient, be admitted to the hospital, have the transplant, and remain at the transplant wing of the University of Washington Medical Center for the next 30 days as an in-patient. She will then once again be seen as an out-patient at the Hutch for the next 80 days or so, and then sometime around May 1st leave Seattle. Whew!

Dr. Storb concludes the consult after he answers our questions about minitransplants, the use of cord blood, the possibility of not having radiation as part of the preparatory regimen for the transplant, and Dani's concerns about fertility. Dr. Storb, in his meeting notes to Dr. Christie on October 21st, says, "The family indicated that we should initiate our unrelated donor search here in Seattle. I conclude by thanking you for referring this delightful patient and her family to us...."

After our consult with Dr. Storb, Jay and I visit the financial office where we are advised of the costs associated with the transplant. Our conversation with the financial representative was positive but sobering, to say the least, and consistent with the information we had already gathered. She explained to us that the cost of the transplant protocol that Dani will need was estimated to be $253,000. This included the expenses incurred from the time the donor search was initiated on October 3rd through the stay at the University of Washington Medical Center Transplant Wing, which Dr. Storb estimated to be about 30 days. This would not include the approximately 70 days of treatment following release from the hospital as an out-patient at the Hutch. Nor would it include the expectation of an additional year of relatively constant follow-up. Approximately 80% of the medically related costs would be covered by insurance. The non-medically related costs of relocating to Seattle for almost four months (transportation, lodging, food, and the other expenses of setting up our living quarters) were not covered under Dani's policy, which was the best that her county school system had to offer. We found this to be consistent with what was occurring already back home.

After this "eye opener," we head downstairs to the blood clinic on the first floor. A smiling technician retrieves Dani from the waiting area. She takes one look at our daughter and she says, "Oh, you are so beautiful." Dani of course, is now all smiles. Five minutes pass and the technician returns Dani to us, saying, "We can't wait for your return. We are going to have so much fun with you here!" Dani, we're sure, by these two statements has decided which medical facility she prefers.

10/19

We leave the Seattle Cancer Care Alliance clinic facility in a very different frame of mind than at the conclusion of our last consultation. Upon reflection, it was not what was said factually that was all that different; it was how it was said, and the confidence with which it was said, that made all the difference in the world. We believed that the Hutch had the attitude as well as the expertise to save our daughter's life. Dr. Storb spoke quite frankly about the perils associated with the treatment Dani required, but he never, never, never mentioned the terms morbidity or mortality. Instead, with each possible and anticipated complication he spoke about the treatments that would battle the complication. Dr. Storb also continually referred to what was proven by the research and how the treatments prescribed were always based upon the data. He went to the white board several times to "teach us" the facts about transplants. His approach to a room full of teachers was right on target. All four of us were impressed by the facility (even Micah, who is not easily impressed), the personnel, the attitudinal set, the positive and professional climate, and the upbeat, friendly environment. Never did Dani feel like just a number; she actually felt like these strangers would become her friends and support her through the trials that await her, just like her new friends at Virginia Hospital Center did for round one of her fight.

In retrospect, how could we expect anything else? Over the last five years we have found the Seattle area to be a friendly, down to earth, and warm place. The Hutch impressed us in that same way. It is a large facility with tremendous resources, but the individualized, personalized care was quite apparent. Before we even step out into the Seattle sunshine, the decision had been made. The Hutch is the place to go for Dani, and Dr. Storb allows us to be cautiously optimistic that a match will be found.

Chapter Seven
Battle Plans are Formed . . .
"People Get Ready"

10/20

On Saturday, we say goodbye to Micah and Seattle and return to the D.C. area. Once home, Jay and I prepare for our Sunday trek to Philadelphia in order to test our respective families. Jay's cousin offers the use of her home as a place for family members to come to have a DNA swab taken. On Sunday morning the 20th, we drive the 156 miles to Philadelphia. We manage to complete this task with our well-known efficiency. Members from both the Shotel and Balin side of our family join us at a cousin's home, with the confidence that one of them will be a match for Dani. Jay drives those same 156 miles back to our home in Gaithersburg later that afternoon. We are exhausted from all of this activity after having sat for 30 days in one hospital room. We may be physically tired, but now Jay and I are cautiously optimistic that a donor will be found, despite the odds against the possibility that one of the 43 family members tested in the past two weeks will become that donor. With Monday morning rapidly approaching, we both prepare for our jobs, trying to fit in our time with Dani accordingly.

Dani's Memory

The week of 10/21

After my first hospital stay, I'm able to come home to my four-bedroom house with my three roommates. It actually becomes "my four roommates" rather quickly. There is no way that Scott is ever going to let me out of his sight (except when he has to go to work). When he goes to work, my mom tries to adjust her schedule so that she can be with me.

Between the two of them I'm taken care of as if I'm still in the hospital.

One day about two weeks after I had returned home, I have had enough. I feel stronger and I want to, at the very least, show my mom that I can care for her as well as myself. I call her at work and tell her that I'm going to make her lunch on that day. She sounds so excited at the news. She is going to be over within an hour, that is, after 8th grade lunch duty ends. It's now time for me to get to work. I go into my refrigerator. Quickly I realize that because I've been in the hospital for a month, I no longer have much of a food supply in my own house. All of the food in the refrigerator belongs to my roommates. I figure that if I borrow a few eggs from the box of a dozen and some slices of bread to make egg salad sandwiches no one would ever notice. But then…I forgot about "chemo brain." Something odd happens to your memory when you undergo chemotherapy. The "Cancer Community" refers to it as "Chemo Brain." I look at these four eggs and can not remember for the life of me how long you have to boil eggs to make them hard-boiled. Feeling strong and stubborn, for there is no way that I'm going to look that up, I begin the task. And so it begins. I fill a pot with water and turn the burner on high. The water begins to boil and I drop in four eggs. I decide that 30 minutes on a hard boil will be a good idea. It wasn't. The eggs are glued to the shell. And they are slightly browned on the inside. At this point I could have called my mom (who was on her way); I could have looked it up on the internet; or I also could have looked into my Joy of Cooking *and found the answer in just a few moments. "No way, I can do this," I think to myself. "I have boiled eggs hundreds of times before." So I begin the process again. This time I start the water at a boil but then when the next four eggs are dropped into the water, I turned the water down to a low simmer for 10 minutes. The eggs turn out runny and gross when I break open the shells. I have now used up 8 of the 12 eggs. I also only have about 15 minutes until my mom arrives. Suddenly it comes to me. I get it right this time. The third time is the charm! And for those of you who don't know…first you boil the water. Then you drop the eggs into the boiling water. Set the burner at a med-high heat for 12 minutes and...voila! You have hard-boiled eggs!*

After our delicious egg salad sandwiches, Dani and I head to Dr. Christie's office for her weekly check-up. After her blood is drawn and analyzed, Dr. Christie responds to our usual slew of questions. This time, we ask about the old carpet and tile in Dani's home. We are informed that we shouldn't take any chances with cleanliness concerns. So we make a decision to purchase new floor coverings for Dani's living room, dining room, hallway, and kitchen. We are assured by Scott and Dani's three roomies that they will now be fastidious in keeping their home clean. Jay and I, of course, don't quite believe them! But we realize that it's virtually impossible to protect our daughter from resuming her life outside of a more sterile hospital-like environment. After all, there isn't such a thing as a "germ-free environment"...especially among five "20 somethings"! Jay and I go out that evening and buy the wall-to-wall carpeting and tile which Home Depot promises to deliver and install the next day. During this procedure, Dani and Phoebe camp out at their former home, our place in Gaithersburg.

10/28
Once she returns to Falls Church and her beautiful new and clean carpet and kitchen tile, Dani returns to what has become "the new normal!" On Monday, October 28th, a new crisis arises when Dani's permanent Groshong Catheter falls out.

Dani's Memory

I wake up this morning feeling pretty great. I have basically slept through the night for the first time since I came home from the hospital. Scott is getting ready to leave my place for his job and he suggests that I get ready for my day as well. He says that he will take Phoebe out and get us some breakfast ready while I shower. This is extremely helpful and I guess he is probably well aware that if he doesn't make me get up now, I would lie in bed for hours. The doctors have instructed me to be somewhat active during my home stays. Scott can be so manipulative. So, I jump into the shower. I pull off the bandages that surround my Groshong Catheter, just like I have been instructed by my doctors. I lean against the shower wall just to breathe in the steam and relax. It feels so good. The chemotherapy has left me completely hairless all over (yes, like an all-over body wax). The hot water touches every inch of my body and I appreciate that so much. I grab the soap and begin to lather up. As I begin to scrub my arms, I notice that it looks like my Groshong has pulled slightly from its original location. The line looks a bit longer. The end of the Groshong now passes below my belly button. It used to just hang right beside my belly button. "Never mind," I say to myself. "I'm pretty sure that it's probably just my imagination playing tricks on me." After all, I'm thinking that the Groshong is linked to an artery that runs to my heart, right? So, if it is actually falling out of my body, does that mean that I am having internal bleeding? Oh my God, IT DOES!!! Not so casually, I look down again. This time the end of the catheter is adjacent to my inner thigh. Oh my God, I'm going to die right here, right now in this very shower!!! I jump out of the shower with soap still all over my body. I quickly towel off and then run into my freezing cold kitchen. I scream to Scott that my Groshong Catheter is coming out and that I am going to have internal bleeding. He sits me down to take a look at it. He agrees that the Groshong is falling out. Now it is down to my knees. He instructs me to breathe slowly and sit down. Movement can only make it come out at a quicker pace. He calls my dad, who of course is the font of wisdom as far as Groshong Catheters are concerned. Scott tells him that he has to go to work, but would feel better if he left me with my dad, than leaving me alone. I then call my doctor's office. I am speaking at an extremely fast pace. I'm trying to explain that my life will be over in a matter of moments. The woman on the other end of the line is extremely patient and listens to every word I say. I finally give her enough time to respond, and she says, "Well, it looks like Dr. Wagner has an appointment available at 2:00 this afternoon. We'll see you then." WHAT? I think to myself. Did she not hear me? Maybe she doesn't understand what a Groshong Catheter is! Maybe I've entered some bizarre parallel universe where a life-threatening emergency is interpreted by a receptionist to be "no big deal." I finally respond a bit unsure, "Okay, I'll see you then." I've never been one to argue. I lie on the couch and watch my catheter loosen with each breath I take. I finally fall asleep. Scott leaves for work as my dad comes to my house to watch over me. When I awake the Groshong has completely fallen out of me. As always, I survive.

10/30

Dani re-enters Arlington for her consolidation chemotherapy. The plan is to have her remain as an in-patient for the duration of the treatment and then have her go home until she gets a fever. Hopefully things will continue to go well and she will be back home by the middle of next week. The doctors are pleased with Dani's recuperation, and are confident that she'll only need two consolidation chemotherapies until she leaves for Seattle. Prior to Dani's admission to Arlington, Joanne, the lead nurse, has been attempting to requisition a private room for Dani. Unfortunately, all private rooms are filled. With apologies galore, Joann places Dani in a room with a very angry elderly lady. This woman is the antithesis of Dani, for she complains about everything. Even though we whisper, she is upset with the noise we make and the number of people who visit with Dani. She tells us quite frankly that she hasn't had a bowel movement in a year, and the doctors can't seem to find a way to cure her of this problem! All of us hope that our collective positive thoughts will help, but we fail. She presses the call button often, complaining about the racket we (Dani, Jay, Scott, and myself) are making. As a result, we advise Dani's friends not to drop in that evening and hope that Joann can work a miracle—and by October 31st, Dani has a private room. Joanne rules!

11/1

Dani's website is up and running! Micah kept his promise to have it up and running by November 1. It posted our first Dani update, which Jay emailed to our friends and relatives on October 23rd. Weekly updates continue for the next seven months or so. Micah created this interactive website not only as a source of information on Dani's health, but also as a resource guide to fundraisers, blood drives, and medical information. But the truth is…the most valuable part of it was the interactive component that allowed people to write words of encouragement to Dani and the rest of us. Every day, Dani would check the website for the incredibly uplifting messages.

Tonight and tomorrow morning Dani will have her third and fourth doses of high dose chemotherapy and then she'll get a day of rest. So far she has had very little in terms of side effects (as the doctors predicted), since she is much healthier generally and in remission this time around. Dani will have doses 5 and 6 on Sunday night and Monday and, if all goes well, she will be home on Monday afternoon or Tuesday. It is expected that she will develop a fever and be readmitted to the hospital about 7 to 10 days after she goes home, as once again the chemotherapy will cause her blood counts to drop significantly. However, as the counts start to rise and her immunity comes back, she should feel even stronger, as she gets closer to the time of transplant.

The bad news today was that, despite the fact that 43 friends and family members spent a portion of their weekend being tested as a possible match for Dani a few weeks back, no one was a match for Dani. Jay, Dani, Scott and I were talking tonight about how neat it would be if one of the many donors turned out to be a donor for one of the 3,000 people that are currently searching for a donor right now in the United States. We also discuss our extreme optimism of a personal blessing occurring…a match for our girl. Now that the search process has been formally activated for a donor for Dani by Seattle, the registries are automatically searched every day, and new potential matches would be added to the list for further screening as they come on line. Of the

4.5 million people currently in the international registry, six have been identified as having the *potential* to be a matched donor for Dani. All it takes is only one person to provide the miracle of life for Dani. Our evening visit with Dani ends with these positive thoughts dancing in our heads.

11/5

It is another good day for Dani. She was released from the hospital yesterday after completing her first round of consolidation chemotherapy. Although she was initially told that she would probably run a fever and be back in the hospital by Friday, after the doctor reviewed her blood work today he said it could be from 8 to10 days before Dani returns to the hospital. It looks like the continuous good wishes and prayers are helping to keep our Dani strong.

11/7

We have the first bone marrow drive at Walter Reed Elementary School in Arlington (Dani's school). We are amazed at the number of people that attend. Reed colleagues man the various volunteer stations. Other colleagues stand in line waiting to be tested. Also in attendance are parents of Dani's students, Arlington County Public School employees, Dani's many friends, and other Arlington community members who have heard about Dani and the bone marrow drive. Gayle and John arrive with what appears to be their entire church congregation. Dani's summer league softball catcher brings her entire women's football team with her. Despite the most valiant of efforts, like bringing in more technicians to assist in the task, and extending the hours of the drive, the Red Cross actually runs out of supplies by 9 p.m.

Over 360 people are screened tonight and 75 more are turned away. This even includes the group of oncology nurses from Arlington Hospital Center. Information is provided to those who were not tested regarding subsequent drives. All of us are in awe of the outpouring of love and support for Dani and the willingness of the Arlington Community to step

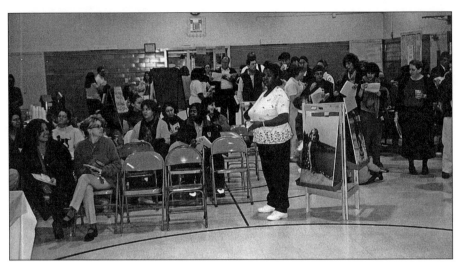

Over 360 people are screened during the Arlington drive!

up to the plate. The Friends of Allison Foundation and the Fair Lakes League supported their efforts by financing the testing at $63, so that all who could be are tested for free. Laurie Alderman, Liz Lichtman, the staff at Reed, and the representative from the D.C. Red Cross and her band of volunteers are exhilarated and exhausted at the same time. It is an amazing thing to witness

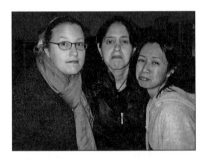

Dani's nurses from Arlington Hospital came to get tested but alas...they came too late!

such goodness. We all leave with smiles on our faces, even more hopeful than ever that a match will be found.

11/9

Dani is having a good weekend and her counts have remained high enough so that she is able to attend Ally Samuel's and Ryan Frank's wedding ceremony tonight. Since Dani was originally supposed to be a bridesmaid, she joins the wedding party prior to the ceremony. This is one of the few times that Dani is on her own in the past two months. We all survive this 15 minute absence. Although a bit unusual, in her effort to support her friend Dani, Ally includes information about being a bone marrow donor in her beautiful wedding program. We are touched by this loving gesture.

11/10

Dani's blood counts continue to drop this week and, although her temperature is still normal, Dr. Christie informs her that it is quite likely that she will be returning to the hospital early this week as a precaution. Dani tells us all that she is feeling wonderful!

11/11

Today, Earle B. Wood Middle School (a Montgomery County public school where I am an assistant principal) hosts our second drive. The PTA president, Susan Hoopes, coordinates this tremendous effort with help from Liz, the Atlas family, the Red Cross, and scores of volunteers. Jay and I get to personally thank Alvin Atlas, Allison's dad, for supporting this drive. A newspaper reporter from the local Channel 8 News (an ABC affiliate) interviews us and then heads to Dani's to interview her. Local newspapers and even a reporter from the Rockville High School News report on this community effort.

We pronounce the drive a success, as 323 additional people are tested. This brings the total number tested to 571 in the two drives held thus far. Over 700 people are screened during the two evenings of testing. Susan Hoopes has been unbelievable in her efforts, resulting

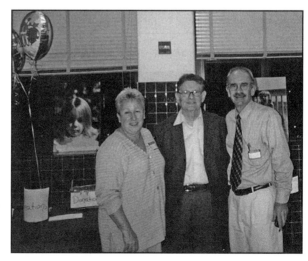

Mr. Alvin Atlas between Dani's parents at the Earle B. Wood Drive

in incredible organization. The "heads-up" call for extra volunteers and testers was successful as almost everyone completed the process of registration and testing in less than 30 minutes. Carol, Bruce, Sandy, Liz and other friends, school staff, and community volunteers help with the registration process. I see many colleagues former and present, community members, former Wootton and Damascus Flames softball families, and even a former boyfriend or two of Dani's in the registration line. We continue to be overwhelmed by the level of concern and support expressed by the community.

We find out today that our Dani is now a celebrity of sorts. She actually becomes "poster person" for National Marrow Awareness Month in the Washington D.C. area with two televised interviews.

11/11

Today an e-mail from the president of Key Elementary School's Parent Teacher Association is sent to Dani (which Jay later posts on her website):

I'd like to encourage everyone to seriously consider this opportunity to truly give the gift of life...and to help you understand that there is very little discomfort attached to the actual donation if you and Dani are lucky enough to be a match. Six weeks after our wedding my husband, Jim, was an anonymous donor for a terminally ill man in the West. The procedure was relatively painless because of the epidural he received (remember, moms how much easier this made childbirth!!) No incision is required. Recovery is fairly rapid, less than 24 hours in Jim's case. (Remember that if stem cells are harvested from the blood through apherisis the process is even less invasive.) Also, please don't hesitate if you are not of Jewish descent. In fact Jim, who is Jewish, was a match for a non-Jewish man. There is always the opportunity for a match. There are no words to express how powerful this event was for

Jim and vicariously for me. The willingness to participate is heroic itself. Take the chance!

In less than two weeks, Dani's website has been accessed by so many people. We receive helpful information, and lots and lots of best wishes and prayers. It is one of the things that highlight each day as we wait for a donor to be found.

11/12

On Tuesday November 12, at 9:00 a.m., Dani posts a message on the website. It reads: *I just wanted to thank everyone for their kind words and thoughts. It means a lot to my family and me to browse through the positive energy and thoughts that you have been sending to us. We appreciate it so much! I love you all! –Dani*

Dani returns to the hospital this evening. She is very pleased with the fact that she was able to hold out for 10 days after consolidation chemo ended, but it is tough work even for an athlete like Dani to function with no immune system. This is all to be expected with high dose chemotherapy. Her temperature is normal and she will need to ride it out in the hospital for a few days until her counts come back. She generally feels good, looks good, and even has a corned beef special for dinner. When Jay writes in the website today, he includes information about a very special fundraiser, "A Night with Dani and the Washington Wizards." Dani and Scott have been busy for the past couple of weeks stuffing envelops in preparation for the second of Dani's fundraisers. The "Friends of Dani" are sponsoring a game as the Wizards play the New York Knicks on Saturday night, December 7th. We've lucked into a situation where a colleague of Jay's has a brother who works in Sales and Promotions for the Wizards. Abe Polin has agreed to help us out by supplying tickets at a significantly reduced rate. People will be able to purchase two tickets for the price of one, and Dani's transplant fund gets $30 of every $50 raised. He's made 500 tickets available to us. It should be a fun evening as all Dani's friends get together. Dani is planning to attend this event. She even is hoping to meet Michael Jordan!

11/13

Over the past few days Dani has her first experience with Neupogen. It is a medication designed to have your bone marrow go into overdrive to produce white blood cells. Interestingly, it is the same medication they give to potential donors to force stem cells out of the marrow and into the blood stream for harvesting for transplant. The goal is to speed up white blood cell growth, and, therefore, get Dani out of the hospital quicker, so she doesn't catch anything (which sounds like a good idea to us)! In point of fact, it works perfectly. Her marrow is reacting the way healthy bone marrow should. However, this explosion of healthy cells causes Dani to feel all achy. She has a heating blanket and heating pads placed on every joint of her body. She is not a happy camper.

11/17

On Sunday, November 17th Temple Beth Ami (our synagogue), in Rockville, is the site of our third bone marrow drive. This drive is organized by our good friends Bonnie and Steve Spivack and Sandy Davis. The volunteers all have familiar faces. Carol and Bruce and their children, Heather, Ari, and Jason, Shawn (Heather's husband), nephew Adam, Jessi (Spivack) and her fiancé, Todd, and an assortment of Dani's buddies man the various drive stations. WUSA, the CBS affiliate in Washington, showed up at the bone marrow drive at Temple Beth Ami, and later at Dani's hospital room to do an interview. Over 300 potential donors showed up on this Sunday despite the chilly, rainy, sloppy, monsoon-like weather conditions.

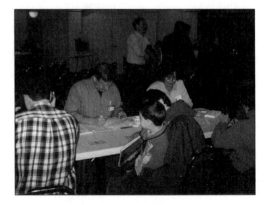

Aunt Carol and Uncle Bruce screening potential donors at Beth Ami

We pronounce the Beth Ami Drive a success! We are once again amazed at the number of people who have come to the three drives. So far over 1,000 people have been screened and 869 additional people have been added to the registry of the national marrow donor program.

Scott brings Dani home from the hospital as the rest of the posse is at the drive. She is no longer neutropenic (lacking an immune system). Unfortunately, the reaction to this quick growth of white blood cells is often compared to having flu-like symptoms, in terms of the way you feel. So Dani has been feeling pretty lousy as the cells multiplied and pain killers and heating pads haven't done much. The awful weather hasn't helped her mood any either. The good news is that the pain is temporary. Phoebe, who has been staying with us during Dani's hospital stay, will return to her home tomorrow, and life can return to the "new normal" for Dani and Scott. They'll focus on the task of continuing to busily stuff envelopes with Wizards tickets. We're all pretty excited for December 7th. The way we figure it, Dani will be in-between treatments and will be able to attend the Wizards' fundraiser. Dani and Scott are optimistic that they'll sell all 500 tickets for the game.

11/23

On November 23rd, 2002, an additional fundraiser was put together by Dave Brubaker, the principal, and several teachers of Earle B. Wood Middle School in Montgomery County, to benefit our daughter and Harry Williams, another assistant principal at the school. Dave and four staff members from Wood (Jeremy Whitaker, Jason Hunter, Steve Orders, and Matt Brubaker) are running as a team in a 50 mile ultra-marathon race along the Appalachian Trail in central Maryland. This team will become a physical symbol of the courage that Harry Williams (Assistant Principal, Wood Middle School) and Dani exemplify in their battles with cancer. Dani is so impressed by their determination to complete this difficult task that she insists on going to cheer the team on.

It is freezing cold this morning. The five runners of Team Wood hit the starting line in Boonsboro, Maryland, at 5:00 a.m. in the darkness, facing a mid-20 degree wind chill. They follow the steep footpaths of the Appalachian Trail. We don't get up quite that early, but we bundle Dani up and drive to the half-way point of the race. There we find Harry, and Dave's wife Judy, his daughter, Judy's parents, and the school's Deaf and Hard of Hearing Team waiting for Team Wood to run by us at the Antietam Aqueduct. Dave and the other members of the team stop when they see us, catch their collective breaths, embrace Dani and Harry and then press on. I'm sure that Dani and Harry's presence refreshes them as they start off again, this time to reach their goal.

We are not the only ones who have come to cheer them on. Throughout the day, many from the Wood MS community come out to the remote race course to offer moral and physical support as the five pass by. Community members are at the starting line at 5 a.m. in the dark and cold to wish the runners well. Several teachers meet the group at the 28 mile mark and complete 5 miles with them. The wives and girlfriends of the runners are there towards the last 10 miles to cheer and support. Finally, the physical education teacher, Rob Pinsky, joins the team at mile 35 and finishes the last 15 miles with them, giving much needed encouragement. Together they all reach the finish line as one, wearing their Wood tee shirts, just before 7:00 p.m. at Williamsport, Maryland. Everyone finishes the race, and no one quits. The finishers' medals are accepted on behalf of Harry and Dani. Those of us who work in middle school understand the great symbolism of this accomplishment, as middle schools epitomize teamwork. This selfless act demonstrates the positive effects that individuals can make when they work together toward a common goal.

The Montgomery County Public School weekly newsletter, *The Superintendent's Bulletin* states:

> *The race was run as a tribute and a symbol to the courageous battle that Assistant Principal, Harry Williams and Dani Shotel, daughter of Assistant Principal, Sue Shotel are fighting against Cancer. The race is over, but Team Wood lives on in*

any group that works together in a positive way to persevere through difficult times. Congratulations to Team Wood on what we consider to be a pretty amazing accomplishment.

Team Wood is successful in raising over $13,000. All of these funds were donated to the various organizations that supported Harry Williams, our family, and other families in need of support.

11/28 – Thanksgiving

Thanksgiving this year is an extra-special one for all of us. Gayle, John, Scott, and his sister, Abby, join us. Philly Mom-Mom sees her princess, Dani, for the first time in three months. Although Dani is quite bald at this

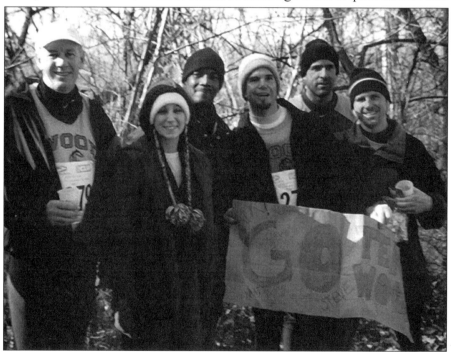

Team Wood with Dani and Harry at mile marker 27 of the 50 mile run

time, Philly Mom-Mom appears not to notice. Dani and I have always secretly felt that she knew all along that her granddaughter has cancer, but as long as she ignores it, it just couldn't exist. Jay's mom always has a "Pollyanna" approach when it comes to her grandchildren!

As is our family custom, we provide a meal for a group of people who wouldn't ordinarily have a home-cooked meal on Thanksgiving Day. Usually we deliver a meal to a Rockville children's shelter that sends its middle school-aged kids to Wood Middle School. Sometimes we feed my mother-in-law's nursing home staff to thank them for all of their care. This year, we deliver a meal to the Oncology wing nurses at Arlington Hospital, who are both surprised and appreciative of our gesture. We feel that if anyone deserves our thanks, they do. I prepare so many sweet potatoes for so many people that there appears to be some sweet potato vapor droplets on my kitchen ceiling! Prior to our meal, we speak with Poppy and Grandmom in Florida. This is the first year in over 20 years that they do not grace our table, as my dad is once more hospitalized for his congestive heart failure. It is a bittersweet conversation. We miss both of them terribly and promise to save a turkey leg for my dad and some perfect chocolate cake for my mom. The meal is served in our living room. We set up three six-foot tables lengthwise to seat all 25 guests. It is a delightful evening, filled with lots of laughter, love, and good food.

11/30

As the month comes to an end, Carol and I plan another trip to Florida to be with both my parents, but to primarily check on my father's care. Surgery is planned for his heart, and we are all quite worried about this. He is glad to hear the good news that Dani is recovering quite well from her first consolidation chemo.

Dani's counts continue to increase. The doctor has said that she will probably avoid any further transfusions and has delayed her next round of consolidation chemotherapy for another week. This means she should be able to attend the Wizards game with her friends next Saturday night. All 500 Wizards seats have been sold and we could have sold another 200 if we had only been allocated additional seats. We also learn today that the Lafayette College alumni group in New York raised over $1,000 for the NTAF Bone Marrow Transplant Fund for Dani while watching

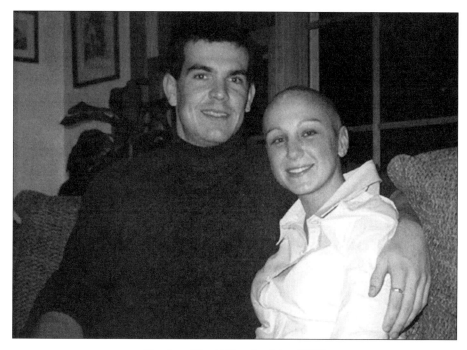

Dani and Scott Thanksgiving 2002

Lafayette beat Lehigh for the first time since 1994. Go Pards!

Despite the fact that we haven't yet had a confirmation that a donor has been found for Dani, we continue to be optimistic that the miracle will occur. So many positive thoughts (from the website's interactive guest book) keep all of us constantly positive. Here are a few samples from November:

From Dani's principal: *Dani, we're behind you 1000%! You are going to beat this leukemia, and by spring 2004 be building a beach sandbox for your 2-year-old class!* ☺ *Radio station 94.7 is going to air public service announcements about your Beth Ami drive.*

From her high school coach: *The web site is great. What a great way to keep everyone involved with your eventual triumph over this hurdle. I'm sure that you are handling it in the same way that you handle everything...with class, strength, and that great smile. I look forward to* *your Beth Ami drive. I hope to be the right match*☺

From Pamela, Dani's second year intern: *Hey Dani! Micah did a fantastic job on your website....You have no idea what an inspiration you are to me (and apparently everyone else you've ever known)....I'm wearing my pearl earrings and praying that my bone marrow ends up being a match.*

From a colleague of mine: *I've known your mom for years because we were both social studies teachers. I remember a time when you were in elementary school and you made your mom a friendship bracelet...she wore it...told us how you made it...and what you said to her. Though I have never met you, I will have you in my thoughts every day. I will help to spread the word about the need for donors. Keep positive thoughts.*

I am a teacher at Jefferson Middle School. I was at the Reed drive yesterday and was SO impressed by the number of people there. So many college students, teachers, people who didn't even know you! And so many people who do that really care about you. The card with the picture of you and your dog is perfect! I have it here with me and will place it on my fridge to remember to pray for you! Stay strong!

I registered with the NMDP when my sister's best friend Allison Atlas had a marrow drive back in the late 1980's. Now I'm a pediatric oncologist at Hopkins, and I take care of many kids with AML. Your site is wonderful and I wish you all the best. If there is anything I can ever do help....Keep up the positive attitude. It means everything.

I saw you on TV and from my experience a positive attitude is 75% of the cure. You are 3/4 of the way home. Keep on kicking butt! Winston Churchill once said, "Never, never, never, never quit." You do the same. We are all counting on you.

From a parent of one of Dani's former students: *Patrick still gets the sweetest smile on his face when your name is mentioned. I truly believe that you will always be his favorite teacher. You have such a gift with children and I am positive that you will...be back to doing what you do so amazingly well. God Bless You!*

I'm Allyson's dad, the guy who saw many of your softball games with the Peaches. It's great fun watching you pitch. I could feel your energy from the mound all the way to the stands.... You'll beat this.

From a dear family friend: *Dearest Dani – Your poem and painting are exquisite – yet they pale in comparison to the person you are. We love you, and you are in our hearts 24/7.*

From Ally, Dani's life-long friend: *Ryan, my dad, Jeff and I were thrilled that you...were able to come to our wedding on Saturday. It was a dream come true to have you there with us....*

...If you remember, I played softball for Quince Orchard. I wish I could be at the Wizards game, But I'm in the Navy deployed in Italy. Please know that you are in my thoughts and prayers...and if I remember the way you pitched then, I remember you being a fighter ☺ Be strong!

From our dear family friend: *Dani.... Every evening I put my Dockers on...they're like slippers at this point. I bought them against your advice when you were about 12 years old. We were all shopping on the Maine coast. I think your dad drove both families in his Ford Pinto Wagon. Well, even though you thought those shoes were "so uncool"; they remind me of you each day. They also remind me of the Shotel family.... Whether its' softball or your most recent battle, the power of your family's togetherness astounds me. Keep up the fight, Dani, because you are a winner.*

From a parent of a former student: *You taught and loved my children in your class last year and we have never forgotten you. I wish I could take the boys to see you…and we could have a Big Group Hug! We have never found another teacher as Wonderful, Patient, and Loving as you.*

From a friend: *I think you have more people rooting for you than the Redskins do.*

From John Schnabel, Dani's resident: *I just heard about your website from Pamela and I wanted to say hello. You are such an inspiration to me and obviously everyone who has remotely heard about you. I can't begin to tell you how much you affected me and my career. You and your family are absolutely the best. Thanks again for the presents. My prayers and thoughts are with you all constantly. Hope to see you soon.*

From a parent of a former student: *Ben woke up today and listened to your voice mail message twice, as he had every day for almost a year. That, "Go Ben, go Ben" message really starts his day off right, with a little swing of his hips and fist pumping the air! Today he said, I wish 'Nesto' take me go see Dani….*

Chapter Eight
A Match, Consolidation #2, and Travel Plans

12/4

Scott and Dani have made separate plans for this evening. Dani will be meeting up with her former roommate. On the previous evening Scott revealed his plans for spending New Year's Eve with his friends and not with Dani. Apparently the discussion did not go well. Dani's e-mail to Scott reveals many up-until-this-point suppressed thoughts: *Let me preface this letter with a couple of things...first I don't mean to come off as a drama queen or needy in this note...if I do I am pre-apologizing for it. Second...you are amazing. I love you. Everything you have done for me within the past 6-7 months has been truly wonderful. I constantly look forward to and plan us spending the rest of our lives together. That being said...let me explain to you what goes on in my head. I think about death too much...I think about not being able to have children all the time. I am so terrified about this transplant...about being away from you...about staying positive. I am tired of talking about cancer...I am tired of doing interviews...I am tired of the first question anybody asks me being, "how are you doing, really? Tell me the truth." I am just tired of it. I hate that you feel guilty when you are out without me. I want you to have fun...*

This brings me to the whole new year's eve/birthday discussion last night...when you first brought up the topic of new years/birthday....I honestly believed that you would choose to go out for your birthday (December 30)...not new years eve. It is still fine either way, but I need to explain how I took this. I have never in my 26 years been alone on New Years Eve. I am usually huge into holidays (not so much this year). I am pretty sure that I can recount what I did for New Years Eve for at least the last 10 years of my life. You had before mentioned that you would spend New Years with me wherever I was (be it in the hospital or at home). You going to 9:30 Club sorta snuck up on me. I am scared to enter this year of 2003, and probably more scared to enter it alone... because it means a whole lot of things that I am not exactly ready for. It means moving to Seattle for four months...it means being away from you...it means having a transplant...it means possible organ failure... it means possible death....I am not ready for any of it. I put on a great game face...I can tell this story numerous times to numerous people... but, it doesn't mean that I am not scared. PLEASE DO NOT TAKE THIS AS A GUILT TRIP...YOU TELL ME TO BE HONEST AND THIS IS ME BEING HONEST. I want you to do whatever you want for both new years and your birthday. I want to see you smile. I have plenty of time to adjust to being alone on New Years Eve. I will get through it like I have gotten through everything else. I just needed to express what was going on in my head...and I will talk to you about things...I just can't stand crying...and that seems to be all I'm doing lately when the subject of my illness comes up around you. I love you so much...you are still my sunshine.

Love always, Dani

Dani and Scott decide very soon after that e-mail that wherever she may be on this very important and symbolic New Year's Eve, he will be by her side. As if a premonition of things to come, their relationship survives this crisis, and they now begin to plan together for the future.

12/5

The final bone marrow drive in Dani's honor takes place at Washington Hebrew Congregation on the evening of December 5th. It is snowing, and that weather phenomenon doesn't bode well for Washingtonians. Burton paces back and forth all during the drive worrying about the possibility of a low turnout caused by this awful weather. Burton and Wendy's son, Adam, even shuttles nearby American University students to and from the bone marrow drive. Dani's buddy Kris Featheringham once more is present to lend a hand as a volunteer. Wendy has arranged that trays upon trays of cookies from the Potomac Deli are provided as a "thank you" for the donors as well as the volunteers. Meanwhile Dani is at her home in Falls Church, keeping warm.

In the four drives scheduled on behalf of Dani, close to 1,000 people are tested. We are aware of more than eight people who were matched as donors to other persons in need of a transplant.

12/6

Good news! This afternoon, Jay gets a call from Colleen Duffy, the Search Coordinator for Unrelated Transplants at the Seattle Cancer Care Alliance, that an acceptable match has been found for Dani. A 30-year-old German male, known only to us as URD, DEAKB 117626 matches Dani on 9 out of 10 characteristics, with the one mismatched characteristic not significant enough to eliminate him as the donor. Under the rules of the potential donor's country, we will not know the identity of the donor until two years after the transplant. While not perfect, it is a nice present for the last day of Hanukah and for Micah's birthday. They will continue to analyze blood from the potential American donor and the donor from Italy to see if we can get a 10/10 match, but for now a recommendation is being made to our local doctor to proceed to transplant as scheduled. The search so far has come up with this one person out of what we believe to be 8 million people currently listed in national and international bone marrow registries. If all goes well, Dani will have a new "birthday" to celebrate at the end of January. We collectively breathe a sigh of relief, and the warmth from our smiles seems to melt the snow.

12/7

Tonight is amazing! Dani and Scott get to host 498 of their nearest and dearest friends and they watch the Washington Wizards defeat the New York Knicks. Even the nurses from Arlington Hospital's Oncology wing are there to cheer on Dani — I mean the Wizards — to victory! After the game, Dani meets with friends in a nearby pub. Jay and I are exhausted and say goodnight to Dani and her buds. Dani hugs us both and assures us that this is just what the doctors have ordered!

Dani, Katrina, and Lisa after the Wizards game

12/8

We learn that two more drives are scheduled in the DC area for December. These drives are specifically in support of PJ Siegel, a 43-year-old single mom, Army veteran, and all-around great lady, and all other patients needing a donor. Jay and I decide to attend, to lend our support both to PJ and the Red Cross. We are so thankful to the close to 1,000 people who were tested in the four drives that were specifically scheduled in support of Dani. We use the website to announce two additional drives scheduled for the Washington area in December that we are aware of to assist those who still wish to be on the registry and save a life.

12/10

Dani re-enters Virginia Hospital Center, Arlington, for her second round of consolidation chemotherapy. It's not quite routine yet. Dani is a real trooper, though. We continue to rise to her expectations! During this time, Jay starts making arrangements for our stay in Seattle. It looks as if our plan is to rent an apartment in the Pete Gross House, which is a building especially for Hutch patients and their families. During our visit in October, Dani was excited about the fact that they even housed a school for the children (either those undergoing treatment or family members).

She tells us that she'll look into volunteering there post-transplant. We are put on a wait list. In the meantime, we make reservations for a two-bedroom apartment at the nearby Marriott Residence Inn. The plan as it currently stands is that Dani and I will reside in Seattle for the duration, with Jay commuting there every other week. Scott is making inquiries about tele-commuting to his job from Seattle. He is surprised and pleased to find that there is a branch of the company he works for in Renton that is about 10 miles from the Hutch. We're delighted that Scott has plans to be with us on occasion as he is a great source of comfort and support for Dani. So Jay creates "Miles for Smiles," a way for friends to donate their frequent flyer miles for Scott's commutes. He finds out that Delta, U.S. Air, United, American, Continental, Northwest, Southwest, Alaska Air, and America West all fly between the D.C. area and Seattle. Jay is amazing. The way he figures it, this management of our affairs is his job; mine is to be the primary caregiver, and Dani has the most important job of all—to win this battle!

12/11

The official notification letter of the match for Dani is faxed to Dr. Christie's office today. Jay brings the copy of it to the hospital that evening. Dani shares its contents with anyone and everyone who enters her room. Who knew that a piece of paper could bring such joy?

12/14

Jay and I attend the bone marrow drive for PJ at her son's middle school, Thomas Pullen Arts Magnet School. We are welcomed by Sharon Gallop from the Red Cross, who is managing this drive, as she did for Dani. Several of Jay's George Washington colleagues and their families get tested after being shut out of the Arlington drive. Sharon introduces us to members of PJ's family. We are united for this common cause.

12/15

Carol and I travel to Florida for a few days to see our parents. Dad is now in critical condition at a hospital in Del Ray Beach. Upon our arrival, we try getting support for both of my parents in terms of attention and improved medical care. There is such a difference between the care and services provided for Dani and my dad's medical care. My dad is almost uncommunicative, and when he does speak with us, he is so unhappy. We both try to provide comfort. Neither of us feels successful in any of our efforts. We have both always been concerned about our parents' medical coverage. It doesn't make either of us feel any better to know that our concerns are justified. We both feel that my dad's poor medical treatment is certainly related to his medical coverage. This reinforces even more our belief that the very best health insurance plan possible is worth the cost. I'm afraid that my parents do not share this belief.

12/16

Dani writes a message to her friends on the website: *I just wanted to let everyone know that I am out of the hospital again. I finished my second round of consolidation chemo; it made me a little more tired this time...but overall...I think my body has fought this stuff pretty well. I wanted to just let everyone know how appreciative I am of all your phone calls, visits, and emails. It is really easy to stay positive with everyone saying such nice things about me. Hee! Hee! Keep it up! ☺ It appears that I will be heading out to Seattle around January 13th... and the transplant is scheduled for sometime around February 6th. I am hoping that some of you will be able to do a weekend trip out there (or at least call me a couple of times). Your positive messages mean so much to me and my family. So...until the 13th it is much easier to come see me in Virginia than in Seattle. I look forward to hearing from you all. Love you all so much, Dani*

12/21

Although a bit achy and tired, Dani continues to stay out of the hospital after her second round of chemo. She receives two units of blood today and has gotten some energy back. Tonight we plan to hold a movie and pizza marathon at our house. Although Dani will probably have to go back in the hospital some time this week as her counts are predictably very low, she will tough it out for as long as she can. She is a bit saddened by the fact that in all probability she will be in the hospital for Christmas Day (which was to be spent with Scott's family) as well as for Scott's birthday (on December 30th). She is hopeful, though, that she'll be out in time for New Year's Eve.

Jay and I spend some time today visiting PJ's second bone marrow drive, which is being held at the Greenbelt Community Center near her home. Once more, we are heartened by the numbers of people, both friends as well as strangers, willing to be part of the national bone marrow registry. Also, just this morning, we receive in the mail the monthly report from the National Transplant Assistance Fund informing us that over 250 people have made contributions to Dani's fund to date. We know that this number is an underestimate, because it doesn't take into account the 500 tickets sold for the Wizards fundraiser. It is indeed gratifying to have first-hand knowledge of the many good deeds done every day that occur without flourish or fanfare.

Today, my parents have been married for 61 years. My mother spends it by sitting vigil at my dad's bedside at Mount Sinai Hospital in Miami, where he has been transferred. This is hardly the way they wanted to spend this special day. We speak to her and she tells us about her memories of when they were first married in 1941. We send our love, and ask mom to make sure she gives "Poppy" a kiss from all of us and a special one from Dani.

12/23

Dani returns to the hospital. She keeps busy by creating a music journal of sorts for Scott's birthday on the 30th. With various colored small pieces of paper, torn from magazine ads, she creates a mosaic self-portrait as a cover for this journal. Jay spends most of the next few afternoons tearing up the ads and separating the torn pieces into colors.

The room begins to take on the look of an arts and crafts facility, as I also bide my time knitting Scott a birthday afghan. We hide both projects when Scott is present. Dani is complaining about a sore butt. Taking precautions, she is treated for hemorrhoids. As the nurses set up the **sitz bath** for her, I regale Dani with my story of her birth, my resulting hemorrhoids, and how the sitz bath became my salvation.

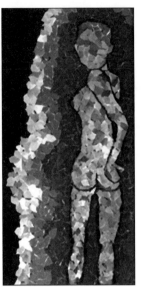

The cover of Dani's present for Scott

Dani eagerly awaits this treatment. Unfortunately, the bath does not have its desired effect, as Dani is still in great pain. We take turns sitting in the bathroom with her, comforting her as she soaks her bottom in the sitz bath and cries.

12/24

Scott's mom and dad have decided that since Dani won't be able to spend Christmas Eve or Christmas Day with

> A **sitz bath** is a warm-water bath taken in the sitting position that covers only the hips and buttocks. It may be used for either healing or hygiene purposes.

them at their home, they might as well bring their celebration to Dani's room. Scott, Gayle, John, and Scott's sister, Abby, and her husband, Justin, enter the room early that evening with their arms filled with tins of specially prepared baked goods for Dani. We are even treated to one of Scott's favorite treats, Gayle's famous cheese straws. Our laughter and chatter bonds the two families this evening. Unfortunately, Dani is still not feeling any relief from the "pain in her butt." Despite this pain, she tries very hard to keep on her happy face.

12/27

Dani is feeling pretty achy today. She has heating pads, a special heating blanket, and several hospital blankets bundled up all around her body. The "hemorrhoid" pain and subsequent sitz bath treatment is dropped, as it is discovered that what Dani is really suffering from is two different infections (**C-dif** and **VRE**), both of which are common occurrences in hospital settings.

> **Clostridium difficile** or C. dif is a bacterium that causes diarrhea and more serious intestinal conditions such as colitis. It is one of the most common infections in hospitals and long-term care facilities. The use of antibiotics increases the chances of developing C. difficile diarrhea. The combination of the presence of C. difficile in hospitals and health care settings and the number of people receiving antibiotics in these settings can lead to frequent outbreaks. C- difficile infections can be limited through careful use of antibiotics and the use of routine infection control measures.

These infections that have caused Dani such tremendous pain are just some of those things that patients can catch when they are hospitalized and their immunities are suppressed. Dani is pretty glum despite the revelation. She doesn't even perk up when my friend, Sandy D, who just so happens to have the world's best laugh, arrives to spend the evening.

> **Vancomycin-Resistant Enterococci (VRE)** are bacteria that are normally present in the human intestines and in the female genital tract and are often found in the environment. Vancomycin is an antibiotic that is often used to treat infections caused by enterococci. In some instances, enterococci have become resistant to this drug and thus are called Vancomycin-Resistant Enterococci (VRE). Most VRE infections occur in hospitals and can be best treated with "designer" antibiotics other than Vancomycin.

About a half an hour passes, when suddenly Dani's very dear friend, Yvonne, pokes her head in the doorway. She announces to Dani that she has a surprise for her, but first Dani has to close her eyes. Of course, Dani obeys. Four of Dani's favorite campers (now in their twenties) appear. Dani cannot contain herself. For the next 2 hours, the five of them entertain Dani. Dani recalls the evening this way: *"Camp," which included James Lizmi, Chris Carmack, Yvonne Townsley, Beth Weinstein, and John McArdle, walked into my room with party hats and horns right after I had taken my evening dose of "knock me out" meds. I had a horrible day before they arrived and was feeling quite depressed. They kicked my sadness to the curb and made me laugh to the point where I almost forgot that we were hanging out in my hospital room.*

We all are laughing nonstop! I can now honestly testify that I do believe that laughter is the best medicine! A smiling Dani bids her friends a goodnight and drifts off to sleep.

12/30

Today is Scott's birthday. Dani has personalized the music journal for Scott so that he can continue to write his songs and poetry. The cover is a mosaic self-portrait, with each page of the journal containing original artwork as a watermark. The inside cover contains a note:

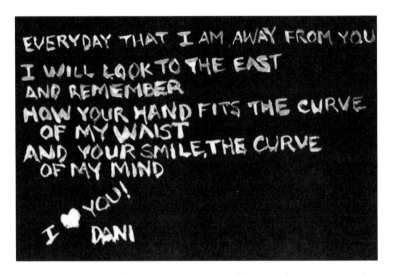

Dani's message to Scott on his birthday

The gift is one that Scott will cherish forever, along with the artist herself!

12/31

Jay, Sandy and I plan to spend a quiet evening at home, since Scott and Dani have a New Year's Eve date planned. Steve and Bonnie stop by to toast to a happy new year filled with good health, happiness, and love. Jay is trying his hand at making chocolate martinis and Sandy and I are his willing guinea pigs. We settle down to watch the movie "*Y Tu Mama Tambien.*" Jay and I had heard so much about this "coming of age" movie that we purchased it earlier in the month for Dani to watch from her hospital bed. For the past week, I had been reminding, actually bugging, Dani to watch the movie. When she didn't, I just brought it home. So we decide that this would be our entertainment for New Year's evening. Imagine our surprise when the very first scene of the film was of two teenagers engaged in sexual activities. This was also true for the second and third scene, and so it seemed for at least 3,000 subsequent scenes. The three of us sit in shock. Then the laughter erupts as I keep repeating that I can't believe that this is the film that I wanted my daughter and her boyfriend to watch. We plan to regale Dani and Scott about our misadventure, but we also decide there on the spot that perhaps it would be best if we keep the video and not bring it back to the hospital!

1/1/03

Dani went back in the hospital on December 23rd and has been patiently waiting for her counts to go back up so that she can go home and get her packing done for Seattle. We are hoping that today would be the day for her departure, but her platelets are still too low and the doctors don't want to take any chances on her getting sick before she leaves for the West Coast.

1/2

Jay goes to her local pharmacy with Dani after she is released from the hospital to pick up meds for her continuing treatment of VRE. The pharmacists now know Dani very well but do not have the prescribed "designer" meds in stock. They send us to another branch of the chain about a mile away, and when the pharmacy submits the prescription to insurance, an "automatic turndown" is made because of the cost of medication. It is $150 a pill. It seems that the human being that has to approve the meds is out to lunch. They do the same at a small restaurant next to the pharmacy, and by the time Dani and Jay get back the prescription has been approved.

1/4 – 6

Carol and Bruce have spent over a week in Florida, spending most of their time by my dad's bedside. Their long distance reports to us are very sad, as the medical procedure performed on my dad is not having the desired results. They also report that my dad doesn't seem responsive to their conversations. Carol and Bruce need to return to Maryland, their family, and their jobs. So Jay and I use this short time we have prior to our relocation to Seattle to visit my parents in Florida. We arrive in Florida early in the morning, rent a car and go immediately to the hospital armed with photo albums of the entire family from the last three years. For the first day of our visit, my dad is pretty conversant with us; he even resumes his normal "demanding" nature. I love it! We painstakingly go through the photo album with him, telling stories as we peruse. It is a wonderful time for all of us.

As the weekend progresses, my dad's condition worsens. We say goodbye to him Sunday evening, and remind him he needs to get better because Dani is waiting to see him real soon. He tells us that he has every intention of being there for Dani.

This was the very last conversation that we had with my dad. We left Florida with the realization that "Poppy" would not survive to see his granddaughter return to her "prime pitching condition."

1/11

Dani decides to throw herself a bon voyage party prior to her departure for Seattle. She invites all her and Scott's friends, our friends, relatives, and colleagues. Her former students and their parents are also invited. That evening, Dani's house is filled with joy and high hopes.

Of course these positive wishes continue throughout this month's cards and e-mails messages to Dani. Below are a few samples:

Her best childhood friend sends a poem from Maya Angelou that reads, *"A women of courage enters a room, and everyone is put at ease. There is something appealing in the way she walks and in the way she holds herself."* She continues in her own words, *"...it captures the grace and courage you have shown so many over the past several months. You have an inner strength and beauty that is rare and not only is it the thing that attracts so many people to you, but it is also the reason you will be able to overcome the obstacles life has dealt you."*

Dani's high school best bud and former roommate writes: *"You and I have been friends since the eighth grade. In the time I've known you three things have remained true: You are kind – there isn't a person you've ever met who doesn't think that; you are a fighter – those days of sports showed me that; and, you have a heart of gold – one which we all strive to match. In knowing this, I say goodbye to you for a little while with a great deal of comfort that the qualities you possess help make you strong...."*

During this time, Dani struck up a relationship with a retired 84-year-old U.S. marine captain who she met in her oncology office as he was also being treated for cancer. Captain Miller sent Dani many cards and gifts. He would often take time to have the oncology office staff and the doctors' write their best wishes for Dani on these cards. "*Friendship*," he said, "*it warms a cold heart*" and "*Some people just naturally bring to mind warmest thoughts and wishes.*"

From a former ninth-grade boyfriend: *"To this day, I have yet to meet somebody as genuine as I remember YOU to be. I must say that you have been on my mind since your BBYO Sweetheart Dance in the ninth grade, and especially after seeing you at our reunion, but in the past few months it hurts to think of you having so many struggles at your plate. You will beat this, I know. I have learned...that with a positive attitude and a good heart every dream is accomplishable. Babe Ruth once said that the only player he couldn't beat was the one that didn't give up. So keep that smashing smile handy and press right on through this...."*

From a Wootton High School Alum: *On behalf of the entire Wootton* *class of 1992, we wish you the best in the coming months....Our class wanted to honor your courageous spirit by donating some of the excess money from our reunion proceeds to your fund. We hope that...this helps you...in some way...beat this challenge and return home strong and healthy. Please know that the Wootton community...is behind you all the way!"*

From Dani's first high school softball varsity catcher: *" The pictures on your website show that your great smile and beautiful personality continue to shine through....My youngest brother had a bone marrow transplant years ago so I know that you have a challenge ahead of you. I also know it is a challenge that you will be able to handle with your determination and positive outlook.*

From a fellow teacher: *"Although I'm sure we've informally met through preschool in-service training, I don't know the wonderful person that so many others who have signed (your website guestbook) know. Upon learning of your need and the Arlington Drive, I figured that it would be a nice thing to do, but that I probably wouldn't attend. Then I was filled with this immense sense that I MUST do something! In the scheme of things, it's not much, but I invited each staff member at Campbell to be tested. I was amazed at how many people attended. The next day I showed my appreciation by inviting them to my class...and gave each of them a...rose to thank them for...their selfless act."*

So on the morning of January 13th, Dani, Jay, and I depart for Seattle packed with enough good wishes and prayers to see us through the next four months.

Chapter Nine
Welcome to the Emerald City

1/13

We arrive at Sea-Tac in the early afternoon. Micah greets us and takes us to the Marriott Residence Inn on Lake Union. We settle into our temporary apartment and we unpack. We check in with Carol in Maryland. She tells us that dad has been moved from the hospital in Miami to a rehabilitation center near mom and dad's home in Delray Beach. His status, she says, remains unchanged, but at the very least because of the proximity to their home, my mother and friends will have no difficulty visiting him.

As we walk through the lobby, we encounter a former law school buddy of Jay's, who is here to receive treatment at the Hutch as well. We also meet Tiffany, a young woman about Dani's age, who will be receiving a bone marrow transplant a few days before Dani. She is accompanied by her mom, Debbie. We become fast friends. Because of its proximity to the Hutch (about .4 of a mile), about 15% of the hotel's guests are involved with treatment at the medical facility.

1/15

After a day of acclimating ourselves to our new surroundings, Jay, Dani, and I arrive on the sixth floor of the Hutch for our initial consult with Dani's outpatient team members. The receptionist greets us warmly and gives Dani a schedule, which begins by having us return to the first floor for a blood draw. When we return to the sixth floor, we are met by Diane Stayboldt, who informs us that Dani has been assigned to the Blue Team. Each team includes the attending physician, the primary provider (either a medical oncology fellow or a physician's assistant) a team Registered Nurse (Diane), a nutritionist, and a scheduler. Diane hands Dani her weekly outpatient itinerary listing appointments and scheduled times, and escorts us to a conference room where we meet with Dr. Eric Chen MD/PhD, a medical oncology fellow. We find out that the attending physicians and primary providers rotate these positions on a monthly basis. Dr. Mary Flowers, the Director of Long Term Follow-Up Care at the Hutch, will be our substitute attending physician (as Dr. Paul Martin is not available for the next week or so). Dr. Chen meets with us, takes a family and medical history, and then has Jay and I wait in the reception area while he examines Dani briefly. His report to Dr. Flowers, written later in the day states, "This is a 26-year-old female in first complete remission for AML…with high risk cytogenetic features (monosomy 7) who will be undergoing an anticipated mismatched unrelated donor bone marrow transplant on February 6th 2003 with Busulfan and Cytoxin conditioning."

He further states that all of her blood pre-transplant labs have been drawn, that she will have a pre-transplant bone marrow biopsy and lumbar puncture on Friday, January 17th, and that, because of her past VRE urinary tract infection, she will have another urinalysis performed as part of her pre-transplant work-up. This initial meeting goes well.

Later that evening, around 11:15 p.m. (Seattle time), I receive the sad news from my mom that my dad has passed away. We are all numb with grief. After a flurry of phone calls with my sister, we decide that Jay, Micah and I will fly home to D.C. on Saturday, attend my dad's funeral in Philadelphia on Sunday, return to our home in Gaithersburg, Maryland, on Sunday evening, and then Micah and I will head back to Seattle on Monday morning to reunite with Dani. Dani, in the meantime, will remain in Seattle with Micah's buddies who will provide companionship.

Dani tells us the next morning that she felt her Poppy's "presence" as she went to sleep on Wednesday night. We told her that her grandfather was just checking that she would be okay. Later on in the day, we hear from my mother and my sister that my dad's presence was felt by my mom and my nephew the previous night. Jay and I recall to Dani what my dad said to us when we visited him in Sinai Hospital a little over a week ago. He told us that he had every intention of being there for Dani. We all feel comforted by this thought that Poppy will always be in our hearts. We would often joke that, this way, my frugal dad saved on air fare. We are glad to have him along for the ride.

1/16

We arrive at the Hutch in the morning for another series of appointments. Our first meeting is with the nutritionist, who advises Dani on foods to eat and foods that are taboos. Dani will be on an immuno-suppressant diet and she can have pasteurized dairy products, but no buffets, deli salad bars, blue cheese, or salads, in a restaurant. She advises Dani to have 32 to 64 ounces of fluids (which include yogurt, soups, and fruit) a day.

The rest of the morning is occupied with more physical exams and a stop at the pharmacy for a new supply of prophylactic **Bactrim** and multi-vitamins. At 1 p.m. Dani, Jay and I attend our first counseling session, and meet with the social worker, Christy, and the chaplain, a female rabbi named Shoshana. Since Dani, Jay and I are the only ones present for this session, we get to discuss our favorite topic…Dani! Christy and Shoshana inform us about the counseling and support services provided at the Hutch. They advise us that their regular support group sessions are held every Thursday from 9:30 to 10:30 in the morning. After this meeting, the three of us decide that we now have developed a standard speech regarding Dani and AML. The three of us also feel that Christy and Shoshana are quite impressed with Dani's coping skills.

At 2:15 p.m., we finally meet with Dr. Mary Flowers, a very tiny lady (Dani thinks she is very cute), and Diane Stayboldt, the Blue Team R.N. Dr. Flowers, with her expertise in long term follow-up care for bone marrow transplant patients, impresses us with her candor and positive attitude. Once more she reviews Dani's medical history from 9/11/02, the subsequent and planned treatments, and the potential short and long term side effects resulting from the chemotherapy and transplant. She does not mince words as she speaks directly about rejection and toxicity. However, she also lets Dani know that "you are in a good prognostic risk group to do well with your transplant because of your age, and the fact that you will be receiving a bone marrow transplant product from a male donor" (which, she says, the research suggests is associated with less severe Graft vs. Host Disease). She further tells us that we want some GvHD to occur because it can be treated. She says, "We want to adjust the good, and eliminate the bad." As our meeting comes to a close, Dr. Flowers reminds us of a famous quote by an unknown author:

> *In order to know tomorrow, we need to do today,*
> *Yesterday was the past.*
> *Tomorrow is a mystery.*
> *Today is a gift.*
> *That's why it's called the present.*

We are all delighted that Dr. Flowers shared this quote with us. The three of us look forward to many more "presents."

1/17

After Dani's blood draw this morning, the two of us go to the fifth floor of the Hutch where Dani will receive a pre-transplant aspirate and bone marrow biopsy. Jay is back at the apartment preparing a eulogy for my dad's funeral on Sunday. Unlike Dr. Christie, the staff at the Hutch pre-medicates Dani to decrease her stress as well as limit the pain. Dani is none too pleased that the aspirate process has to be repeated despite her complete cooperation. We decide to inform our team nurse and fellow about this.

Later on in the day, the two of us attend a class on "Managing Care at Home." We take all the helpful hints of the instructor quite seriously and are attentive students. As the class ends, Dani is bundled up and we walk down the hill to the Marriott. Dani spends the afternoon sleeping.

Dani's Memories

1/18 – 1/20

I wake up Saturday morning, and I am pleased that the pain from the aspirate and biopsy has eased. Micah, my mom, and dad leave for Sea-Tac Airport but not before they make sure I know what to do just in case something happens. I feel great—I kiss them goodbye, tell them to give Grandmom a big hug, hand them a letter to give to her, promise that I am okay, and proceed to get ready for an adventure. I remember that the REI has its flagship store right down the street from the Marriott. After all, it will be good exercise. Little did I know how much exercise it will be. First I have to climb the .4 of a mile hill to the Hutch. Then I turn right and REI is just a hop, skip, and a jump from the Hutch. WRONG! I walk, and walk and walk...uphill, for what seems like forever. I am exhausted by the time I get there, so I turn around and walk all the way back to the Residence Inn. I spend the afternoon sleeping. Later on in the day, Micah's friends, Cameron and Beth, stop by. I invite them to stay for dinner. I decide to treat them and order delivery take-out from one of the fancy restaurants, which is across the street from the hotel. The dinner is quite expensive. I'm pretty sure I'll be in big trouble with my parents when they come back.

Sunday comes and goes without any drama. I think about Poppy a lot, rest, and look forward to mom's and Micah's return. On Monday, I wake up, walk up the hill to the Hutch, have my blood drawn and return to our place at the Marriott, which is starting to feel like home.

My dad's death instantly returns us to the real world, and away from the parallel universe where the only thing that matters is Dani's well-being. Heading east from Seattle takes the whole day. With a stop in Minneapolis to change planes, and with a three hour time difference, we return late Saturday night to our home in Gaithersburg. After laying out our clothes for the funeral the next day in Philadelphia, we attempt to get a few hours sleep.

The next morning, we leave for the funeral; Jay will drive us to and from the funeral. It is a bitter cold day. The funeral is attended by friends and family alike. Both Bruce and Jay deliver beautiful eulogies filled with great stories of my dad and his strong work ethic, as well as his love and devotion to his wife, kids, grandkids, other family members and friends. After the service, we go to the cemetery to lay my dad to rest. Then we all return to my brother Ken's home, where the family will sit S*hiva* (in Jewish tradition, this is a seven-day period of formal mourning observed after the funeral of a close relative). We are all comforted by condolences offered to us. After spending about three hours at my brother's home, Jay, Micah and I get back in the car and drive back to Gaithersburg. On our way back, we remember that Dani's camp buddies are having a fund raiser for Dani at a local Irish Pub. Micah volunteers to drop us off at home and represent the family at the fundraiser (what sacrifices the boy makes). We arrive home about 9 p.m., Micah heads to the party, and Jay and I go to bed.

As Jay will be spending the next few days in the D.C. area working at G. W. U., he drops us off at the airport early Monday morning. Later on that afternoon, Micah and I arrive back in Seattle. Dani looks none the worse for our absence, and we get mentally ready for week two of the pre-transplant regimen.

1/21

Dani and I arrive at the Hutch at 9:15 a.m. and we are greeted by our physician's assistant, who informs us that Dani's bone marrow donor is cleared. Dani and I both are surprised at that announcement, as we thought that he was cleared on December 6th (the day we were informed that a 30-year-old German male had been found to be a close enough match for the transplant to proceed). Dani is then told that, according to Germany's regulations, Dani will have to wait for two years after her transplant before she can communicate with him. There are many stipulations placed on this first communication as well: she can write him without identifying herself; she can send a photograph of herself, but it cannot include any clues to her location; and the communication is done through the Matched Unrelated Donor offices at the Hutch. We're also informed that Dani's blood type will change with the transplant from O positive to A positive, and that because of this blood type change, she probably will need a plasma exchange, using apherisis a day or so prior to the transplant. Once more, Dani and I are stunned by this medical phenomenon. The physician's assistant further explains that Dani's O positive blood's plasma may have some anti-A blood titers or antigens, which would reject the A positive bone marrow or stem cells without giving them the opportunity to engraft in Dani's body. We both accept this news as just another step in the long process of healing.

The next scheduled meeting of the day is with the pulmonary specialist. Dani receives several tests that check and provide base-line data on pulmonary functioning, so they can better monitor her vital signs after transplant. The specialist attempts a special type of blood draw on Dani's left wrist and fails. Dani screams and cries from the pain caused by this failed draw. The specialist is successful on the second try with her right wrist. Several other tests are completed in what is called an atmospheric chamber. Her lung volume, lung capacity, and oxygen flow are tested. Dani "passes" the tests. Hooray! Before we leave, the specialist wraps both wrists, which results in many strange and pitying looks from the people we pass by during the day.

That afternoon, Dani and I attend a food safety class and learn what foods are okay and what foods we'll need to stay away from (i.e. sprouts, certain cheeses, uncooked vegetables, etc).

We go from that class to the Managing Care Class. In this class I'm given a huge loose-leaf binder, which tells us both about what is expected of me, Dani's primary care giver, during Dani's 100 days post-transplant. Dani assures me that we'll both be all right. Dani is now comforting me!

At 4:15 that afternoon, we meet again with Eric, the Blue Team's oncology fellow, for a spinal tap. Dani informs Eric of her misadventures from her previous **bone marrow aspirate and biopsy** and the pulmonary blood draws. Eric reassures her that he's pretty good at this procedure. A few minutes later, Dani confirms Eric's assessment. Exhausted, we both march down the hill to the Residence Inn.

1/22

Dani begins her day with an appointment with the ob/gyn. She chooses to go into the office alone. When she returns to the sixth floor waiting area, she appears pretty distraught, as the ob/gyn has told her that, from her knowledge base, no one can become pregnant after receiving Dani's upcoming chemotherapy protocol. If a pregnancy does happen to occur, the data suggest that there is a greater likelihood of a relapse of the cancer. Dani has heard this all before but still asks to speak to a fertility specialist. Ever optimistic, she still is hoping for a miracle.

As if she hasn't experienced enough pain, Dani's next appointment is with the gynecologist's husband, who happens to be a dentist. Of all of Dani's appointments, this one, strangely enough, is the one she dreads the most. Fortunately, all that occurs during this consult is an X-ray of her mouth and more base-line data gathering for the Blue Team. Unfortunately, Dani is scheduled for another dental appointment tomorrow.

We spend our afternoon in a nutrition class, where we are once more inundated with information about the importance of good nutrition. We are told that Dani's protein needs will be higher during the period of transplant and engraftment, as it is essential to strengthen and repair any organ damage that may have occurred from the high dose chemotherapy. We're also informed that we may need to increase the fat intake during treatment. We're educated about the benefits of complex carbohydrates, what foods to eat if constipated, what foods to eat if she has diarrhea (apple sauce, oatmeal, bananas, and rice), what vitamins help to convert food into energy (B), which vitamins promote healing (C, Iron, A, and E), and which vitamins will help prevent nutrition deficiencies (multivitamins). Dani finds out how important weight maintenance will be, and that she will, in all probability, have some weight gain (because of fluid retention) as well as weight loss (caused by muscle loss and the lack of sufficient calorie intake during the treatment). The dietician also shares some helpful hints about eating during treatment.

With regard to foods:
- Savory and sour flavors are most favored
- If smells are bothering her try eating cold foods or even keep the fan on while cooking
- Eat crunchy, chewy foods as well as foods that appeal to you visually

To combat a poor appetite:
- Eat and drink frequently
- Keep snacks within easy reach
- Take a walk before eating
- Keep a meal schedule
- Have several easy to microwave frozen food meals on hand

To curb nausea:
- Eat small amounts of food often and slowly
- Make saltines a part of your diet
- Drink fewer liquids with meals
- Eat food at room temperature
- Pre-medicate before eating
- Don't force yourself to eat
- Rest after meals, but don't lie down

Dani and I marvel at how much we are learning in our "parallel universe classes" and how important it will be for us to "ace" all the classes.

1/23

Dani wakes up terrified, for today she has to return to the dentist. She predicts that this appointment will be worse than the chemotherapy. She is pleasantly surprised when the dentist and hygienist's treatments are all pain free. The dentist will prescribe a Mycelex cream for mouth sores and Mycelex lozenges (troches) for throat soreness.

The day proceeds with more tests (i.e., a mugascan) as well as a patient and caregiver group meeting. Dani and I find ourselves to be the only two participants meeting with the social worker (Christy) and the chaplain (Rabbi Shoshana). Our last meeting scheduled for the day is with the pharmacist. She presents us with a chart listing the drugs, purposes, dosage, and times per day to dose, and sits down with us with a huge tome in front of her. Her agenda is a simple one. She will be informing us of the drug treatment Dani will be following for the next few months. Going down the chart, she describes each drug, its purpose and possible side effects. She then opens the giant book and shows us each drug. Dani is hoping that the pictures of the pills are magnified but they are not! Some of them are huge. Dani mentions that she is not the best pill taker and some of them may make her gag. The pharmacist notes this comment and says that they can provide her with smaller, single strength pills but will have to increase the number because of the smaller dosage. Some of the drugs she introduces us to include:

- Cyclosporine – to help prevent transplant rejection and GvHD. Its' side effects include nausea, elevated blood pressure, kidney malfunctioning, and high blood sugar counts. This is a major medication, and Dani's Cyclosporine levels in her blood will be checked twice a week. The pills are huge and they really stink. The pharmacist says that she hears that a lot of patients say that it's not so bad if you take it with chocolate milk

- **Prednisone** – a steroid used to suppress the immune system. It will be taken initially in large doses and the doses will very gradually **taper**. Side effects include what has come to be known as moon face, mood swings, muscle atrophy, hyperactivity, and increased appetite

- Bactrim – a prophylactic antibiotic to help prevent infections

- Busulfan – out-patient high dose chemotherapy pills, which cause extreme nausea

- Ativan – an anti-nausea drug, which will need to be taken 45 minutes prior to the Busulfan
- **Dilantin** – taken as a precaution against seizures from the chemotherapy medication

As the meeting draws to a close, the pharmacist hands us a fairly large plastic tray that includes seven smaller plastic containers, one for each day of the week. Each container has five compartments according to the time of day each drug will be dispensed (a.m., mid-morning, lunch, afternoon, and p.m.). We count the number of pills Dani will initially be ingesting each day. By our count, the number is sixty-four! Amazing! Dani comments that it is a good thing that Scott has taught her an easy way to swallow her pills (put the liquid in your mouth first). As we say good-bye to the pharmacist, she lets us know that drugs may be added or subtracted from Dani's protocol on a weekly basis, and that it will be my job as primary care-giver to dispense them correctly. An awesome task!

As we walk down the hill, we continue to discuss the number and size of the pills, and we promise to work together to make sure we follow the protocol to the letter.

1/24

It's Friday, and today we are scheduled to meet with the Blue Team for our weekly progress report. As a result of a random test, all of Dani's chromosomes appear normal, and there is no evidence of leukemia. Dani comments that this must mean that she is no longer at-risk and that she can go home! Collectively, the team shakes their heads from side to side, and Eric continues with the report. Once Dani is hospitalized, she will have another temporary catheter inserted in her shoulder/neck region in preparation for the plasmapherisis. Dani once more raises the issue of fertility. The attending physician states that, in order to make the transplant safer, the prescribed chemotherapy protocol, along with Dani's chromosome abnormality cancel any chance of possible pregnancy. Eric says that prior to her hospitalization, the team wants Dani to meet with a fertility specialist who can address her options for having children. His plan is to schedule this appointment as soon as possible. The team wants Dani to be sure that this issue has been addressed thoroughly prior to her hospitalization.

Once back in the apartment, Dani's mood improves as she remembers that Scottie will be arriving tomorrow and will remain in Seattle for two weeks.

1/25 – 1/26

Scott arrives on Saturday, and together the three of us, with Micah's input, plan our Super Bowl party for Sunday, January 27th. It is an important day, not because of the two teams playing, but because it will be the first day in a month that Dani will be allowed to eat dairy products, as her VRE prevention treatment and subsequent prescription has ended. We prepare a cheese-filled menu of chili with cheddar, nachos with cheddar, salsa, and sour cream, Buffalo wings with blue cheese dressing, and cheese cake. Disgusting, yes, but the menu more than satisfies her lust for dairy products.

1/27

As Scott commutes to the suburban Seattle branch of the company he works for in Renton, Washington, Dani and I prepare for her visit with Dr. Mark Khan, a University of Washington fertility specialist. His offices are elegant, with walls filled with hundreds of photos of beautiful and precious children. Dr. Khan meets with us and briefly reviews Dani's medical history before he begins to discuss fertility treatment options. He emphasizes to Dani the importance of her receiving the transplant prior to beginning any form of fertility treatment. Throughout our meeting he repeats this message: Dani should not delay this life-saving procedure for any reason. He tells her that if they were to freeze embryos (a process completed with married couples), one must first have two months of stable cycles. As Dani's AML with chromosome abnormality places her at high risk, timing of the transplant is crucial. Another non-option would be to remove an ovary and freeze the tissue. This experimental procedure has not yet been utilized with humans. To date there have been no pregnancies from this procedure. Even if this procedure could be used now, his concerns would be: the possibility of reintroducing leukemic cells back into Dani's body; the amount of time that it would take for Dani to heal from the surgical procedure would further delay the transplant process; and there would be no guarantee that Dani's body would be able to use the immature egg cells once replanted.

With these possibilities discounted, Dr. Khan then speaks to Dani of the options available to her after her treatment and remission. He speaks about in vitro fertilization (with a donor egg) and adoption. He then answers our questions. He says that he has had patients on a Cytoxin chemotherapy regimen who have become pregnant, but this has only occurred if the patient's uterus responds to hormone therapy. He also says that pregnancy does put stress on the body, and the research is inconclusive as to whether pregnancy can cause a relapse of leukemia. He also explains that since Dani's genetic make-up will have been altered post-transplant, this will be a non-issue (unless the donor egg carries the abnormal mono-chromosome 7). But all this is supposition; and the bottom line, Dr. Khan clearly states, is "Get your treatment as quickly as possible, knowing that you have the option of either receiving a donor egg or of adoption."

With all of her questions answered by one of the nation's top experts in fertility, Dani says goodbye to Dr. Khan. We head back to the Hutch on the shuttle bus that runs back and forth from the University of Washington campus and medical complex, and I try to offer Dani words of comfort, but she can't accept them. She cries on my shoulder for the entire trip back. When we return to our apartment she closes the door to her bedroom and awaits Scott's return from work.

Later on that evening, we all agree that we will not delay the transplant for any reason. We are reminded of Dr. Christie's primary goal of saving our daughter's life first and foremost.

1/28

Today we meet with the attending physician. He reviews all the tests, and even though Dani's bone marrow and chromosome tests confirm that she is in remission, and her flow cytometry tests have no abnormal white blood cells (blasts), he tells us that the high white blood cell count alone from September 11th warrants this transplant. He then confirms that Dani will most likely have a single apherisis run a few hours before the transplant, as Dani's blood type will be changed to that of her donor's, i.e., A positive. He then tells her a bit about Donor # 117626's medical history, and Dani is both amazed and thankful for several other similarities. (Neither has ever had HIV, hepatitis, syphilis, or CMV in their lifetimes.)

The doctor pronounces that being that the mismatch of the donor's contribution is ever so slight, "the rejection risk is very small."

> Approximately one-third to one-half of the general population is exposed to **CMV** or **Cytomegalovirus** in their lifetimes, particularly urban dwellers. Patients who test positive for CMV prior to transplant are twice as likely to develop a CMV infection post-transplant, the most dangerous of which is CMV pneumonia.

The next item on the agenda involves Dani's chemotherapy protocol prior to the transplant. The doctor tells Dani that on Wednesday the 29th Dani will take Dilantin (a drug to prevent seizures). She will also begin to take Zofran (a pill to prevent nausea), in preparation for the outpatient chemotherapy (Busulfan pills) that Dani will begin on Thursday morning. Dani will be taking Busulfan for three days (Thursday, Friday, and Saturday). We will be spending most of those three days, he tells us, in the blood draw lab where they will be testing the toxicity levels hourly. Sunday will be a chemo-free day. He informs Dani that on Monday she'll enter the University of Washington Hospital and receive Cytoxin intravenously for the next two days. He lets Dani know that some patients need a bladder catheter during this time but she will not. On Wednesday, she'll have no treatment and will feel as though "she is coming out of a fog." He predicts that by late evening of February 6th or early in the morning of the 7th she'll receive the transplant. The last thing he tells Dani is that, in order for all this to occur, she must submit the consent forms first. I write this down in large print in our notebook, "CONSENT FORMS— BRING THEM!"

The consent forms that the doctor alludes to were put together by Jay prior to coming to Seattle and basically amount to a "living will." He had done this once before for his mom when she entered a nursing home. Dani and I review them one more time later that afternoon. Dani has put off completing these documents until the last minute, as they give specific instructions about her care should she become "terminally ill, unconscious, or otherwise unable to communicate" her wishes. Dani requests that:

- "Food and water be artificially administered, even if it would also have the effect of prolonging her life
- All comfort care be provided, even if it would also have the effect of prolonging my life
- All additional life-prolonging treatment be provided, including blood, cardio-pulmonary resuscitation, diagnostic tests, dialysis, drugs, respirator and surgery"

In completing these forms, she also appoints Jay and me as healthcare agents if she becomes unable to make healthcare decisions for herself. Dani signs the forms, and together we place them in our Hutch tote bag, which includes the ever-important notebook, bottled water, and granola bars. Without much discussion we prepare to pick up Jay for what will be the first of his many "commuter" flights to Seattle on the 29th. Jay has set up a schedule at work where he will be at the office for five days, fly to Seattle on Saturday, telecommute while in Seattle for the next five work days, and fly back to D.C. on the following Sunday.

1/29

It's raining more than the usual "Seattle mist" this morning. We pick Jay up at the airport (Dani drives) and head over to the Hutch for our appointment with Diane, the Blue Team nurse. Diane enters the examination room and asks Dani, "Are you ready for your adventure?" We all answer in the affirmative and then Diane once more explains the Dilantin and Busulfan regimen that will begin later in the day.

We've decided that, since for the next few days or so Dani will be a bit under the weather, tonight we should celebrate Jay's birthday, two days early (pre-Dilantin and pre-Busulfan)! The kids have told us that they would like to treat us to a celebratory dinner at one of our favorite restaurants, Roy's, which is part of a chain owned by Roy Yamaguchi. It just so happens that my parents (prior to my dad's passing) gave us a generous gift certificate to that very restaurant. Since we have not used the gift certificate, we offer it to the kids and they happily accept, as it will help them pay for what promises to be a delicious and rather expensive dinner. After we dine, the check is presented to the kids, who pay for the meal (with a bit of help from the gift certificate). Jay and I offer thanks to the kids and they graciously accept our appreciation. At that very second something quite eerie occurs. My funeral button (a black button with a torn black ribbon that a mourner wears in the Jewish faith to signify the designated month of mourning) inexplicably pops off of my blouse and lands on the table. We laugh and agree that once more Poppy's presence is felt as he too wants to be included in our appreciation of the fine meal. We return home to the Marriott ready for the next step of our adventure.

1/30

At 8 a.m., we arrive at the Hutch's blood draw lab's waiting room. Dani's vitals are taken (BP106/70, weight 55.2 kilos) and she takes her first dose of Busulfan. Since she's feeling a bit nauseous (Dani believes that it's from the Dilantin), she takes some Ativan to combat the nausea. By 8:30 a.m., Dani has blood draw #1, and by 9 a.m. she has blood draw #2 and also takes the prescribed Bactrim (anti-biotic preventing pneumonia), Fluconasol (anti-fungal), Alpurinol (anti-biotic), **Acyclovir** (anti-viral), and a multi-vitamin. The draws continue: #3 at 9:30, #4 at

10 (Dani feels dizzy), # 5 at 11, #6 at noon, #7 at 1, and finally #8 at 2 p.m. (Our pill count is now up to 27 pills every six hours!) With the day one regimen of blood draws complete, we head back to our apartment.

1/31 – 2/2
The regimen starts over again early this morning, as at 1 a.m. Dani takes the Ativan in preparation for the 2 a.m. dose of Busulfan. We are not surprised when Dani wakes us at 2:46 a.m. with a vomit pan in one hand and a fork in the other hand. Our job is now to search through this gore for undigested particles of the Busulfan. When we find none, we all return to our respective beds to sleep.

The next morning, we celebrate Jay's birthday by hiking up to the Hutch and repeating yesterday's blood draw scenario. When we finish with the blood draws, we head upstairs for our 3 p.m. meeting with the Blue Team. Dani describes her dizziness to Diane and rates her nausea as a 2 on a scale of 1 to 5 (with 5 being the most severe). We all then report that Dani's appetite is just fine. Then the doctor tells us that Dani's most current draws show that her blood contains antibodies that will attack the donor's A Positive blood, so the plan is to go ahead with the scheduled plasma exchange apherisis prior to the transplant. With that final information passed on to us, we thank the attending physician and Eric for their support, as Dani's team membership will change as of 2/1, when she will have a new attending physician and a new physician's assistant.

On Saturday and Sunday we briefly return to the Hutch for a single blood draw in the lab, and then head upstairs to the clinic to have Dani's vital signs taken. We get to spend most of the weekend relaxing, speaking on the telephone to family and friends, and preparing for Dani's hospitalization on Monday morning. We find out on Sunday that a larger two-bedroom apartment will become available to us in the coming week. (We had previously decided to remain at the Marriott rather then move to the Pete Gross House, when an apartment also became available there this week.) We're told that we will be able to move into it by February

6th or 7th. Even though this complicates our plans a bit (as this is the proposed time for the transplant to take place), we figure that we'll be better off in the long run with a larger apartment. So we agree with the management to make the switch. The day continues without any crises occurring, and we all go to bed early that evening knowing that tomorrow, February third, will be a busy one for all of us.

So much has happened since we first arrived in Seattle three weeks ago. It goes without saying that the cards, letters, phone calls, packages and messages from the website have kept us connected with our friends and family. The thoughtful and poignant messages continue to have a profound positive impact on Dani and the rest of us. We are especially gratified by the kindness of my parents' friends in Florida. As a tribute to my dad (Dani's "Poppy"), these generous friends make contributions to Dani's Transplant Fund. We're all sure that "Poppy" would be pleased by their loving and helpful words and gestures.

Other encouraging notes from the past 3 weeks also appear on Dani's website:

A family friend says: *"I first entered the Marrow Registry about a decade ago. Never did I imagine that someone close to me might benefit from that simple act. For as long as I have known you, you have been an incredible radiant source of energy and inspiration. This holds true now more than ever."*

Team Reed (Dani's school colleagues) send a group message: *"On the night before your hospital stay, your friends from work want you to know that we think about you ALL of the time. On the eve of your 'new birthday' after the students are dismissed, we will all join hands in 'a circle of support for our favorite colleague, Dani.' We will be sending our collective positive energy, compassion, courage, and most of all... Love. Although we won't be singing 'Kumbaya' at this time, we're all pretty sure that you'll be able to receive all of our positive energy. Hang in there, kiddo, we're all with you for your big day!"*

So with lots of love, hope, best wishes, and the best medical attention in the world our journey continues.

Chapter Ten
Plan B

2/3

Dani, Scott, Jay and I arrive on the seventh floor oncology transplant wing of the University of Washington Medical Center at 8:30 a.m., and we are met almost immediately by Corrine, our hospital Silver Team nurse. Corrine strikes us as a committed, take-charge kind of person. After reviewing the rules of the oncology transplant wing, she tells us that the VRE infection has not yet totally cleared in Dani and, as a result, we will be practicing "reverse isolation" to protect the other transplant patients. She explains that we must all be gowned when we leave Dani's room to go to other parts of the seventh floor, as a precaution against spreading the infection to other patients. In addition, Dani's door has to be closed, and we cannot use the laundry room facilities on the floor until the infection clears. None of us are terribly happy with this message and for that matter we are not too happy with Corrine, the messenger. However, it doesn't take us long to warm up to her and appreciate her advocacy for her patient, her efficiency, her warmth, and her sense of humor. Within an hour, Corrine has Dani settled in her bed and supplied with vitamins, Mycelex troches, potassium, nausea meds, **Mesna**, and Kotex pads for Dani's never-ending menstrual cycle. As she leaves us, she announces that our attending physician, Dr. Paul Martin, and his Silver Team associate, Betty Stewart, a physician's assistant, will be arriving shortly.

While waiting for the Silver Team to arrive, Dani takes her doses of Bactrim, Acyclovir, **Fluconazole**, and Alpurinol and decides to take a walk around the seventh floor. Dani and Scott put on their hospital gowns and circle the oncology unit four times. The transplant wing is located in the Medical Center on the University of Washington campus, and is about a ten minute drive from the hotel. The view from the seventh floor is not as spectacular as the sixth floor of the Hutch, but on a clear day you can see Mt. Ranier, more than 60 miles away, from the window of Dani's room.

Dr. Martin and Betty Stewart arrive shortly after Dani and Scott finish their walk. Dr. Martin answers all of the questions that we have regarding the upcoming Cytoxin chemotherapy, the plasma exchange, and the reverse isolation procedures. Betty is instantly endeared to us as she agrees to find out exactly how restricted we will be by "reverse isolation."

When the team members leave, Corrine hooks Dani up to the IV and begins the dosages of Zofran, Mesna, Decadron, and the chemotherapy drug Cytoxin. Within an hour of the Cytoxin administration, Dani's temperature rises, she feels nauseated, dizzy, and tells us that her head feels like it is going to explode. She is immediately dosed with Phenergren and given an ice pack for her headache. Corrine slows down the Cytoxin drip but Dani doesn't feel much relief. In fact, now she is also experiencing joint pain. By 6 p.m., Dani takes her first dose of morphine for the pain. She complains that this small pill, placed under her tongue, "tastes terrible!"

As Dani's day draws to a close, she reports that her throat is getting scratchy, but that she is no longer feeling dizzy. The good news of the day is that Dani will not have to have a catheter. The bad news is that her period has started once more. With Day 1 of the hospitalization almost over, we discuss the most current important news arising from the recent broadcast of "Joe Millionaire." It appears that Evan (Joe Millionaire) has chosen Zora and Sarah as the finalists for his upcoming decision-making show. With that finally settled, we all breathe a sigh of relief, kiss Dani goodnight, and the three of us head for our home away from home at the Marriott. It is a quiet ride as each of us seems to be thinking that the next 30 days will be no walk in the park for our Dani.

2/4

By the time we arrive at Dani's room in the morning, Dani has already been visited by the Patient and Family Education Coordinator and the hospital-based social work intern. She has also received a phone call from Grandmom and two from Uncle Bruce. Whew! Later on in the morning the Silver Team visits with Dani and discusses the upcoming surgical procedure necessary for the plasma exchange apherisis. The surgery is scheduled for after 9 p.m. this evening. Dani is told that she may not eat after 2:30 p.m. in preparation for the insertion of the temporary catheter into her neck. Dani is for the moment quite sad. She announces to no one in particular, "I just want to go home!"

The social work intern, with her big eyes and caring demeanor, is not successful in getting Dani out of this funk. After she leaves, however, Dani has a laugh at the intern's overly sympathetic approach. In fact, throughout Dani's stay in the hospital, this intern's affect continues to amuse Dani…as Dani rejects her every offer of support.

As the intern leaves, Corrine rushes into the room with the news that the line won't be inserted until first thing tomorrow morning! Dani

> **Titer** is a measurement of the amount or concentration of a substance in a solution. It usually refers to the amount of medicine or antibodies found in a patient's blood.

is relieved. However, 6 minutes later, Corrine reenters and tells Dani she is back on for surgery tonight. Betty stops by and lets us know that the plasma exchange will take two days to exchange Dani's O plasma with its anti-A titers to A plasma. The goal will be to get Dani's anti-A **titers** down to below 16. Currently they are at 256. (Titers are measured in a scale that goes from 16 to 32 to 64 to 128 to 256 to 512, etc.)

Dani's chemotherapy continues as do the dosages of Phenergren and morphine. In the late afternoon, a vascular technologist performs a sonogram of Dani's neck to determine which side to insert the line. After he leaves, Dani doses with morphine again to "take the edge off." The surgeon stops by and tells us that the earliest time for surgery will be at 8:20 this evening. When he leaves, Corrine sets up the post chemotherapy hydration, and tells us that Dani will take the rest of her meds later on this evening, after the surgery.

Dani is taken downstairs to surgery at 7:30 p.m. At 9:00 p.m. the surgeon calls us in Dani's room and tells us that Dani wants a pizza when she comes back to the room! Her wish is our command, of course. Soon after we place the order, four male attendants (we're not sure why this number was required to move one patient) return Dani to her room from post-op. By 9:30 that evening Dani has her pizza, and has us vote for Julie D'Amato as our "American Idol" "choice of the week." By 10 p.m., Dani throws up the pizza. Poppy would have said that her big eyes (wanting all that pizza) got the best of her! Dani reports that she feels okay. The nurse gives Dani her meds, and with that we say good night and have another quiet ride home…as tomorrow is another day.

2/5

By 9 a.m., already dosed with **Fentanyl** and Ativan, Dani is ready for the plasma exchange. The technician for the apherisis process arrives at the same time as Dr. Martin and Betty arrive. The doctor and Betty are equally impressed with Dani's appetite. They both check her mouth and the newly inserted line and depart. The apherisis

> **Albumen** is a simple water-soluble protein found in many animal tissues and liquids.

technician sets up the equipment for the plasma exchange. She tells us that they'll first infuse **albumen**, which will act as place holder until Dani's O plasma is out of her blood system. Once that procedure is complete, the A plasma will be infused. This process has to occur because Dani's Type O blood plasma is incompatible with the new blood products that will enter Dani's body, as a result of the upcoming bone marrow transplant from her Type A donor.

Within 45 minutes of the start of the procedure, Dani announces that she feels awful! She is given some Benedryl, Phenergren, and Tylenol to ease the aches and pains. By 1 p.m., approximately three hours after the process begins, Dani announces that she has to go to the bathroom. As the apherisis technician made no provisions to have a commode (portable toilet) to be in the room, she unhooks Dani from the machine and has her go to the bathroom. She informs us that the pause mechanism on the apherisis centrifuge only lasts for three minutes. After that the machine will have to be restarted. Unfortunately, Dani is not in "tip top" softball season physical condition, and she does not make it back by the three minute deadline. When she finally does get back into bed, the centrifuge has stopped. The plasma exchange technician goes into a panic as she is unable to restart the machine. She calls her nurse manager, who quickly arrives and is able to start the centrifuge. While all this is happening, Dani announces that her heart is hurting. We call Betty, Dani's physician's assistant. In an instant the room is filled with hospital staff. I look over at Scott, who appears quite calm, so I take my cues from him and remain (on the outside at least) a calm presence as well. Betty suspects that Dani's calcium level has dropped, causing the chest pain. A test proves Betty to be correct. By 1:30 Dani is given a calcium drip and reports, to those of us who have been holding our collective breath for the past 20 minutes or so, that she is feeling much better…"not 100%, but much better." By 4 p.m., the process is completed, at least for the day. It will, in all probability, and as predicted, be repeated tomorrow, with one change, the addition of a commode placed discretely in the corner of Dani's room.

Later on in the afternoon, Betty tells Dani not to worry if she doesn't feel up to eating or exercising. The hospital staff, she says, will take care of Dani's nutritional needs if she isn't eating. Betty also wants us to keep Dani's fecal samples for further VRE testing. We're hoping that we will soon be taken off the reverse isolation that greeted our arrival.

Before we head home that night, Dani is visited by Shoshana, the Chaplain from the Hutch. We are all comforted by her presence. As she is about to leave she asks if she can say a prayer for Dani, and we all think that that's a good idea. We all give her our Hebrew names, but there is one problem. Since Scott is Methodist, he does not have a Hebrew name. "No problem," says Shoshana. She gives Scott the name "Shiya." She says it means, "Gift of God." She says her prayer in Hebrew and then translates it into English. Shoshana will visit us often and we are always comforted by her company and her prayers. We always marvel however, that her Hebrew prayers are much shorter (about 30 seconds) than her subsequent English translations (about two minutes). Nevertheless, we look forward to these moments.

As if invigorated by Shoshana's visit, Dani completes two laps around the hallway circuit before she returns to her room. Although she has a bit of a temperature, Dani's vital signs taken from a lying down, sitting, and standing position are quite good. We depart for home after midnight when Dani falls asleep.

2/6

The day begins officially with Dr. Martin and Betty's visit. Dr. Martin says that he hopes for a better day today than yesterday. We laugh and totally agree with him! He tells us that Dani will receive a transfusion today, as her hematocrit is at 24, and it should be at a minimum of 26 for the transplant. He then tells us the good news…that Dani's anti-A titers went from 256 down to 64 as a result of yesterday's treatment. Today with the second apherisis, the titers should come down to below 16. With all our questions answered, they depart, and the blood transfusion begins.

At 2 p.m. a new apherisis technician arrives, and by 2:45 the final plasma exchange process begins. She predicts that the apherisis should conclude by 7 p.m. The afternoon passes quietly with the requisite blood drawing, med dispensing, and vital sign taking. Before Jay and I depart for dinner in the hospital's cafeteria, Dani becomes nauseous after having her dose of morphine. She informs Betty that the Ativan is not having the desired effect and asks for Demoral instead. With that bit of business taken care of, Jay and I head downstairs for dinner. We return in about 30 minutes to absolute chaos. The apherisis technician has reported to Dani, Scott, and Betty that Dani has received O plasma rather than A, as someone placed the wrong pharmacy order. She says, quite matter of factly, that they'll now have to repeat the process without the albumen step. We are all incredulous, and this latest statement makes even less sense. Betty contacts the head of the Apherisis Unit. She reports that the technician caught this error with only one liter of O plasma left. He informs Betty that the process should be restarted, with albumen given prior to the A plasma. At the end of the call, he informs Betty that Dani's donor bone marrow is now in San Francisco, after traveling from Germany, and should arrive at Seattle's Sea-Tac airport within three hours. A blood draw taken shortly after the conversation reveals a hematocrit level of 32 and we anxiously await news of what is sure to be an elevated ratio of anti-A titers. At 8:30 p.m. the third plasma exchange is about to begin. Prior to its start we have Betty place a call to Dani's attending physician, Dr. Paul Martin. Together, Jay and Scott have a conference call with him. Meanwhile, back in the hospital room, a miserable Dani is waiting to take her usual array of medications plus the additional pain and nausea drugs. Jay and Scott return to the room and tell Betty, Dani, and me of their phone conversation.

At 9:10 p.m., prior to beginning the emergency apherisis, the technician receives a call from the Director of Blood and Blood Component Services, Dr. Linenberger. He informs her that the apherisis will not be necessary, and for her to halt any preparatory steps at once. Apparently, the blood draw reveals that Dani's anti-A titers instead of going down went up to 512, twice what it was when the process began yesterday. They will now use an alternative strategy (red cell depletion of the donor marrow) to separate out the red blood cells from the stem cells, when the marrow arrives later this evening. Jay has Betty call Dr. Linenberger to ask whether this red cell depletion strategy gives Dani a jump start on the engraftment process, or if we have lost the advantage that the plasma exchange would have provided. The answer is quite interesting, and at the same time, fuzzy. The doctor says that there are times when the plasmapherisis process cannot bring the titer count down, so that they perform this Plan B (red cell depletion) on the donor's bone marrow.

At this point we are all pretty anxious...Dani especially. She repeats and repeats, through tears, that someone needs to get the (temporary) line out of her neck—immediately, if not sooner! Betty agrees and proceeds to remove it right then and there. A bit more comfortable, Dani finally rests as Jay, Micah, Scott, and I settle in for the longest night of our lives, awaiting news of the marrow's arrival.

2/7 – Day 0 – Dani's New Birthday
Shortly after midnight, we're finally informed that the bone marrow has arrived and will be transported to the Hutch's Blood and Blood Products Unit for red cell depletion. Dani is being prepped for the transplant, which really just amounts to a single bag transfusion. She is given Cyclosporin and **magnesium**, as the medications she is now taking decrease the body's supply of magnesium. We're told that it will take at least four hours for Dr. Linenberger to personally deplete the red blood cells from the bone marrow. Jay, Scott, Micah, and I alternately pace and sit.

At one point, Scott and Dani have some alone time while Jay, Micah, and I seek out alternative sleeping arrangements and goody-laden vending machines. While we are on our family crusade, Scott presents Dani with a note that not only expresses his love, it also puts a smile back on her face:

Today is…an important exciting day. You changed and enlightened my life more than I can tell….I always wondered about love at first sight, though I might not have been instantly in love (though I thought you were…adorable when I met you), I was hooked and deeply smitten by the end of that first wonderful day we spent together at Merriweather Post….I can't imagine being happier or being with someone more perfect….Through the years, I learned what I was looking for in a woman….I realized I was looking for kindness, inner beauty as well as a hot exterior, interest in the arts, strong family roots, outdoor lover and travel enthusiast, great similar network of close friends, dedication and love of a chosen career, love of kids, undying love for one's significant other, putting others before yourself except in dire circumstances, a best friend whom I tell any and everything...no holding back,...a lover...only she who turns me on, and someone I want to spend the rest of my life with. Well, Dani, you filled these items and many more.... I knew when I first wanted to introduce you to my parents that this was forever! I love you so much and am excited to be with you and excited to be a part of such a special event tonight! I love you, Scott

When the three of us finally return to Dani's room, we find her much calmer. Although, it is said, "actions speak louder than words," these beautiful words seem to be having a very powerful impact on our daughter. She is far less agitated than she was a few hours ago. In fact, she appears quite content, and with Scott by her side, dozes off. Jay, at this point, decides to head to the hospital lobby to try to nap, as there are large comfy sofas there. We promise we'll find him if anything develops.

It's not until 5:55 a.m. that the bone marrow arrives, at last... pretty unceremoniously. Despite the enormity of the event, Dani's vital signs are normal. At 6:40 a.m., the donor's marrow begins to flow into Dani's body. Dani actually sleeps through this miraculous event.

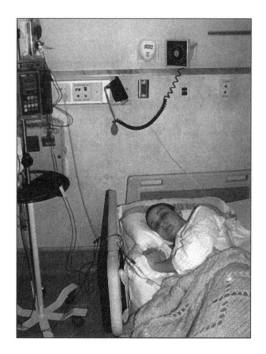

Also exhausted, Jay, Scott, and I depart for the Marriott, leaving Micah sprawled across three chairs to keep an eye on his sister. We'll return to the hospital in a few hours.

While Jay, Scott, and I are at the Marriott, Dani and Micah receive a visit from Dr. Gernsheimer, the Director of Transfusion Services at the Hutch. She sits down and is

Dani sleeping through the transplant

about to explain what has just transpired. Micah, being no dummy (and also having terrible handwriting) hands Dr. Gernsheimer the famous "notebook," and asks her if she can write down what she is saying. He explains that his mom insists that we keep careful records of what is happening medically to Dani. Not only does the doctor explain the process to Micah and a somewhat "out of it" Dani, she even draws pictures. In a nutshell she explains that the Hutch prefers using plasma exchange to rid the patient's body of antibodies that might cause rejection of the donor's red blood cells. She says that they get a bit nervous about manipulating a donor's bone marrow and the risk of losing some of the stem cells that need to engraft. For that reason, they prefer to take away the patient's plasma containing the antibodies that would potentially attack the donor's blood products.

When Dr. Gernsheimer leaves, Dr. Martin and Betty drop by to see how Dani is doing. In their presence she puts on a happy face and even eats half of a banana. Dr. Martin tells Dani that they'll stop by later on, to let us know how many stem cells were retrieved after the red cell depletion process. The team departs, and Dani throws up the banana, probably expressing her true sentiments about the past 48 hours!

Jay, Scott, and I arrive shortly before noon. Dani and Scott walk two laps of the hallway circuit before she receives three visitors. Dr. Martin (Dani's attending physician), Dr. Gernsheimer (The Director of Transfusion Services), and Dr. Linenberger (Director of Blood and Blood Component Services) have come to tell us, as Dr. Martin puts it, "your luck has just changed." He tells us that they recovered 3.56 million stem cells as a result of the stem cell depletion process. (They didn't tell us how they counted them!) He tells us "Usually we are happy when we recover two million cells. This is the best we could hope for." He then continues, "With this number there is a greater opportunity for engraftment." He tells Dani that tomorrow she'll begin to take Methatrexate (and again on Day 3, 6, and 11 post-transplant). Methatrexate is a drug that kills rapidly dividing cells. He apologizes to Dani saying, "Yesterday was a disaster. I think we are back on track." He then informs us that tomorrow Dr. Mark Stewart, the Medical Director for the Seattle Cancer Care Alliance, will become her new attending physician on the Silver Team. He leaves and Dr. Gernsheimer says that she hopes, with this good news, Dani will gain some confidence. She also tells Dani that she has had no donor transfusion negative reaction. She then introduces Dani to the man who stayed up all night to perform the red cell depletion process on the donor's marrow, Dr. Linenberger, the Director of Blood and Blood Products Services. He is so excited to meet Dani. He tells her that 99% of the donor's stem cells were recovered, and this "Plan B" did not compromise the procedure at all.

We thank both doctors for their personal attention to correct what truly could have ended in disaster. We tell them how much we appreciate them coming to Dani's room and sitting down with us to explain how, despite a couple of significant snafus, lemonade was made from lemons! We also let both doctors know how much we appreciate our physician's assistant, Betty Stewart, especially how she reacted to each "crisis de jour." The doctors then ask us for any questions or comments. Jay and I both enunciate how the problems of the past two days, in our opinions, demonstrated how the Silver Team assigned to Dani's care did not communicate effectively with the independent Apherisis Unit team. If lines of communication were more open, a member of the team (we were sure) could have assisted the technician in room set-up (and provided a commode), and in double-checking the medication needs of the patient during the apherisis process, as is done with all transfusions Dani has received prior to this event. With this communication process in effect, the inappropriate plasma would have been caught prior to infusion! They listen to our comments, and agree that this feedback is valuable to them. They assure us that they will continue to focus on improved communications with the various components of the Seattle Cancer Care Alliance (SCCA).

After the doctors leave, the five of us agree that both Dr. Gernsheimer and Doctor Linenberger heard our concerns. We are pleased that a director from each of the departments came to provide personal explanations and make amends for additional discomfort that was caused. They had voiced that they hoped that their explanations would restore Dani's confidence in the process. Dani is reminded of Dr. Storb's comment, back in October, that if something doesn't go quite right, their job would be to fix it. Dani is feeling confident enough to complete four more laps around the seventh floor after the doctors leave.

Later on that evening, we celebrate Dani's new birthday (February 7th) with a Baskin-Robbins ice cream cake. Dani is thrilled with the surprise celebration. She notes that she is quite pleased to be an Aquarius, as she didn't like being a Cancer (her June 22nd birthday sign)!

During the cele-bration, Jay gives Dani a very special birthday card, one that she will cherish forever. He writes:

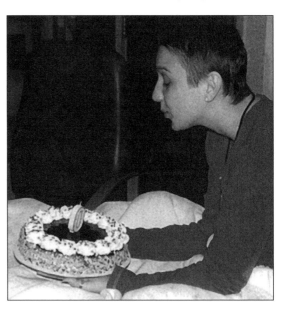

Happy Birthday, Dani!

My dear daughter,
On your original birthday, you and Mommy had to work really hard. It seems that no "birth" day is an easy one. We are all working as hard as we can, but in the end you are the one who has to work the hardest. You obviously know that we wish we could make this process easier for you…but the only thing we can do is be there with and for you in whatever way we can. This we will do. We love you very much…more than we can ever express…certainly more than I can ever express. We will be strong for you…and you are stronger than we could ever imagine.
Love, Dad

Jay's beautiful words leave us all a bit misty-eyed, but smiling. The brief new birthday celebration ends shortly after Dani opens all of her birthday cards. We all say good night to Dani, and go home to try to get some catch-up rest. Dani, we are sure, is having sweeter dreams tonight.

Each of us knows that there are going to be some tough weeks ahead and many bumps along the road, but we also know now that Dani is well-prepared for all of the challenges she will be face. During this week, we all receive many wonderful e-mails, cards and letters. These notes are as powerful as any medication that Dani receives. As usual they touch us all and continue to inspire Dani:

Dani's cousin Heather writes: *Your spirit is beautiful, graceful and strong. Your ability to make people feel welcome, included and loved is rare. I have admired you always but now more than ever….*

From our dear friend, Steve: *As Dani's very important day approaches, I wanted to send you this short note. I think about Dani and her courageous battle every single day. I can't put into words the emotion I feel every time I think about what you all have been going through since September 11th. As I know you know, Dani is an inspiration to me and everyone who has come in contact with her. She has so positively affected so many lives with her spirit, good humor, and sweet disposition. Any time I have to deal with professional and personal challenges both big and small, I think of Dani and the whole Shotel family and realize in the scheme of things my problems are not so serious at all…. With all our love….*

From a Team in Training coach: *Hi! I am one of the DC TNT coaches and have truly been touched by your story. Your amazing strength, courage, and determination are contagious! Here in DC, you have many TNT friends training in your honor! While the miles we pound pale in comparison to your journey, I hope it helps to give you additional endurance to continue the fight! Keep up the great spirit….*

From another TNT coach: *Just want to let you know that you are in my family's thoughts and prayers. My 13-year-old daughter Marissa finished treatment for acute lymphoblastic lymphoma four years ago, so we know the battle you are fighting. I have done several marathons to raise money for lymphoma/leukemia research and am now a coach with TNT. People like you and my daughter are a true inspiration and stories like yours make me more determined that ever to do what I can to end these terrible cancers. You have such a winning spirit and you will surely be in our hearts as we continue training and fundraising. I wish the very, very best to you and your family....*

From a cancer survivor:*...I was in my oncologist's office yesterday and saw a flier for the second upcoming Wizards game fundraiser. After visiting your website, I wanted to send my prayers, strength, and smiles to you to help throughout your miraculous transplant journey. I was just at the Hutch last week for my one-year post-MUD transplant follow-up and am happy to say that it all went well. You are truly in the most wonderful hands out there in Seattle and your donor is one of your angels here on earth! Stay strong and positive, the things you are and will go through are only temporary and the days are brighter ahead! Take care and smile even if you don't think you can!*

From Dani's favorite Arlington Hospital nurse:*...Congratulations on the smooth transfusion – I am so happy that everything went well! I told everyone at the hospital that you were getting your transplant today, so you were on everyone's thoughts and prayers. I know they're taking good care of you over there, but don't forget your favorite nurses in Arlington....*

From an old softball buddy:*...Stay strong and keep fighting. Here is a quote for you by Elizabeth Kubler-Ross:*

People are like stained glass windows
They sparkle and shine when the sun is out
But when the darkness sets in
Their true beauty is revealed
Only if there is light from within

Tiffany writes to Dani one week after her own bone marrow transplant:....*I know you have had quite an adventure over the last four months, but the same drive, energy, and love for life, will carry you through this transplant to a successful recovery. Not only are my prayers and thoughts with you – the day we met, I spoke of this energized woman that I met to my friends. They ask me daily how you are and send their prayers as well....Happy birthday and a successful and speedy recovery.*

Liz writes: *The best things in life aren't things at all. They're people like you! I can't help thinking that in some hours your transplant will happen. Finally here!! And...luckily by the time you get this...it will be a thing of the past! On the road to recovery....sure it may be <u>tough</u>, but that's what you are. You're not little, you're not a weakling, but you're one of the strongest people I know. It's amazing how many people you've inspired. Just today I read some 20 messages on your website from people running marathons – they don't even know you! But...they're running in your honor. Needless to say, lots of people are pulling for you.... So close to the finish line – almost breaking through the banner!! Okay girly, hope you're doing well. I'm thinking about you lots and lots and know it's all going to be fine in the end. Keep truckin' chica!*

A birthday card from Jay and me: *You are truly our sunshine, our happiness, our smiles, and our love!*

Chapter Eleven

Banana and Root-Beer Ice-Pops and the Button

Post-Transplant

2/8 – Day 1

Dr. Mark Stewart, the Medical Director for SCCA is Dani's new attending physician (We're still pretty amazed that even the various titled directors of the SCCA take a month rotation as an attending physician). We are all instantly drawn to his smile, positive attitude, and sense of humor. More importantly, Dani really appreciates his straightforward communication skills. He arrives with other members of the Silver Team Saturday morning. He announces to Dani that today is Day 1 post-transplant, and that there doesn't appear to be any unanticipated negative after-effects from the transplant. Dani puts on a big smile, but lets him know that she is feeling a bit achy and nauseous. She is dosed with many anti-pain and anti-nausea meds and also uses two heating pads; one for her achy back and one for her stomach, which appears tender. Despite the various aches and pains, Dani manages five laps of the transplant wing hallway, with one hand on her IV pole and the other hand firmly protected by Scott.

2/9 – Day 2

Dr. Stewart arrives in the morning and announces that Dani is finally VRE-free. Despite this great news (as we all can now stop using the reverse isolation practices), Dani doesn't feel so good. She announces that she has no desire to eat, and she continues to have what seems to be the period that never ends. Later on in the day, she tells us that her urine is now burning. A urine test is taken and within 11 hours of us all being off of reverse isolation, we're now on it once more, as Dani's urine tested positive for VRE.

2/10 – Day 3

Dani walks four laps prior to Dr. Stewart's a.m. visit. He is glad to hear that Dani is still eating, and after reviewing her vitals once more, issues a positive report! Dani, on the other hand, reports that she still has a lot of burning when urinating and continues to bleed. The doctor appears unconcerned and says that the **Levaquin** should stop the burning caused by the urinary tract infection.

After Dani's morning shower, Betty and Corrine enter the hospital room. Betty tells Dani that, at this point, she is susceptible to many infections and that "your body is filled with bugs!" Corrine adds her wisdom to this conversation by suggesting, in the most un-medical way possible (so that we can all understand her), "your woo" (we think she means urinary tract) "is taking precedence right now." Even Dani has a good laugh at this statement.

Dani continues her regimen of pain killers, antibiotics, and anti-nausea meds. She even continues to gargle with salt water to try and prevent the dreaded mucositis. By dinner time, she tells us that she is starting to feel better and requests that we watch the Robin Williams movie "Patch Adams," where he portrays a real-life doctor who uses humor as part of his patient's treatments. Dani gets to watch about 30 minutes of the movie before she falls into a medication-induced sleep.

2/11 – Day 4

Dr. Stewart arrives this morning wearing a bowtie and Dani comments how handsome he looks, prior to reporting how she is feeling. She tells him her mouth is sore, she has diarrhea, her urine is still burning, and she still has her period. He, in turn, forewarns her to be good about her mouth care, that she soon may be out of reverse isolation, and that the site where the temporary catheter was inserted (for the plasmapherisis) is healing nicely, and he lets her know that she will be put on **PCA** or Patient Controlled Analgesic today. This will allow Dani to use a push-button, which will release pain meds to her body as frequently as every seven minutes. Dani is most grateful for this, as "chemo's big guns" are taking their toll on our daughter. As he leaves us, he turns to Dani and says, "STRONG WORK DANI."

Despite the encouraging words, Dani is in pain and is hardly eating. The only so- called foods that she can swallow are root-beer and banana flavored ice-pops, as all the other "citrussy" flavors burn her mucositis-effected throat. She receives a transfusion of O Positive red blood cells (the universal donor variety), and enjoys a visit from Micah and his friend, Kat, before attempting to sleep.

2/12 – Day 5

Dani has a terrible night as a possible reaction to the transfusion adds one more problem to her high dose chemo-wracked body. Her shakes, chills, and nausea continue in the morning. Still Dani is given another unit of blood. She develops a slight rash and vomits.

Corrine comforts Dani with her soothing words and her medical prowess. She tells us that Dani is doing well and we have to believe her, as she has a lot more experience in these matters than we do. She states that narcotics frequently make people itch, which is Dani's new symptom for the day. She also informs us that Dani's body is sensitive to the newly transfused red blood cells, and that from now on she will pre-medicate Dani with Benedryl .

When Dr. Stewart stops by he tells her that he has authorized Dani to begin **TPN**, or Total Parenteral Nutrition later on in the day. Through IV Dani will now be

> **TPN**: Total Parenteral Nutrition is used for patients who cannot or should not get their nutrition through eating. TPN may include a combination of sugar and carbohydrates (for energy), proteins (for muscle strength), lipids (fat), electrolytes, and trace elements.

provided with the necessary nutrients. At this point, she is off solid foods, including her root beer and banana ice pops! He also tells Dani that she is finally off reverse isolation (we've heard that before)! We are not sure that she cares very much about who has to wear hospital gowns and where they have to wear them!

2/13 – Day 6

On his early morning rounds, Dr. Stewart informs Dani that "everything is A-OK!" A bit later, Dr. Gernscheimer, the Director of Transfusion Services at the Hutch, visits Dani for the third time and informs us that, from now on, Dani will be only given **leukoreduced** blood products when she is given transfusions,

> **Leukoreduced** red blood cell units contain leukocytes in a specifically reduced amount. The blood is filtered to make leukoreduced red blood cell units. Leukoreduced red cells are usually effective in preventing certain types of transfusion reactions for most patients.

because of her negative reaction to the recent blood transfusions. We appreciate the fact that she chose to share this information with us directly, and agree that this personal attention is more than likely related to the plasmapherisis issues of several days ago. We continue to be impressed with the "hands on" approach that the various SCCA directors have with their patient, Dani.

Uplifted by both doctors' visits, Dani posts a message on her website for her "fans."

Hi all!

I apologize for the mass message...but, I wanted to write everyone and tell you how I'm doing. First off...if you haven't already heard the transplant ran pretty smoothly. I actually slept through it. I now have strong German blood in my body...and couldn't be prouder. I have also now joined some of my favorite people as the zodiac sign of Aquarius, and have decided to drop my old birthday sign of Cancer! I have had enough of cancer for this lifetime. Liz stated that I was always a closet Aquarius anyhow. Thanks to all who have taken the time to write me through email and/or letters. I still feel so close to all of you by getting mail everyday. I'm also so excited that some of you have planned trips to visit me in Seattle. I look forward to sharing some face time and smiles with you. Now, to catch all of you up on

the latest news. I am now on day 6 (post-transplant). My doctor has told me that I have been doing "strong work," and is really pleased. Now, for the really great news (as if my transplant going well wasn't enough)....Before I left the D.C. area, I entered two of my paintings in a gallery show that is beginning this Saturday, February 15th. They were both accepted and will be displayed at the Khoja gallery in Arlington off of Lee Highway and George Mason Drive for a few weeks. If you get the chance to go and see them...please do it...so, you can tell me how talented I am. :) Anyhow...love you all! I look forward to hearing from you.
Love always,
Dani

2/14 – Day 7

Despite the fact that Dani can release pain killers into her body every seven minutes, she awakens in great pain as the meds are not released while she sleeps. By the time Dr. Stewart arrives on his rounds she is quite "medicated." He tells Dani, "Predictably, this is the toughest part. You've done, knock on wood, very well so far. Your bilirubin has come down and all other parameters are good. Your kidney and liver functions are fine." He looks in her mouth, and continues, "It's looking kind of rough right there, but you sound really good." When Dani reports that she has a tender tummy, no sour taste in her mouth but lots and lots of extra mucus, Dr. Stewart tells Dani to "hang in there," as she will be having visitors this weekend (Jay who left Seattle on Sunday (2/9) will be returning with Liz). He then exchanges videos with us. We lend him "My Big Fat Greek Wedding" and he lends us his very favorite movie, "Moulin Rouge." Before he leaves, he complements Dani on her new haircut (as she is once again bald from the high dose chemo). Dani smiles and nods off.

By mid-day, Corrine informs us that the pain meds will now be released into Dani's body as she sleeps in the evening, through an IV continuous feed. Three more positive events occur by early evening. Jay and Liz both arrive from the East Coast and a massage specialist arrives to give Dani a "gentle massage"! All are greeted with big smiles.

Dani's smile continues when she receives some very special messages in the day's mail, as today is Valentine's Day. Dani, as usual, is delighted to read these messages:

Phoebe, Dani's chocolate lab (and a very gifted dog at that) writes: *To the Scooper...from the Pooper! I miss you – When are you coming home? Can I get a treat? Can I go out? Will you play with me? Isn't it time to eat? Can we go for a walk? I need some water! I'm hungry...I'm thirsty...I'm bored...What's that smell? xxoo*

Dani's former student Ben's mom sends this note: *The day of your transplant, Ben listened to your "Go Ben" voice mail message and said, "Dani get all better today! I go see Dani tomorrow?" He still thinks that you are just up the road and doesn't understand that you are so far away. He listens to your voice message every day and asks for you all the time. Happy Valentine's Day from your biggest and littlest fans!*

Scott has remembered Valentines Day as well, and has created a scrapbook of photographs and messages especially for this day. Each photo has a special meaning for Dani and Scott. The photos span the time that they have been together, from the very first date to the present. Even though he can't be by Dani's bedside on this special day, he makes sure that Dani knows that he is thinking of her every second of every day...and especially today.

2/15 – Day 8
Betty is off today, and her substitute Marc informs Dani that she will have to put up with about one more week of throat sores. But he asserts that, right now, Dani is cruising through post-transplant reactions. That's easy for him to say!

Liz spends the day with Dani. She has brought a special video with her. Knowing that she would be visiting Dani during a pretty rough time, she created a spectacular 30- minute production, where she poses as a street reporter and interviews people on the street about Dani Shotel. These random "people" turn out to be several of Dani's friends and family (i.e., Scott, Carol, Bruce, Sandy etc.). Using only public transportation and her bicycle, Liz has traveled across the D.C. metro area to put together this tender, yet hysterical, composite of well wishes. Dani will watch this video often, reacting with laughter and smiles to its messages. Laughter is indeed the best medicine, as Dani seems to be feeling better.

Later that evening, we begin watching "Moulin Rouge." Fortunately for all of us, Dani falls asleep about 15 minutes into the movie. It doesn't take us much longer to realize the character portrayed by Nicole Kidman has TB, or some similar fatal disease and that she will, in all probability, not make it to the end of the film. We stop the film, rewind it, and wonder what Dr. Stewart was thinking! Dani continues her well-deserved deep sleep as we leave for the evening.

2/16 – Day 9

Dani awakens with yellow eyes. A blood draw reveals an elevated bilirubin of 2.8. This,

Bilirubin: a pigment that is produced from the breakdown of red blood cells.

according to Dr. Stewart, is no big deal, but since this is a function of the liver, her bilirubin will be checked more frequently. The normal bilirubin range is 0.1 to 1.2 milligrams per deciliter (mg/dl). When we are told that the medical personnel anticipate these damaging "bumps in the road" and consider them to be "routine," we can only pray that we never again will have to deal with an unanticipated "bump." He then tells Dani that her body has been "insulted" by the chemotherapy, and this could lead to something called Venal Occlusive Disease (**VOD**), which is chemotherapy-induced liver damage. He also notes that her liver is a bit tender. He adopts a watch-and-see approach to this latest problem. As he says goodbye to Dani he motions me into the hallway.

He tells me that he wants me to put the video "Moulin Rouge" aside, as Nicole Kidman meets with a tragic ending. I smile and tell him what had occurred the previous evening. I then head back into Dani's room, retrieve the video, and return it to a "what was I thinking?" Dr. Stewart. I console him by telling him that it was really a nice gesture, and after all, it's the thought that counts!

The best news of the day comes a bit later on, when Dani decides that it's time that she once again tries an ice pop. The attempt is not successful, however, as she can't swallow without tremendous pain. You can't blame a girl for trying!

2/17 – Day 10

Dani wakes up and immediately summons her nurse Corrine, as she cannot swallow. She also reports that she is constipated, and she has some surface stomach pain. Betty arrives and believes it may be that Dani's bowel is inflamed. She calls for a film of Dani's abdomen, and will recommend that they introduce **Dilaudid** for the pain. She tells Dani that her liver is stressed, but that she is not concerned. Maybe the fact that we are from the East Coast and, by nature, appear more anxious than the general West Coast populace, makes us think that a "stressed liver" should cause some concern! But Betty's low key and confident approach manages to keep us calm, despite the seriousness of these reactions to treatment. She says, "This is what the transplant does. You're in the valley right now, where you should be." She reminds us that during Dani's initial chemo treatments in Arlington, in September, Dani's liver was also "stressed," and says that the same thing is happening this time, but with the high doses of chemotherapy required for a transplant, her liver has to work even harder. She questions Dani to make sure that her fluid output is okay, and when Dani responds in the affirmative, Betty moves on to her other charges, and Dani and I decide to take a walk. As we are doing our "lap" in the hallway, we run into Dr. Stewart. Dani tells him that things are good but she is not sleeping through the night. He tells her that when he continues his rounds and visits with her in her room they'll continue this discussion.

About an hour later, Dr. Stewart arrives by Dani's bedside. He agrees that the Dilaudid is a good idea for Dani's pain, and will also be checking for signs of VOD. Dani reports that she has no pain in her abdomen and she doesn't feel bloated, although she is constipated. She has back pain, is passing gas, and, to add insult to injury, a heavy period returned yesterday. After hearing this, Dr. Stewart agrees to speak with the pharmacist, regarding the benefits of Fentanyl versus Dilaudid. He also mentions to Dani that her liver experienced little dysfunction during her previous chemo treatments, but, to be safe, he agrees to do an ultrasound. Her bilirubin level is now five times normal at 4.9. He tells Dani that VOD, the disease of the liver, occurs with high doses of medicine, such as the chemotherapy she received, and that left alone, the liver, an amazing organ, will heal on its own. Corrine and Dr. Stewart discuss whether the Fentanyl could be contributing to the VOD. Corrine thinks that this generally does not impact the liver. Dr. Stewart then reiterates that the high dose of chemotherapy is causing the liver reaction. It appears as if the agreed upon treatment to keep Dani comfortable, alert, and sane is to gradually introduce Dilaudid. The goal, they both agree, is to get Dani's pain score down to a 2 or 3 out of 5. Presently, Dani reports the pain to be about a 4! Dani tells Dr. Stewart that she feels full all the time. He tells her that they will get some answers after tomorrow's ultrasound. He leaves Dani with what has now become a standard comment, "Strong work, Dani!"

Before Dani receives a platelet transfusion in the afternoon, two positive things occur. First Dani receives Benedryl as a pre-medication for the platelets, which hopefully will prevent an allergic reaction to the transfusion. Secondly, and maybe even more important than the Benedryl, is that Dani consumes her first non-TPN food…she actually eats a banana-flavored Popsicle the normal way—by mouth!

2/18 – Day 11

Day 11 post-transplant begins with a bit of excitement. Dani's blood draw shows a white blood cell count of .20, which suggests an early sign of engraftment. Her white counts had declined steadily since the chemotherapy and today they appear to have begun to recover. Despite the good news, she reports to Dr. Stewart that her pain is at a level of 6 on a 5-point scale, and when her meds kick in the pain is reduced to about a three. She also tells him that her tummy is sore. Dr. Stewart explains that the ultrasound will show whether this is caused by sludge (the byproducts of all that the chemo has destroyed) in the gall bladder or liver damage caused by the chemotherapy.

An hour after the ultrasound, we get our answers. There appears to be sludge in Dani's gall bladder. The test also shows that Dani's spleen is normal in size, her right and left kidneys appear fine, and the flow from the gall bladder looks good as well.

So much for the good news. By 2 p.m. Dani tells Corrine of her swelling feet, numb lips, and that she also feels feverish, nauseous, and dizzy. Corrine readjusts Dani's legs and head on the bed, and informs her that her elevated blood pressure (142/100) is the result of her liver working overtime. She tells Dani that she is "not worried" because right now Dani's body is a bit overloaded. She also advises Dani that blood pressure meds will now be added to her medication regimen.

Within minutes of Corrine's visit, Betty stops by and notifies us that Dani will now be given **Ursodiol** to combat the sludge in her gall bladder. Betty tells us that this drug comes from the bile acid produced by the Chinese Black Bear, and has been used for centuries to fight liver disease. She then comes clean and tells us that the Ursodiol is now man-made, so that no bears had to give up their liver for the medication. She also informs us that Dani being on TPN adds to the sludge. Once on this drug, we are told, the gall bladder should clear up within four days. Betty also feels that Dani's swollen ankles aren't too bad but will dose Dani with a bit of Lasix, which will hopefully reduce the fluid build up in her body. Before she leaves, Betty tells Dani that the except for the fact that her liver is affected (higher than normal bilirubin), her kidneys look great, and everything else is normal.

How right Betty is. Within one hour of Dani receiving a dose of **Amlodipine**, a blood pressure medication, Dani's blood pressure begins to come down.

2/19 – Day 12
A pretty bad night for Dani. She throws up throughout the night and has to be given some **Nubain** for continued pain and itchiness. The morning doesn't bring any relief. She vomits at least five times before we see Betty. Betty believes the nausea will decrease if we can make some adjustments to some of the medications. She further points out that there is probably some liver damage, and because of that, Dr. McDonald, a gastroenterologist, will meet with Dani later on in the day. Despite the nausea and the resulting vomiting, Betty is quite optimistic, as Dani has no fever and does not have VOD…yet!

Throughout the afternoon, Dani remains nauseous and has some stomach pain. A medical intern stops by and tells us what he thinks the pain could be caused by. We decide that we'll wait for the gastroenterologist's opinion. At 5:30 p.m. Dr. MacDonald stops by. He is a most impressive man. He gives us all an excellent explanation of what is happening in Dani's body, an explanation we can all understand. He even draws pictures for us. He puts his hands on Dani's belly, and tells us that there are two possible issues at play here. There is a moderate possibility of VOD. He guesses that Dani's bilirubin is close to as high as it will get (it is now at 8.2!), and that it should begin to head back down on its own over time. We can't quite believe how he can make this statement with such conviction, just by laying his hands on Dani's tummy! The other more likely scenario, he believes, is that Dani has a bit of GvHD of the gut. He reiterates what the oncologists have previously said, that a little GvHD is a good thing, as it shows that Dani's engrafted cells are fighting any cells that they do not recognize, including any remaining leukemic cells or other potential fast-growing cells. Unfortunately GvHD can attack good cells as well, which is why Dani will be on immune suppressant medication and other medications to control the GvHD. A little bit of GvHD is a good thing, but too much is not. Normally GvHD shows up on day 20 post-transplant, but because it appears that Dani's donor cells have engrafted early, the sore tummy could be an early stage of GvHD. He tells us that he'll consult with Dr. Stewart and Betty to decide what the next step will be. We are all comforted by Dr. MacDonald's explanation and predictions and wonder how "on target" he will be.

2/20 – Day 13
Believe it or not, as Dr. McDonald predicted, Dani's bilirubin is down this morning to 7.2 (only seven times what is considered a normal count), Dr. Stewart reports. He smiles, shakes Dani's hand, and gives what is now his standard assessment—"Strong work Dani!"— before he leaves us to continue his morning rounds. Unanimously we decide that Dr. McDonald deserves the "coolest doctor of the week" award.

Later on that morning, Dani is visited by the SCCA nutritionist, who speaks with us about Dani's future diet. She informs us that Dani should gradually try food, but food without fat or fiber…food like ice pops, water, Jello, broth, Gatorade, diluted juices, melon, bananas, canned fruits, pasta with butter, and baked potato. She tells us to be cautious when trying dairy products, as Dani could become lactose intolerant post-transplant. (This bit of information about dairy products could have saved all of us, especially Dani, a lot of anxiety in the months to come if we had remembered it. In October of 2004 Dani developed a cough that continued for almost a year-and-a-half. She consulted with many specialists until, late in 2005, an allergist determined that Dani had developed an infant-like allergic reaction to dairy products). Still later in the day, a discharge planning nurse stops by to confirm her meeting with us on 2/21 at 1:00 p.m. Although Dani doesn't feel quite like kicking up her heels, she delights in hearing the conversation turn to the word "discharge" for the first time.

2/21 – Day 14
As I enter Dani's room, I am greeted by the big news…Dani finally

pooped! This news is shared a few minutes later with Jay and then Dr. Stewart, who appears pleased by this announcement. He tells Dani that she is doing great, as her bilirubin count continues to go down (5.0) and her blood counts continue to increase. When Dani announces that her mouth pain is gone, Dr. Stewart begins to speak about taking Dani off the many pain medications she has been on. This, he says, brings Dani another step closer to leaving the hospital. He tells Dani that her goal this weekend will be to switch over to oral meds and to begin eating… real food and not just ice pops. He discloses that there is a higher rate of GvHD among mismatched transplants, but not to worry as "everything is going in the right direction."

At 1 p.m. the Discharge Planning Nurse stops by to detail Dani's post-discharge routine. She informs us about the "Pump" class we'll both take prior to discharge. This portable IV machine will help us to infuse any intravenous medications and other fluids that Dani requires. She also tells us about a long-term follow-up care class that we'll be taking soon. The nurse then conveys to us that, on our discharge day, we'll meet at the Hutch with the Blue Team, and at that time they'll determine how often they want to see Dani. She hands us a laminated sheet that informs us what conditions signify a medical problem and what to do about them. I then begin to note a list of "To-Dos" for the first two weeks post discharge:

- First week or two…lay low
- Use common sense
- The biggest risk is a virus so wash hands frequently, let someone else open the door, or push the shopping cart
- Wait a couple of weeks before you use the gym
- Wipe counters, and equipment down with antiseptic cloths
- Don't travel more than 30 minutes away
- Keep bathroom exceptionally clean
- Only vacuum the apartment when Dani is out of the room
- As Dani is a candidate for some GvHD of the skin, liver, gut,

or mouth we need to take her temperature twice a day
- Exercise through the fatigue improves long term outcomes

In addition, she tells us that Dani will probably leave the hospital on some immunosuppressant meds. Before she leaves the room, she informs Dani that the following goals must be met prior to her discharge from the transplant wing at the University of Washington Medical Center:

- She must be totally off TPN and eating a bit
- She needs to convert to oral medications
- Nausea needs to be controlled with oral medications
- All vital signs must be stable
- GvHD and diarrhea must be limited

After a quiet afternoon, Dr. McDonald stops by. He reports that Dani's medical condition is not getting any worse. He tells us again how the liver has the primary responsibility for filtering out all of the old blood products from Dani's old bone marrow as well as the massive doses of chemo that were used to rid the body of leukemic cells. "This," he continues, "is hard work for the liver, but the liver is an amazing organ that tends to heal itself when given time, and that is exactly what is beginning to occur." He still has the same thoughts as he had on his first visit on 2/19. He believes that Dani has a bit of GvHD in her tummy, and that this is kind of okay. His only question is whether we want to confirm this diagnosis through a biopsy. He is pretty sure her liver disease is not getting any worse, and that by the nature of her lower bilirubin counts (now at 5.0) it actually appears to be better. He advises Dani to "hang in there," and that "Dr. Stewart and you will have to decide when you've had enough pain." With that mixed message, Dr. MacDonald departs.

We're not sure what happened next, whether it was medication or pain-induced, but shortly after Dr. McDonald leaves, Dani finally has a "meltdown." It probably wouldn't have lasted very long. However, minutes after Dani begins crying, in walk her dad, brother, housemate

Matt, and college bud, Topher. Overwhelmed by everything and anything, Dani sobs for what seems to be an eternity. After having traveled thousands of miles to see their good friend, Dani, both Matt and Topher seem to pretend that her behavior is quite normal, so they pull up two chairs by Dani's bed and make themselves comfortable. Their patience pays off, as within a few moments our girl Dani puts on a happy face and welcomes her guests!

2/22 – Day 15
Dani's vital signs are great today. She also has no fever or rashes. We tell Matt and Topher it's all because of their visit. Even her bilirubin is down to 3.8. Unfortunately she is also having a lot of diarrhea (which her nurse refers to as GvHD diarrhea). There is also the possibility that another infection has entered Dani's body, so once more tests are run on Dani's stool and urine for signs of infection. As the morning progresses into the afternoon, Dani begins her regimen of switching over from IV medications to oral meds. It seems that every fifteen minutes she is taking a pill of one type or another. Matt and Topher offer witty commentary with each pill pop, nurse visit, or bathroom experience. Still later in the day we have an equipment failure that at first shocks, but then becomes new material for their comedy routine. The end of Dani's Groshong Catheter actually falls apart. As Matt and Topher look panic stricken, Micah and I assist Dani in the clean up. The faint of heart need not apply for this job.

Totally exhausted, as she should be, Dani falls asleep. Apparently, all these events have also put a strain on Matt and Topher as well. Jay, Micah, and I steal quietly out of the room to have our dinner, leaving our three sleeping beauties to their dreams.

2/23 – Day 16
It's no surprise to any of us when Dr. Stewart comes into Dani's room gowned once more. Dani has tested positive for C Diff once again, and its reverse isolation time again for the "Friends of Dani." Undeterred

by this inconvenience, Dani continues her visit with her friends and the day turns out to be relatively uneventful, as Dani is entertained by her buddies.

2/24 – Day 17

Matt, Topher, and Jay leave early in the morning to catch their planes back East. In their place Dani's life long and recently married friend, Ally, and my life long friend, Helene, arrive in the afternoon. Since this will be a "Jay is back in D.C." week, the three of us girls plan to camp out at our Seattle home at the Marriott. The two of them are just what the doctor ordered for both Dani and myself, as both are selfless in their love and support (and funny as well).

Unfortunately, Dani is still in substantial pain, is having a hard time eating, and it's difficult for her to enjoy the company of our two dear friends. The doctor thinks that a transfusion of A Positive irradiated leucoreduced platelets will help. He also plans another **endoscopy** to determine the underlying cause of the discomfort.

2/25 – Day 18

Dr. Stewart continues to be positive about the "strong work" ethic of our Dani. On his morning visit he announces that a steroid, prednisone, will be introduced to keep Dani immuno-suppressed, so that her newly developing blood system will not beat up the rest of her body too badly. In essence, it is designed to control (along with the Cyclosporin) the GvHD that now appears to be showing up in her body. He informs us that that this may raise her blood pressure. He also has ordered an increase in the hormone medication she is receiving, to attempt to control her ongoing period. He tells us that this dosage may agitate her, impact her sleep patterns, and affect her mood. We are beginning to feel like Dani is a television commercial for every side-effect the manufacturers have to tell you about when medications are advertised. We're not sure we can take all this good news!

2/26 – Day 19

Every day Dani is in the hospital a blood draw is taken and a two page printout becomes available about nine a.m. The morning begins with a white blood count that has jumped from .5 to 1.25. Although a long way from normal, it reinforces the good news about the initial success of the transplant. There is no question that Dani's new blood system is taking hold, but that along with it will come the possibility of GvHD side effects.

We are told that Dani will begin the prednisone dosage today as part of her treatment protocol. To Dani, this is just another day and another drug, as she has yet to experience the effects of prednisone. Not all transplant patients are placed on steroids, but with GvHD a near certainty at this point, the doctors have no choice. Steroids are often associated with athletes and their attempts to run faster and jump higher. Not so with prednisone. It actually does the opposite. It destroys your muscle tone and changes your physical appearance. It also increases your appetite drastically. It is a mixed bag for sure, but necessary at this point.

Today Dani seems to have a new set of symptoms that are, more than likely, not unrelated to her new blood system engrafting and the accompanying battle being waged for control of her body and its immune system. She has stinging eyes, a swollen tongue, and vivid dreams. She also tells us that she is feeling "a little weird" today. We laugh about this statement and inform Dani that she has always been a little weird. She is not amused, nor is Corrine, her nurse and protector, who doses her with some Benedryl.

Later on in the morning, Dani is visited by an oral surgeon who is monitoring Dani's mouth and gums for signs of GvHD. The doctor notes that Dani's upper gums in the front of her mouth already have a "glossed-over" effect, however subtle. This, she says, is a sign that the tissue is breaking down and healing itself. She also sees a sore beginning to form in the front of Dani's mouth. All this is related to GvHD. When Dani mentions how dry her mouth and lips are, the doctor prescribes a topical steroid cream for Dani's daily use as part of her dental hygiene.

All this and so much more have become the "new normal" of Dani's daily regimen.

Dani decides that she would like some "girl friend" time with Ally. She arranges for Micah to take Helene (with me tagging along) on a sight-seeing tour of Seattle, as the day is quite beautiful. Reluctantly, Helene and I leave Dani's bedside. Later on Dani tells me how special this time with Ally was.

When we return, Ally reports that there is no need to worry…that the blister by Dani's central line (Groshong) is just irritated skin caused by the tape surrounding it, that Dani's steroid treatment will be intravenous for about seven days, and then converted to oral meds, that Dani still has not had a bowel movement (Day 3), and that Dani received platelets today. Ally states this news all so positively in her sweet, little voice, that one might think all this is fabulous news. Her tone almost makes us forget the circumstances that surround our precious Dani.

2/27 – Day 20

With news of another impending snow storm on the East Coast, and all eyes glued to the Weather Channel on Dani's hospital room TV, both Ally and Helene revise their travel plans, so that they can beat the storm home. They cut their visit short and arrive in Philly later on that day. They both call and report that the massive storm that was predicted is just a "dusting" of snow. Both Dani and I feel that this visit by our two best friends was just what the doctor ordered.

Speaking of doctors, the newest member of the Dani fan club, Dr. Stewart, tells Dani, "clinically, you're fine," despite the fact that it's the fourth day without a poop! He advises her to take more naps and eat more, now that she is on the steroid prednisone. He tells her that there will be some side effects resulting from this treatment.

Doctor Stewart then advises us to try Etta's (a seafood restaurant) down by Pike's Place once Dani leaves the hospital. We, as always, appreciate his wise counsel and promise to follow his recommendation.

2/28 – Day 21

Despite the fact that Dani reports to Dr. Stewart that she feels "nauseous in my head," the doctor continues to be pleased with the "strong work" Dani is doing (especially when she notes that she had a bowel movement this morning)! As a result of her positive vital signs, he tells Dani that she is now totally off of TPN and is no longer on blood pressure medication. He reminds Dani that her goal is to transition to oral meds so that she can return to her Seattle home as soon as possible. Dani's white blood count has jumped again to 2.9 approaching the normal of 4.3 to 10.0.

Later on in the afternoon, Dani is visited by the transition nurse, and together they discuss the side-effects of the steroid prednisone. She says that steroid-induced diabetes can occur, and because of that, the staff at the hospital will be monitoring her blood sugar four times a day. Other side-effects include restlessness and sleeplessness, mood swings, and weakness in the muscles of Dani's legs and arms. Because of this muscle-weakening reaction, she advises Dani to work on her cardio exercises. She concludes her visit by assuring Dani that it's possible that within 10 days, the prednisone dosage will begin to be tapered off (a process that may take up to two more months). After she leaves, Dani mentions that she's surprised that the nurse never mentioned "moon face" as a side effect. Prior to Dani's hospitalization, in our first three weeks of visits to the Hutch, this one condition was quite visible in other transplant out-patients. It's the primary side effect that Dani is dreading. Along with one of

> A patient on steroids will tend to put weight on around the face and trunk but lose it from the arms and legs. This gives the characteristic **"moon face"** which is exacerbated by the loss of hair from the chemotherapy. This change of fat distribution simply reflects the normal role of adrenal steroids in controlling the handling of food stores.

the more nasty side-effects of the Cyclosporin, the growth of thick, dark facial hair, Dani is reluctant these days to look in the mirror. Suffice it to say that one's physical appearance after transplant doesn't make one feel any better, even someone with the ego strength of our Dani.

3/1 – Day 22

Dani's weekend is highlighted by the visit of her college roommate, Cat, and her husband, Fitz. Dani has taken great pride in the fact that she is the one who introduced Cat to Fitz during their freshman year together at Lafayette College in Easton, Pennsylvania. Together, the newly married couple has traveled thousands of miles just to spend two very short days with Dani, catching up and discussing the "good old days" between Dani's frequent naps. Later in the evening, they both get to hear the now famous Dr. Stewart pronounce that Dani is living up to the Superman cut-out image that is posted on Dani's hospital room wall.

3/2 – Day 23

Dr. Stewart arrives bright and early this Sunday morning and predicts that Dani will probably be out of the hospital by tomorrow. This is the news that we all have been waiting for! To say the least, we're a bit stunned by the news, as Dani isn't feeling great today. She reports the she feels pressure in her ears when she is standing up and walking. Corrine thinks that, on top of all the other painful reactions to the various treatments, that Dani now has caught a sinus infection.

Cat and Fitz arrive a bit later in the morning, and Dani brightens up and shares the good news with them. Jay, Micah, and I use this time to slip away from the hospital for a couple of hours to plan for Dani's homecoming back to our apartment at the Marriott. The three of us have spoken about surprising Dani to celebrate her discharge in a very special way. In the nearby neighborhood of Fremont, the Seattle version of Haight-Asbury, San Francisco, there is a statue placed in the center of the community. The statue includes five life-sized adults, with one of them holding a baby. The community often embellishes the statue with balloons, ribbons and signs to commemorate various events: birthdays, anniversaries, graduations, etc. We have decided to do just that to rejoice in Dani's new beginning. So, with that goal in mind, the three of us go off on a treasure hunt to find items such as a Supergirl t-shirt, an American flag, a German flag, boas, paper flowers, balloons, poster board, markers, etc. Our plan is to create a scene that includes the three of us, Dani's German donor, Dr. Stewart, and baby Dani. Within a couple of hours, our mission is accomplished, and we return to hospital.

When we return, we discover that Dani's blood pressure is elevated (136/100), she is feeling achy, and is having difficulty breathing. Corrine tells us that the consensus of the Silver Team is that these ailments are the reaction to Dani being weaned off of the pain-killing narcotic Dilaudid. The doctor orders another blood culture along with another urine sample to confirm the diagnosis. The five of us continue to keep Dani company, as this dreary rainy day turns into night. As Cat and Fitz have an early flight back to the East Coast in the morning, the five of us exit the room around 9 p.m. Dani sleepily bids us all a good night, and we wish her the same.

3/3 – Day 24

Unfortunately, it is not a very good night for Dani, and as a result, her night nurse consults with Corrine. They both agree that they will recommend that Dani remain in the hospital at least one more day.

When Dr. Stewart visits, he is glad to hear that Dani's pain from the previous evening has lessened, as she reports "no tender tummy today!" Dr. Stewart thinks that it is possible that the pain meds are causing the cramping pain, so he orders a sustained-release pill. He agrees with the recommendation of the two nurses, not just because of the pain Dani experienced last night, but because once more our girl has tested positive for C-Diff.

The stomach pain reappears at around 4 p.m. Dani also reports that she is nauseous, has joint pain similar to the after-effects of neupogen shots, and has loose bowel movements, as well as cramping. Dr. Stewart remains pretty firm in his opinion that most of this is the body reacting to being tapered off of the intravenous narcotic. None of this opinion is making Dani feel any better.

When she finally falls asleep shortly after 8 p.m. (we think for the night), Jay and I leave the hospital and return to the Marriott to do Dani's laundry. Imagine our surprise, when the phone rings in our apartment at about 8:45 p.m., and it's Dani on the line crying, "WHERE ARE YOU?" Quickly, we change our plans, get back in the car, and return to UW Hospital. Within 15 minutes of the phone call, Jay drops me off at the hospital and returns to the laundry that awaits him at the Marriott, while I head up to Dani's room to provide some additional comfort to our daughter. I'm back in the room by 9, a record-breaking time, even for our "Indy 500" Jay! Dani tells me that when she awoke and found us gone, she got scared. We have known for these past few months that even with anti-anxiety meds, Dani experiences her most terror-filled moments in the late evening. For the past month, Dani has dealt with this by talking with her night nurse. This evening…that was not to be "the fix." I remain by Dani's side until about 11:15 that evening, when she assures me that she is fine now and that I can leave. She then nods off into what I hope will be a peaceful sleep.

3/4 – Day 25

When Dr. Stewart arrives this morning, we ask him why, for the past three days, Dani has had pain at approximately the same time (4 p.m.) and why she is experiencing such severe joint pain. His best guesses are that the pain is a result a combination of the pain meds taper and the C-Diff infection. He also believes that the joint pain can possibly be Cyclosporine-related, along with the reaction to the growth of Dani's new white blood cells that is taking place in her bone marrow. He tells us that he will consult with Dr. MacDonald (Dani's magical gastroenterologist) as to whether the pain is C-Diff-related, GvHD, or a combination of both. As he leaves, he tells me that the team continues to be extra-cautious with Dani in light of the pre-transplant events (although by this time we are all convinced that this special attention to detail is given to all its' patients, and that it is exactly this care that makes the Seattle Cancer Care Alliance the world's foremost blood-related cancer treatment facility).

3/5 – **Day 26**

When Dr. Stewart arrives this morning, he informs us that Dani will have an endoscope today to determine once and for all what is causing this persistent infection (GvHD or C-Diff). As he leaves, Corrine marches into the room and hands me not one but two enema kits, and informs Dani that before she has her Lower G-I scoped, she needs to give herself two enemas! Dani and I are just about speechless by this announcement, and we plead utter ineptitude in implementing this task. Together, we convince Corrine to show us how it is done. She does, and then Dani and I (at this point we're beyond being grossed-out) are successful with the second. Together we hope that this is one mother-daughter experience we pray never to share ever again!

The endoscope test finds nothing major besides a bit of GvHD of the stomach, so the plans proceed for a 3/6 departure for our Seattle home at the Lake Union Marriott Residence Inn.

Despite this great news, normal vital signs, and abating stomach pain, our girl is quite weepy, when she breaks the good news to Scott (who is back on the East Coast). We attribute this weepiness to any of several reasons, which include, but are not limited to: sheer joy, drugs, home-sickness, missing Scott, and/or the fear of leaving the safe haven of the hospital where her every need has been attended to.

Later on in the afternoon, Dani is visited by a health care supervisor from Providence (out-patient) Medical Services. She instructs the two of us in the proper operation of the portable IV pump, and shows us how to fill out order forms for the many varied medical supplies that Dani will need once she is out of the hospital. Although Dani has confidence in my abilities, I am a bit anxious about having to accept complete responsibility for the dispensing of Dani's medications and operating any necessary equipment. And, as of March 6th, Dani's day-to-day healthcare would be in my hands…and quite frankly those two hands were shaking at the thought! It was now Dani's turn to convince me that we would do just fine! After all, the Hutch was just up the block from our apartment, and specialists would be available to us 24/7; and in addition, both Dani and

Micah had survived my mothering skills for many years. Still it was quite over-powering knowing that it would be up to me to insure that every pill (of the 60 or so daily) had to be dispensed at the exact time; that I had to make sure that all of the medical equipment, supplies, and living space be kept clean; that Dani drinks, exercises, sleeps, and eats properly; that she arrives to each medical appointment on time; and, finally, that a positive environment surrounds Dani at all times. Dani is quite good at convincing me that she has complete confidence in me and knows that I can do it!

3/6 - Day 27

This is it! Today is the day! Dr. Stewart announces, as he enters Dani's hospital room one last time, "We're on the launching pad. Go for it!" With that said, he departs. As Dani prepares for her exit from the University of Washington Medical Center, she is visited one last time by the transition nurse, who warns us not to put the Cyclosporin in the pill box, and not to take it prior to the blood draw (but after the blood draw), so that they can get an accurate level of the amount of medication in her body. Dani, Jay, and I tuck this last bit of information into our already overloaded medical information base. We thank her for her support. We share one final moment with Corrine and then give her a hand-made afghan, lots of hugs, and words of thanks as we leave the seventh floor oncology wing. We are excited and frightened at the same time.

Micah pulls the car up to the front of the hospital and the three of us carefully tuck Dani into the back seat, and begin the next chapter of our "family adventure"…the healing.

As we head back to the hotel, Jay tells Dani that we need to make a stop. Rather than continuing down Eastlake Avenue toward the hotel, we make a right turn at Lake Union and drive towards Freemont, following the North side of the lake. We stop in front of what is known as "Waiting for the Interurban" or the "Freemont People." The decorating of the statues of the five adults and the child was completed by Micah and Jay before they came to the hospital this morning, and Dani reacts with tears of joy, release and relief. The concrete people that folks decorate for weddings, birthdays, and anniversaries have now been lovingly prepared for Dani. It is a special moment for all of us, as they announce that Dani has indeed done strong work!

Dani's Memory

There is something that will be difficult for anybody to understand who has never been locked inside for a month. When you are kept inside breathing air that has been re-circulated and sterilized over and over again...when you see the outside only as an additional photo hung on your wall through a window...when you get accustomed to being in a bed while friends and

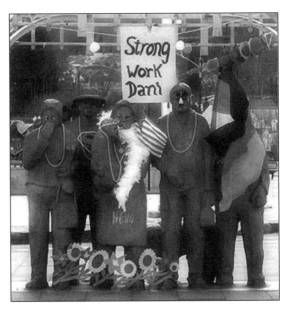

The statues in Freemont dress up to welcome Dani home from the hospital!

families visit you...you somehow forget what it is like to take a step outside, to breathe in fresh/polluted air, to walk inside and outside as you please. When one is released from a hospital, you take nothing for granted. The day I was released from the hospital after my transplant, I took nothing for granted. I took a step outside and saw my father pulling up in his rental car. I don't remember what the car was, what the view was, only the feeling of freedom rushing through my blood. It was exhilarating. I quickly jumped (well it felt like I had jumped) into the car, fastened my seatbelt and pressed my face up to the car window. It was like I was a 3-year-old, taking in everything, so nothing would be forgotten or unseen. I remember talking, and talking. I was so excited about everything I was going to do now that I was out of the hospital. All of a sudden it felt like I got the wind knocked out of me. I couldn't speak. I could only cry. We pulled up to my favorite Seattle landmark. In the town of Freemont, there is a statue. It is one of the more bizarre statues that you will ever see. It is a life-size statue of random people. The individuals in the statue are always decorated by local Seattleites wishing someone a "Happy Birthday" or a "Congratulations" type message. We pulled up to this landmark. The figures of the statue are holding quite an original statement...but, one that I have been hearing daily from my favorite Seattle doctor, Dr. Mark Stewart. The sign said, "Strong Work Dani!" Each figure was decorated with something that directly related to me, my loved ones, or to my treatment: I always wear pearl earrings as I admire the beauty and simplicity of them; the boas somehow represented my flashy side, which I believe I inherited from my Philly Mom-mom; of course the German flag represented my donor; and the infant wearing the Superwoman tee-shirt is me with my new life. My father and brother had decorated these statues earlier that day, only to have me ride by it upon my release. I think I cried the whole way home...it was a good kind of cry.

Chapter Twelve
Out and About

Thirty-plus days of Dani's stay at the University of Washington Medical Center has finally come to an end. Now she can begin the next round of her courageous battle in the comfort of her home away from home, our apartment at the Marriott. At this point in time, Dani's return to "normalcy" begins in earnest.

My job has changed a bit, from the public school administrator and the expert multi-tasker, to a singularly-focused primary caregiver. Jay, already the experienced commuter, flies United like it was the Washington Metro (a routine of eight-and-a-half full days with us and five-and-a-half days back on the East Coast). Not too organized by nature, he somehow manages to combine his work, communication efforts, and detailed research, while providing comfort to his family at all times! Scott hangs in there as Dani's guy. He telecommutes from Seattle and works at the Renton branch office when he can. He, too, manages to combine work with care. When on the east coast, he speaks to Dani several times each day, and keeps her informed of the news from her friends. He also holds another sold-out Wizards Basketball Game fundraiser, attends others, and plans for future fundraising events. Brother Micah seems to have a magical way about him, as he somehow manages to show up for dinner every night just as we are about to sit down to eat (without even calling and asking when dinner will be)! He often brings a friend or two along and keeps Dani and myself attached to the world outside. Even though Jay and I have been "empty-nesters" for over 4 years, being together in Seattle almost seems like "the good old days" when the kids were growing up…only this time the experience is a bit more intense!

Dani and I become devoted fans of morning television, as we schedule Dani's a.m. blood draws and other appointments, so as not to interfere with Regis and Kelly. We all try to live "normal lives." We have weekly "American Idol," and "24" gatherings. We watch television and see the Iraq War unfold before our eyes. Dani devotes herself to daily exercises so that she can walk with her head held high. She works on focusing, but has trouble reading more than 10 pages of a novel or magazine at one sitting. The Cyclosporin causes some shaking in her hands, so she decides to work on controlling the shakes by taking on a knitting project. She has also made a pledge to herself that she will always take extreme care in her grooming and dress despite how terrible she feels or how long it takes to accomplish. Sitting in the waiting rooms at the Hutch, she has seen way too many sick people, and has decided not to be one of them! Our daily routine is pretty normal — doing lots of food shopping, reading e-mail, talking on the phone, exercising, and watching TV, except that it also includes taking lots and lots of medications…four sometimes fives times a day, having intravenous fluids run through Dani's body, courtesy of our mutual efforts to operate the portable IV pump, cleaning the Groshong Catheter, preparing and eating extra large meals for Dani's enormous steroid-enhanced appetite, and together taking daily expeditions up and down the hill to the Hutch. Our family's devotion to one another has never been as strong! We all settle in…and make the most of it.

3/6 – Day 27

We come home to our apartment at the Marriott, have a quick lunch, and head up the hill for our initial post-transplant appointments at the Hutch. The hill is a lot steeper than Dani remembers it to be, but she makes it just fine. We meet with the nutritionist, Kerry, and learn details about what Dani should and should not eat. Dani has her vitals taken and she has lost some weight. Kerry does not appear concerned as she suspects that her appetite will increase with the prednisone. Later on in the afternoon, we meet with our Blue

Team's physician's assistant and nurse. They both comment on how great our girl, Dani, looks and that her blood counts are now at or near normal levels. They remind us that Dani needs to take Ativan prior to getting "hooked up" with the IV pump. We make note of that.

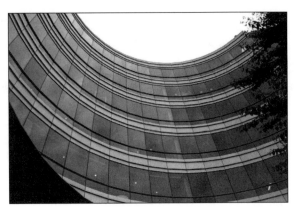

The view of the Hutch from the hill

That evening Jay posts an announcement on the website that folks have been anticipating…that "Dani's finally out!" He explains that Dani took a few extra days to transition from IV meds to tablets. He thanks people for their best wishes and prayers and says that whatever they're doing on Dani's behalf should be continued, as it seems to be working! With their support, and some from the doctors in Seattle, he writes that hopefully our girl will return to the East Coast by mid-May.

After dinner, I excuse myself and go to Dani's bathroom, which has also become our pharmacy and medical supply repository. Prior to the transplant, we were presented with a pill box—and not your ordinary single container pill box. This "Cadillac" of pill containers was about 8 inches in length and a foot wide. It contained seven removable plastic containers each with five closable compartments. Each row was labeled with the days of the week, and each compartment was labeled with a time of the day (i.e., a.m., mid-morning, noon, etc.). So my job each night is to look over Dani's most recent medicine list dispensed weekly by the Blue Team and place the exact number and dosage of pills, which included a variety of steroid, pain, nausea, anxiety, preventative meds, etc. The only meds that weren't included in my assignment were the Cyclosporin (which needed to be kept separately, away from other drugs) and the **Premarin** patch (a birth control medication used to stop Dani's monthly flow while she was immuno-suppressed), which Dani replaces weekly on a spot on her lower abdomen. I check and double check this list and the pill count. Quite frankly, this is the task that makes me most nervous. I really don't want to be responsible for any medical mistakes. I continue this process every night for the next two months, and I never lose that nervousness.

Before we go to bed that evening, Dani and I set our respective clocks for 5:15 a.m., in order to begin the intravenous saline solution. This will be our first time using the portable IV pump. At this time, we also remove the IV bag from the refrigerator so that its liquid contents can be at room temperature when it enters Dani's body the next morning.

3/7 – Day 28

Dani and I both get out of bed before our mutual alarms go off and rendezvous to make preparations for our first mom and daughter attempt at infusing a saline solution through Dani's Groshong Catheter using the portable IV pump. We quietly assemble all the equipment in Dani's bathroom (Jay is still sleeping) and begin the task. We're both pretty nervous about this…and with good reason, because after several attempts at following the directions, the only thing I accomplish is breaking a piece of equipment that attaches the bag of magnesium-infused saline to Dani's Groshong Catheter! A bit panicked, I call the 24-hour medical service line for help, only to find out that the lesson we had received (and the directions we had followed) on operating this IV pump was for connecting the pump to a "Hickman" Catheter (Dr. Hickman is a member of the SCCA staff) and not a Groshong Catheter (which is much more common on the East Coast). The out-patient medical supply company was unable to provide us with the necessary connector, but we are told that the Hutch pharmacy would make the necessary supplies available to us later on in the afternoon. I am told not to worry, that Dani would be okay; she should continue to drink lots of fluids, and that I can pick up the supplies at 4 p.m. this afternoon. Our initial panic is relieved a bit. Jay continues to sleep through this mini crisis, as Dani and I attempt to do the same.

Later on in the day, Dani's friend Yvonne arrives. She will be staying with us for the weekend. Dani is very excited about this visit. Yvonne is just what the doctor ordered for Dani. Together, the two of them will have some "girl time"! However, she arrives with the sole purpose of helping all of us out, and that doesn't just mean Dani! The first thing she does is volunteer to head up the hill on her own to the Hutch pharmacy to receive the correct new supplies for connecting the pump to Dani's catheter. We're all pretty impressed with Yvonne's willingness to help and "can do it" attitude. It also doesn't hurt that Yvonne is also a physical therapist. When she returns with the necessary supplies, Dani, Yvonne and I huddle in the bathroom and manage to get the saline solution pumping into Dani's body. Hooray!! For the record, for as long as Dani uses this portable pump, I am reduced in rank, to that of Dani's assistant. My job now is to get the saline out of the refrigerator so that it gets to room temperature, make sure the bathroom area where we are working is clean, set up the supplies, and squeeze any air out of the saline solution bag. Dani completes the more serious task of connecting the IV line to her own catheter.

Our good friends Bonnie and Steve arrive this afternoon as well, and also plan to provide a brief respite and lots of comfort to Jay and me. They even manage to rent a room at our Marriott very close to our own apartment. This visit is perfect. For the first time in a longtime, we give Dani some time to spend independently with Yvonne, while we spend time just being carefree, even if it is for only a few hours each day. The seven of us (Micah arrives just in time for dinner, naturally) have a celebratory dinner, which includes some incredibly fresh Alaskan King Salmon.

3/8 – Day 29

The day begins with an uplifting e-mail from a good friend:

A couple with whom we are friendly went to one of the Marrow Drives for Dani after I forwarded them your email. A few weeks later, he was contacted that he was a potential match, not for Dani, but for a woman in Chicago. It turns out that after much testing and further evaluation, he is indeed a match for this woman (who is 45 and has leukemia). She will get the transplant in the next week or so. I thought you might want to know that your e-mail, in large part, probably helped to save someone's life.

What a great way to begin the day.

3/9 – Day 30

We spend a pretty quiet weekend with our respective friends. Jay and Yvonne head back East by mid-day on Sunday, while Bonnie and Steve remain until Monday morning. In the late afternoon, after Dani has her second dose of prednisone and becomes dizzy. I call the 24/7 Hutch help line and I am advised that Dani should drink more fluids and have .5 liter more of the saline solution. As if by magic, the dizziness abates.

3/10 – Day 31

It's Monday morning. Dani and I rise bright and early (she holds off on taking the Cyclosporin until after her blood draw, as directed by the team) and head up the hill to the Hutch for the blood draw. She is greeted by the receptionist today, and every day, with a big smile. We hardly wait a minute before one of the technicians collects her from the waiting area. There are several of these technicians and each one is more upbeat than the next. She is welcomed back to their little world in the rear of the suite. Dani enters the lab smiling and chatting amiably with the tech. While I wait for Dani, I begin to notice the other arriving, departing, or waiting out-patients in this reception area. A few are wheeled into the area; several walk in very, very slowly; many have a grayish hue to their skin; some arrive in their pajamas, and, no one is smiling. To me this only reinforces the strength of Dani's resolve not to give in to either the illness or the resulting treatments.

After the blood draw, Dani and I head upstairs for her series of appointments with the Blue Team. Our first stop is with Kerry, the nutritionist. From the moment she met Kerry, Dani felt an instant camaraderie. Her advice to Dani is sound, and when she tells Dani what she should be eating, I write it down as part of my shopping list. Kerry advises Dani to drink milk, make nuts, eggs, tuna, and salmon a part

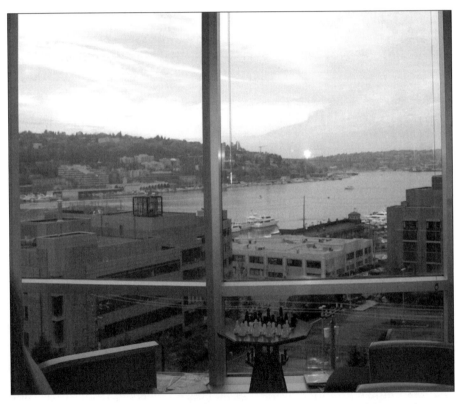

The view of Lake Union is a relaxing site from the sixth floor of the Hutch as we wait for Dani's appointments with the "Blue Team"

of her regular diet, take one Viactive calcium chew a day, and drink 48 ounces of water in addition to the bag of saline each day.

Later on in the day, we meet with the members of the Blue Team. Our new monthly attending physician has changed to Dr. Fred Appelbaum, Director of Clinical Research. I remember that he was my first contact with the Hutch in early October 2002. My opinion of him quickly formed then as a warm, friendly, caring, confident, and extremely competent physician. Back in October, he told me that Dani was the perfect candidate for a bone marrow transplant, and that it would take about three months to find a donor for her. My initial impression of Dr. Appelbaum stands. He "kibitzes" with Dani about his friendship with one of Dani's Arlington oncologists, Dr. Meister (as children, they grew up on the same block), and his love for baseball. Dani immediately is taken by this connection, as she begins to tell him about herself and her days as a fast-pitch softball pitcher. After a few chatty moments, the two of them get down to business. Dani reports that the hefty Premarin dose has kept her from bleeding; but she isn't sleeping well, is quite restless through the night, often waking up in a cold sweat. He tells her to take two Ativan (anti-anxiety) and no Ambien (sleeping) medications at night. Dr. Appelbaum reports that some blasts were noted on the a.m. blood draw but there were none by the afternoon draw. He believes that this is caused by the Cyclosporin and that they might be good blasts. He tells Dani that she is having "very vigorous" engraftment, and when that happens "we sometimes see blasts in the peripheral blood." He tells us not to worry about this, as we'll know better when Dani has another bone marrow aspirate…tomorrow. Not to worry…bone marrow aspirate…who's he kidding? He also lets us know that Dani's bilirubin count is better, and that probably by the end of the week they'll begin to taper Dani off of steroids. He explains to Dani that some effects of prednisone include hyperactivity, emotionality, and increased appetite. We both nod, because Dani appears to be the textbook case on side effects of prednisone.

After having answered all of our questions, we say goodbye to Dr. Appelbaum and the other members of the Blue team who have crowded into the examination room. Dani and I walk the few blocks down the hill and return by mid afternoon to our apartment at the Marriott.

3/11 – Day 32

We return to the Hutch early this morning for the dreaded bone marrow aspirate. Already forewarned of Dani's prior experiences with these draws, Dani is assigned two techs rather than one for the procedure. Diane, our Blue Team nurse, frankly tells Dani, as she walks to the room where the aspirate will be drawn, "Nothing's a cakewalk!" Somehow this doesn't ease Dani's nerves, but the shot of Fentanyl given to her before the procedure begins certainly does! Dani has me be with her during this procedure. I continue to be amazed by her strength (Fentanyl or no Fentanyl)! I believe they took at least two specimens of bone marrow. Both techs report to us that they got a very good specimen. We're both glad to hear this, as there is no way Dani would repeat this procedure again today! We're told that Dani should remain in the room and rest a while before we leave the Hutch. The techs then tell us some extremely important information; they tell us where a secret stash of snacks is located. We are delighted to have this new information as the prednisone has increased Dani's appetite 10-fold. Before we head back down the hill and return to our apartment, Dani ingests two packets of Lorna Doone cookies, one container of cranberry juice, and 10 ounces of hot cocoa. A half hour has lapsed since the medical procedure and Dani says she's feeling fine. We leave the Hutch and head for the Marriott, but instead of going to our apartment, we opt for a change of venue and read magazines in comfy chairs by a fireplace in the Marriott's lobby. Dani reports some discomfort from the aspirate, but nothing she can't handle at this point.

3/13 – Day 34
We return to the Hutch for Dani's blood draw and a meeting with the Blue Team. Dr. Appelbaum reports with a smile that Dani has some hyperactive marrow, and that new young blood cells are forming rapidly, thus causing some joint pain.

Dani shows Dr. Appelbaum some sores that have developed around and under the medicinal tape that holds the Groshong Catheter tubing in place. Dr. Appelbaum continues to reassure Dani that all this is contact dermatitis, and, again, she should just treat it with some medicinal salve and it will go away. He explains that her skin has become extremely sensitive as a result of the treatments she has received. Confident that this new reaction is "no biggie," Dani says goodbye to Dr. Appelbaum and the rest of the Blue Team.

3/14 – Day 35

Dani continues to do well. Her blood counts are essentially normal and her new marrow seems to be having a good time in her body. Dani likes to brag that Doctor Appelbaum called her new marrow "exuberant to match her personality"! Today is an exciting one for both of us. Laurie Alderman and Lena (Dani's teaching assistant from Reed) and my buddy, Sandy D., are visiting the two of us. In preparation for their visit, a bundled-up Dani actually does a little food shopping with me today. We are very careful of germs, and we never leave home without our supply of Clorox Wipes and Purell Hand Sanitizer! After we complete our shopping, we head back to our apartment (our transportation to and from the food market is provided by a Marriott shuttle bus). Dani and I are very excited about the visitors coming to our humble abode! We can't wait!

When Laurie and Lena finally arrive, they drag a large cardboard box into our apartment, which contains a very special delivery. The teachers at Dani's current school, Walter Reed Elementary School in Arlington, Virginia, intuitively sense that Dani needs a little bit of extra sunshine to brighten up her days. So they have students create "get well" cards for Dani. Even the "Peeps," Dani's class of 2- and 3-year-old special-needs pre-schoolers under the careful guidance of their teacher, Miss Irene, make a "welcome home, Miss Dani" wall-hanging for Dani. Dani is delighted to be surrounded once more by her colleagues and students' best wishes.

While Laurie and Lena regale Dani with school news, Sandy D. arrives. Sandy is spending the night with Dani and me before heading off to her cousins' tomorrow night. Laurie and Lena have rented a room in the hotel for the weekend. After Laurie and Lena leave, we have the cot for Sandy delivered. We all become hysterical with laughter just trying to figure out how this cot unfolds. Weak with laughter, we are about to give up, when miraculously the cot just pops open. As Dani finishes up her evening meds, the three of us come to the agreement that "laughter still is the best medicine."

3/15 – Day 36

Today is a big day for Dani. The Blue Team has agreed that if the weather is nice, they see no reason why Dani can't be outdoors. She is told to take it easy and not to over- exert herself. Bearing this advice in mind, Dani makes reservations for Laurie, Lena, and herself to have lunch out, and then take a fun-filled 90 minute tour of the city on an amphibious World War II vehicle called the "Seattle Duck Tour." It is a glorious Seattle day (sunny and 50 degrees) and Dani had a great time being out. She takes it real slow and steady, sits all bundled up on the vehicle between Laurie and Lena, and does just what the doctors have ordered; Dani stays away from crowds, sick people and little kids, and has her Purell handy!

Meanwhile, Sandy and I spend time together, dining at one of Dr. Stewart's favorite restaurants, Etta's, and shopping at one of my favorite Seattle boutiques. Later on in the afternoon, Dani, Sandy, and I rendezvous back at the apartment. Jay has also arrived for his next eight-and-a-half-day stint. Lena and Laurie have made other plans for the night (we think it involves a casino), so it's just the four of us for the evening. An exhausted Dani regales us with her afternoon adventures. As Jay, Sandy, and I sit listening to our girl, we notice that Dani's face is beginning to swell right before our eyes. The much dreaded and steroid-induced "moon face" has finally arrived. None of us mention it to Dani…she will notice it soon enough!

3/16 – Day 37

Dani, Micah, Jay, Sandy, and I spend the afternoon together wig shopping. It is a horrible experience for all of us, but is especially depressing for Dani. The very accurately titled "moon face" has totally transformed her beautiful, petite face. The good news is that Dani continues to have the inner strength to see beyond this "bump in the road." She teaches us all a lesson by accepting a "this too shall pass" attitude.

3/17 – Day 38

We begin our weekly routine by saying goodbye to Sandy and then heading up the hill for the early morning blood draw at the Hutch. This is followed by a meeting with Kerry, Dani's nutritionist. Kerry tells us that the prednisone increases activity, so that it now makes sense that Dani's appetite has increased. She tells us that Dani needs to have more phosphates (like nuts, eggs, and meats), as well as potassium (as found in oranges, V-8, potatoes, nuts, spinach, avocado, bananas, and apricots, to name a few foods). Kerry is pleased that Dani is tolerating foods. At this point, Dani is everything a mother could ask for. The daughter that never finished a meal is now eating everything that is placed in front of her.

Our next appointment is Dani's clinic visit with the Blue Team. Diane reports to Dani that not only are her vital signs great, but that her bilirubin is now normal! We are thrilled. Dani reports that she was able to stay focused and read a book for 15 minutes last night, and the team agrees that this is pretty "cool."

3/18 to 3/20 – Days 39 to 41

The routine continues. Blood draw and appointments with the Blue Team three times a week. Dani has other appointments scheduled as well: gynecologist, pulmonary specialist, dentist, nutritionist, etc. We plan our daily schedule around our weekly Hutch appointments. Besides these appointments, Dani and I head to the exercise room of the Marriott every morning, where Dani uses the stationary bicycle and the treadmill. Before she uses any piece of equipment, I wipe it down with a Clorox Wipe. We really do practice what has been preached to us about making sure Dani's physical environment is a good one. Meals are a big deal now, more than ever before. Dani's favorite lunch (which becomes Scott's favorite as well) is homemade tomato soup with cheese quesadillas. If we're not at the Hutch in the afternoons, we plan an activity like walking or food shopping. We even begin to take advantage of the

Marriott's shuttle bus service when Jay's not around, to visit museums or just shop. But the important thing is that we have settled in. It's not easy going but we try our very best to make it a pleasant time.

Dani's nights are the worst. The anxieties that she felt after her diagnosis in the fall have not gone away. In fact, her nightmares have gotten so intense that she begins to write them down. She actually wakes herself up and forces herself to write of sea-filled canoes, being soaked in what she thought was water but turns out to be blood, being hurt, falling onto a group of chocolate Labrador puppies, being in the hospital, having difficulty reading out loud, going to a bad party, and other nightmarish events. It's a good thing that the Marriott leaves a note pad and pen by each bed. In the morning, we both try to make some sense out of these dreams. Because of these nightmares, and lots of joint pain that seems to be the most severe at night, Dani and I decide to keep our cell phones on our respective night stands when we go to bed at night. Even though our bedrooms are right next to each other, and the fact that I have become quite the light sleeper, I have missed hearing Dani's sweet quiet voice calling for me. Now if Dani needs me, all she has to do is call my cell phone. Modern technology is amazing!

Despite these nightmares and the weakness and continuous joint pain, the Blue Team is pleased with the progress Dani is making. In fact, on our Thursday clinic visit, Dani's doctor said that she is doing "spectacularly." We suppose that compared to others going through the same thing she is doing quite well.

3/21 – Day 42

Dani manages to pedal for 9 miles on the stationary bicycle in the Marriott's exercise room (she has been picking up one mile a day). She's having a good day despite the constant cold drizzle and dark grey skies. So we decide in the afternoon to make a short visit to the Seattle Aquarium. Micah joins us and points out the many varieties of starfish found on the northern Pacific coast. We all enjoy this new adventure and return to our apartment to prepare for a special dinner. The Sisterhood from our synagogue in Gaithersburg, Maryland, Temple Beth Ami, has ordered for our family a Shabbat (Sabbath) dinner. It is delicious. We feast on the traditional challah, matzah ball soup, sweet noodle kugel, roasted chicken and all its trimmings, and a wonderful dessert. They enclose a note wishing us a peaceful Sabbath and a "complete and speedy recovery" for Dani. We are so pleased by this act of kindness.

3/22 – 3/23 – Days 43 and 44
My cell phone rings very early this morning. It is Dani calling from the next room. Her voice is weak and I can hardly hear her. Without waking Jay, I go to Dani's bedroom. She is crying as she tells me of her joint pain in her legs. The pain is so intense that she can't even cover her legs with a sheet or a blanket. We call the 24/7 Fred Hutch emergency number. We are advised to continuously dose Dani with Oxycontin and to use **Oxycodone** for the breakthrough pain as needed. We try using the heating pads like we did when Dani experienced joint pain after receiving her neupogen shots as part of her consolidation chemo protocol, but Dani is unable to have the weight of the heating pad on her knees and ankles. We eventually place the pad underneath her knees and alternate this with her ankles as well. Between the drugs and the heat, Dani experiences some relief, but the next two days seem to test her resolve. After several calls to our Blue Team help line, we find out that Dani might be overdoing it a bit (like the nine mile stationary bike ride that she took on Friday), as her white blood cells have decided to migrate to her knees causing some pretty significant pain. We are comforted a bit to learn that this pain is indeed part of the consequences of recovery. In addition to this, it seems that the tapering of the steroids will cause her muscles to become easily inflamed as well. Dani spends the weekend in bed, only daring to go outside of her bedroom with either Jay or myself assisting her.

3/24 – Day 45
The pain continues through the night. Dani is up early for her walk up

the hill for the routine blood draw and appointment with the Blue Team. We have written down questions to ask Dr. Appelbaum regarding Dani's joint pain. He seems puzzled by the fact that the pain is worse at night. He concurs with the decision and dosage recommended for the pain killers. He thinks that the pain could be caused by a variety of factors, including the steroids, Dani's over-activity, the Cyclosporin dose, Dani's hyperactive bone marrow, or even just plain movement. He also decides that the time is right for Dani to begin physical therapy, to restore her muscle tone that has been destroyed by a combination of chemotherapy treatments and the steroid prednisone. Dani will meet with the physical therapist on Thursday for an evaluation.

The visit with the Blue Team (aided by the diminishing joint pain) has restored Dani's spirit. We make our weekly plan to go to a yarn shop (Dani thinks that a knitting project will help her control the hand-shaking caused by the Cyclosporin), go food shopping, see a movie, write a few thank-you notes, and visit Seattle's art museum, to see a special exhibit of the paintings of one of Dani's favorite artists, Jacob Lawrence. We both look forward to the week ahead.

3/27 – Day 48

Dani meets Andréa, the physical therapist. Andréa appears to be Dani's age and has long, flaming, curly red hair. She greets us warmly as she confesses that Dani is only her fifth patient. As she writes down a bit of Dani's health history, she also informs us that she teaches at Micah's alma mater, the University of Puget Sound. Dani and Andréa instantly connect. Dani reports to Andréa that she has severe muscular weakness, walks slowly, feels that she is often off balance and is at risk of falling, has pain in both knees, has trouble getting off of the toilet and in and out of the Marriott shuttle van, and is currently using a chair in the shower. Dani tells Andréa that she wants to regain her strength, and is willing to follow Andréa's exercise plan exactly to accomplish this goal. Andréa concurs with the doctors and explains that the steroids have, indeed, weakened Dani's hips, knees, and ankles, and also have caused some atrophy of Dani's quadricep muscles. Pleased with Dani's commitment, she warns Dani that if her blood platelet count drops to below 20,000, her exercise should be limited to walking; and if it drops below 10,000, she is to discontinue exercising completely. Andréa sets a few short-term goals, including taking one flight of stairs without the use of the railing and without the subsequent knee pain. She advises Dani to always take the stairs to our apartment as a form of exercise (it's a good thing that we're on the second floor)! For the long-term, Andréa is looking forward to Dani completing cardiovascular exercises three times a week, walking up and down two flights of stairs without the use of the railing or knee pain, and that her fatigue rating will decline to a 1 or less out of a possible 10. Andréa suggests that Dani begin to wear hospital stockings during the day to reduce leg and ankle swelling, and instructs her on how to walk up and down the stairs. Ever "coachable," Dani agrees to follow every bit of Andréa's advice, even when it comes to wearing those unfashionable thigh-high hospital hose. We leave Andréa feeling very positive. Andréa agrees to see Dani initially three times a week. Dani can't wait to begin Andréa's prescribed exercises.

After our meeting with Andréa, we meet with the Blue Team. Doctor Appelbaum tells us both that Dani is "doing great!" We speak about reducing IV hydration, continuing the IV magnesium intake, and whether or not the patch or the pill is more effective in controlling Dani's period. We celebrate with the news that Dani's creatinin level is now normal and that she can now discontinue taking the drug Ursodiol. On our way out of the SCCA, we pick up a flyer for a special program planned for April 7th from 3 to 5 p.m. The program is entitled, "Look Good, Feel Better." We decide to put that event on our calendar as well. Walking down the hill after the appointments, Dani and I agree that today has been a pretty good day.

3/29 – Day 50
Dani writes a note on her website:

Hello all! I'm so sorry that I have not been in touch! Everyone has been so great about keeping me informed, sending me wonderful letters, emails and packages. I wanted to let you know how thankful I am for all of you. So...let me get you all updated. The past week has been a little more difficult than previous weeks (but in a very different way). I ended up having some complications with joint pain due to over-hydration, steroids (that actually decrease muscle mass), and over-working out last week. But...have no fear...I now have my very own physical therapist that I will be consulting with 3 times this week, they have decreased my hydration, and I have begun a slow-but-steady taper off the steroids. My dad is arriving here in about an hour...and Scott is getting here later this evening. I am hoping for a great week with all my visitors. Scott and I have our first official day date (in a very long time planned for tomorrow/Sunday). We are going to the Hyatt for brunch tomorrow morning (12:00)...and then are going to see the movie, Chicago. *I am really looking forward to it. My mom and I have been getting along fabulously. She may be up for an award. She has been the most amazing caregiver ever!!!!! Her cooking has kept my belly quite full, and her patience with my fatigue and emotional ups and downs has been amazing. I get to see Micah all the time. He comes over almost every night. He hasn't eaten like this in years. He looks great and his friends have been amazingly supportive and caring. Today is day 50-post-transplant. This means I'm halfway there. May 18th is Day 100 (supposedly the day I can go home). Fingers crossed everyone! I love and miss you all! I can't wait to see you! Happy spring to everyone! Love always!*
Dani

Dani underplays her reaction (the joint pain and muscular weakness) from the transplant to her fans. She fails to mention: the meds that make her anxious, cause vivid nightmares, mood swings, and sleeplessness; the steroid that causes "moon face," an increased appetite and diminished muscle strength; and, the other meds that cause unwanted coarse dark hair to grow on her shoulders and face. This is a difficult time, even for someone as positive as Dani. The encouraging visits from friends (both Dani's and ours), the e-mails, and cards that continue for this next phase of recovery take on an even greater importance.

Perhaps one of the most inspirational e-mails arrives from a teacher (molecular biology being his specialty) who works at Dani's high school alma mater, Wootton High.

Hi Dani! I hope this e-mail finds you feeling well and improving. You have all of our well wishes and love for a full recovery. Today we did something special for you. During the past week, Wootton students have come to know you through the USA-Channel 8 video clip, your poems, and sheer courage. Today, during homeroom each student received a colored nucleotide and wrote a message to you. Then they found their complimentary basepair and created a paper helix. Each homeroom brought their helix down to the Commons to construct a giant DNA double helix. The finished product actually goes around the Commons twice. I will send you the pictures next week. I can't tell you what a wonderful feeling it was to have so many people doing something for someone they don't know. You have a tremendous gift – the power to touch peoples' hearts. My eyes are filling with tears because my wife lost her sister to Leukemia and it really feels good to do this for you! Anyway, we raised more than $1300 for the NTAF – Dani Shotel Fund. Our hearts and prayers are with you and your family. We want to have a ceremony here at Wootton on April 7 on your behalf as we celebrate DNA Week. Students for Wootton's DNA Academy will present a check to the NTAF at that time. Hopefully members of your family can attend. Regards and may God bless you, Sanford

3/31 – Day 52

Our Monday morning begins with our usual walk up the hill to the Hutch for Dani's blood draw and her appointment with the Blue Team. However, today Scott and Jay join Dani and me. Dani is all smiles after her blood draw (just because she enjoys the technicians so much), despite the joint pain she had last night. By the time the four of us enter what is now a very crowded examination room for Dani's appointment with Dr. Appelbaum, Betty, and Diane, the results of the blood draw have been made available. We all cheer with the news that Dani's white blood cell count is up to 13,000 (normal is considered 10,000 to 14,000). Dani then reports about the nightly joint pain, although she tells Dr. Appelbaum and the team that she was able to go back to sleep last night. She also reports that she's on no pain medications during the day, and is only taking Benadryl to ease stomach pains; her sleeping pattern at night seems to be improving; and, her skin has taken on a mottled look. Dr. Appelbaum explains to us all that the mottled skin is probably a result of the Busulfan chemotherapy treatment (from two months ago). He says that this treatment often causes a bit of sunburn and, like sunburn, it too will peel. He also cautions that this could also be a bit of skin GvHD. He advises Dani to begin to use Eucerin Skin Cream to moisten her skin and to keep Betty informed of any other GvHD–like conditions, such as dry eyes, a sore mouth, or continued skin irritation. With that said, we are all pleasantly surprised to learn that from now on Dani will only have one Blue Team visit per week. Beginning on April 10th, Dani's new attending physician will be Dr. Claudio Anasetti (he was the doctor who actually wrote the unique radiation-less protocol for Dani's medical treatment here in Seattle).

4/2 – Day 54

Dani visits Andréa, the physical therapist, this afternoon with Scott. She tells her, "I'm doing so much better. My knee pain has really decreased" (she rates it at a 3 out of a possible 10). She also reports a fatigue rating of 0 out of 10 (meaning that she is experiencing no fatigue), despite contradicting herself by reporting that earlier in the day she decided to clean up the kitchen by herself after making lunch, and that she was so fatigued that it actually took her 30 minutes to recover and resume her activities.

Andréa listens intently and advises Dani to continue tossing the rubber ball (for cardiovascular build-up) for at least a minute and a half without fatigue, resting about 30 seconds and then repeating the exercise; walking; following the prescribed therapeutic exercise routine; and wearing the lovely hospital-issued hose. She has quickly become another member of the Dani Fan Club, as she is amazed by Dani's motivation.

4/3 – Day 55

After her routine 8 a.m. blood draw at the Hutch, Dani (with Jay in tow) arrives for her 8:30 a.m. PT appointment with Andréa. Ever the coach, Jay is willing to assist Dani in any exercise that Andréa recommends. Dani reports to Andréa that she is currently experiencing zero fatigue but mentions that she has a bit of soreness in both her calves and her knees (she rates it at 2 out of 10). With that said, Andréa has Dani complete her therapeutic exercises (sitting and standing for 10 repetitions as well as balancing on each leg with support). For balance exercises, she has Dani go up and down two flights of stairs at the SCCA without the use of the railings. As Dani experiences some fatigue, Andréa advises Dani to do this activity more slowly for safety purposes. But Dani cheers as she is told that she has just met the short term stair goal. Andréa warns the extremely motivated Dani not to overdo the physical therapy exercises to the point where the therapy becomes the cause of muscle or knee soreness! Dani agrees, and along with her dad say goodbye to Andréa and head back to our apartment at the Marriott.

Later on in the afternoon, we (Jay, Scott, and I) visit with the Blue Team with Dani. As if she needs an answer, Diane then asks, "How is the star of the Blue Team doing? You are the healthiest person on this team!"

Dr. Appelbaum decides to keep Dani on IV magnesium plus protein twice a day, but promises her that, pretty soon, he'll switch this to pill form. As our appointment comes to a close, Dr. Appelbaum mentions that the prednisone taper may cause Dani increased anxiety. Dani assures Dr. Appelbaum that she has a cure-all for that. She then advises the team

of the medicinal benefits of our old family cure-all, "Ugga Mugga."
This combination of warm milk, vanilla, and a bit of sugar, Dani reports,
often calms her down and soothes her stomach. Dr. Appelbaum smiles,
nods and comments that if Dani experiences any additional anxiety, dry
eyes, irritated skin, sore mouth, pain, etc., she should let Betty know,
just in case the Ugga Mugga doesn't do the job completely.

We all say goodbye to the members of the team and thank Dr.
Appelbaum for his kindness and his care. The four of us then head down
the hill collectively feeling pretty good.

4/4 – Day 56

We cancel Dani's physical therapy appointment with Andréa today as
Dani is experiencing some severe knee soreness. We are assured by
Andréa that there is no cause for alarm. Dani spends the day resting.

4/7 – Day 59

In the afternoon, Dani and I head up to the Hutch for her "Look Good,
Feel Better" seminar. Jay and Scott went back to the East Coast yesterday,
so for now it's just the two of us girls in the apartment. We enter the
seminar room and are greeted by three presenters. We find out a little
bit more about what to expect for the next 2 hours. One woman will
teach us about make-up application; another will demonstrate how to
use headscarves to cover baldness brought on by treatment; and, finally,
we'll learn about wigs. With that said, introductions are made. Cancer
patients as well as caregivers introduce themselves. In total there are
about eight women in various stages of cancer treatment attending this
seminar. Despite her "moon face" and baldness, Dani still appears to be
the least affected by the ravages of her cancer. We sit, listen, chat with
the other participants, who until now have been strangers, and play with
makeup, scarves and wigs until the seminar ends. As we walk down
the hill, neither one of us is too upbeat. What we suppose was designed
to encourage more positive attitudes of the women who attended, only
brings an inexplicable sadness to us both. Not only does Dani empathize

with these women, but, as is her nature, she also feels sympathy for them — for what she believes is worse than the hand she was dealt.

Later in the evening, Dani and I speak to Jay who reports to us about the DNA assembly program, in which the Students of Wootton High School, Sanford Herzon, and the DNA club presented Jay with a check for the National Transplant Assistance Fund (NTAF), as a result of their "DNA for Dani" fundraiser. We continue to be so pleased with all the support we have received, as well as with the various events that are being held to raise awareness and funds in Dani's name, to help researchers find cures for the many varied blood cancers that exist.

4/8 – Day 60

In the afternoon, Dani and I head up the hill for her PT appointment with Andréa. Dani reports that she is still having some knee pain, especially at night. Despite this, she tells Andréa that except for Friday, when she was experiencing severe joint pain, she was able to complete the prescribed physical therapy exercises every day since our meeting four days ago. Andréa's assessment is that Dani is progressing with exercises and strength, and also notices that Dani's swelling is decreasing and her endurance is improving as well. With that good news, Andréa suggests that Dani may want to increase her therapeutic exercise reps up to 20, if she can tolerate that many. Andréa approves of Dani's independent use of cuff weights, as she continues her exercise routine in our apartment. Feeling quite proud of Andréa's assessment and challenge, both Dani and I head back to the apartment.

4/10 – Day 62

After her morning blood draw, Dani heads up to Andréa's office. Even though she reports that her status is "good," she also mentions increased pain for the past two nights in both knees and ankles (she rates the pain as 9 out of 10 on the pain scale). Dani describes it as a deep throbbing pain. After some cardiovascular exercise ball tossing with Andréa, Andréa notes that she is concerned with Dani's decreased endurance. She tells us both that Dani really needs more cardio exercises, but because of the knee and ankle pain, playing catch might be the safest cardio exercise choice, in order to ensure that the therapy isn't the cause of Dani's joint pain. Dani reassures Andréa that she believes all this joint pain is the result of the steroid taper. I'm pretty sure that Andréa is as amazed as I am with Dani's determination. Before we leave Andréa, she tells us that her goal is to have Dani increase her cardio capacity (with the ball tossing) and monitor her weight lifting. She believes that with the progress Dani is making, Dani's physical therapy appointments will be decreased in frequency, if Dani meets all the goals of the program (which will be assessed at Dani's next session on April 15th).

Later on in the day we meet with the Blue Team. As Dani and I enter the examination room for today's Blue visit, we are greeted warmly by Diane, who is waving a paper with Dani's a.m. blood draw results in front of our faces, as she beams and says, "Perfect counts!" Dani then shares with Betty and Diane her current "gas" problem. Betty suggests that Dani go off milk products (like Ugga Mugga) for a bit, and discusses having Dani take some anti-gas medications. Betty then documents the medications that Dani is currently taking. Betty adds to the list a time-release pain patch of Fentanyl to control Dani's joint pain. She informs Dani that she'll also gradually add magnesium pills to her list of meds, even though Dani will still be on IV magnesium. Eventually the need for IV anything will come to an end. We both are happy with this news. Betty shares in our happiness. She tells Dani, "You're doing fabulously! It's so very nice and gratifying to see." She and Diane both agree that by day 75 post-transplant, Dani will once more have hair growing on her head! As we are laughing, the door opens. Betty introduces us both to Dr. Anasetti, Dani's new attending physician. After a few minutes reviewing Dani's current status, he too comments on Dani's health as he states, "You look good to me. You're doing wonderfully." As we walk down the hill, we both agree that this was not a bad visit at all!

4/11 – Day 63

Today Andréa introduces weights to Dani's exercise regimen. This addition will help Dani's muscle tone return. Dani continues to follow Andréa's prescribed physical therapy plan religiously. With each day, I notice her physical strength improving.

4/12 – Day 64

After a "not so good" night, Dani wakes up to a beautiful sunny Seattle day. Today is special not only because Jay is arriving, but also because Dani's former professor, Dr. Michael Castleberry, is in town for a conference and is taking us out to lunch. We have a wonderful time with him, as he later relates to Jay in an e-mail sent on April 14th:

....her hair may be different and her chipmunk cheeks may be a touch more full this week, but the eyes are pure Dani and boy do they glow!!! She is an awesome kid, you...should be INCREDIBLY proud of how she lives her life reflecting the values she learned from her family. I'd like to believe my kids and my family would handle something big like this even half as well. And Dani...well truly...even for someone who got to know her pretty well as a young adult, she is just beyond belief! Wow! It's easy to see how feelings of pride in your child's ability to cope with anything and everything life tosses her way can translate into complete confidence that it will all work out the way she wants it to — because she wants it to!!!

During our lunch with Dr. Castleberry, Dani sadly informs him that, because she will be immuno-suppressed for at least a year after her return to the East Coast, she will be unable to work directly with students. So in his e-mail to Jay, he further comments:

...I think she's sad but resigned to having to steer clear of kids for a couple of years, but I am also interested in getting her into some teaching for us (at GWU)...when she is strong enough immune-wise....

When she sees that the age of the 'kid' makes no difference, that she is still the same 'teacher', it may help her until she can get back to kids.

Dr. Castleberry concludes his heart-felt note with a commentary on the "new" Dani, as it is obvious that he has never had the opportunity to dine with someone on large doses of prednisone.

...And BOY...can that girl eat!

4/15 – Day 67
Dani has Jay join her for her physical therapy appointment with Andréa. She tells Andréa, "I feel pretty good," and was able to sleep last night without pain, but admits that she is still using a pain patch, but is tapering off her use of oral pain meds. She boasts that she is now able to complete her physical therapy routine two times with 20 reps each time. She admits, however, that the second set of reps is more difficult. She also lets Andréa know, "I tripped this morning, but it wasn't a big deal because I was trying to walk a little with the weights on my ankles." Andréa and Jay just shake their heads.

Andréa then has Dani go through her exercise routine. Dani goes up and down four flights of stairs without using the railing, losing balance, or fatigue. She also completes a series of forward and backward heel-toe balance activities without a loss of balance. For cardiovascular exercise Dani will now be riding the stationary bike for 6 minutes daily. Andréa instructs Dani to increase the use of weights by 1 pound a week if she is able, and to gradually increase her cardiovascular exercises from 10 minutes to 1 hour at least three times a week. She cautions her about the importance of completing the proper warm-up and cool-down routines as part of her exercise program. Andréa then congratulates Dani on passing all short-term and long-term physical therapy goals. She says that despite the continued knee and ankle pain at night, "Dani's strength, balance, stairs completion, pain levels, swelling, and fatigue levels have all shown very good improvement!" With assurance that Dani will continue her physical therapy regimen independently, Andréa sees no further need for formalized physical therapy appointments. Even though this is great news, we are a bit sad to leave her. Dani's strength, balance, and confidence have continued to improve with Andréa's expertise. For that reason, our departure from her tiny office/exercise room is bittersweet.

4/16 – Day 68

Dani receives a note from a college buddy and former softball teammate, Andrea Cubbage, today. She tells Dani that she will be running with Team in Training (TNT) in Alaska on June 21st for the Leukemia and Lymphoma Society. She tells Dani that Dani's courage and "can do it" attitude has inspired her to complete this marathon. In her enclosed fundraising letter, Andrea closes with, "…running in a marathon will be a challenge, but it is nothing compared to the challenge that Dani and others who battle this disease are forced to confront on a daily basis." Once more, we are amazed by the love, support, and willingness of friends and family to get involved in this ever-important cause of raising funds for research to eradicate blood cancer, not just in Dani, but in the entire world.

Today marks the beginning of Passover. Usually our family celebrates the first night of Passover with a Seder (evening ritual meal) at my sister's house, where she prepares a feast, and Bruce leads us in telling the story of Passover. Tonight being so different from all those other years of family Seders, I have decided to put one together. Jay assists me in the preparation for our own Seattle Seder with our son and daughter and family friends. Jay's job is to go on-line and find some Passover songs as well as the story of Passover for us to read prior to the feast. We have shopped for the matzah, gefilte fish, horseradish, and other special Passover items. Jay and I have also decided to add a bit of humor into this year's special Seder. So besides the children's songs that he has found on the Internet that commemorate the holiday (incidentally they are sung to the tunes of the Brady Bunch and Gilligan's Island theme songs), we also find the same ice Popsicle brand that Dani had while in the hospital. The reason for purchasing this specific brand is that each Popsicle stick has a riddle/question printed on one side with a humorous answer on the reverse side. So as we proceed through the Seder ritual story telling, we come to the spot where, as custom would have it, the youngest member of the family asks the traditional Four Questions (e.g., Why is this night different from all other nights?). When we finish with this, I solemnly pass a Popsicle stick to each person at the table and have them recite the six additional questions. Our children and our guests are delighted with the slightly irreverent Seder. This small family gathering somehow makes it easier for us to not miss the family and friends that would be gathering around my sister's table tonight quite so much.

4/17 – Day 69
We're not so sure if it was the cheese steak that Dani had for lunch, or the Seder supper, but Dani threw up last night. However, the good news was that she was able to fall back to sleep and rise well rested in time for her blood draw and Blue Team appointment. After the blood draw, Dani, Jay and I head upstairs to have our weekly visit with the Blue Team. Kerry, Dani's nutritionist, joins us. Before we meet with Dr. Anasetti, Betty gives Dani the good news…Dani can begin to use a depilatory cream (i.e., Facial Quality Nair) to remove unwanted facial hairs. Dani is beside herself with joy! She further adds to her good mood by announcing to us that it looks like Dani is "losing a bit of your tummy." She also informs Dani that she should begin to reduce her Oxycontin dosage tonight. As we discuss Dani's tapering off of prednisone, Kerry comments that, as the steroid dosage decreases, so will Dani's appetite. Both Kerry and Betty agree that they can almost predict that Dani will go home without a catheter line in her chest. With this additional good news, Dr. Anasetti enters the examination room. With a little prodding by Dani, Jay, and me, Dr. Anasetti tells us how Dani's "radiation-less" protocol was able to occur. He says that through studies they have found that chemotherapy alone has fewer long-run negative reactions for "good risk" patients. He further adds, "By moderating Busulfan we feel

comfortable that patients like Dani will do better. This new protocol of determining Busulfan levels is cutting edge...and that to date it shows an overall benefit of decreasing morbidity, toxicity, and rejection." As he leaves the room, his parting words to us are, "A good start is better than the wrong start." We could not agree more.

After he leaves, Betty reviews with us the plan for tomorrow. Dani will begin the day with a bone density scan at 9 a.m. From there, we'll head to the Triage Unit downstairs for a blood transfusion of two units of red cells. I note this down in my date book. Dani then shows Betty and Diane that the white line of her Groshong Catheter appears loose, and they both agree that Dani needs to head downstairs right after this appointment to get the line repaired. So as Jay heads back to the apartment, Dani and I go to the Triage Unit to have the white line of her Groshong replaced.

This time neither of us panics. We have learned that with time, the various parts of the catheter will require a bit of a "tune-up." We've also come to realize that the Groshong Catheter is rarely seen in West Coast medical facilities, especially here at the Hutch, where Dr. Hickman is on staff! Anyhow, suffice to say, very few people here have much knowledge of the Groshong Catheter. In fact, the staff even appears a bit nervous working with this extremely beneficial form of catheter. So we are not even the least bit surprised that the white line gets changed only after our attending nurse carefully reads the enclosed directions. Pleased with the results, we head back to our apartment to join Jay.

When we return to the Marriott, Dani sits down and writes an e-mail on her website to her friends:

Hello all!

First of all today (Thursday) is my mom's birthday...so, we are looking forward to a day filled with good foods and smiles. Everyone here is in good spirits. Yesterday I spent most of the day resting...but, I have been quite busy lately. For those of you who have any background in special education you will be interested to hear that I passed all my

I.E.P. (Individualized Educational Plan) set physical therapy goals with 5s (the highest rating) on Monday. I have graduated from PT. This does not mean that my body has regained all of its strength, or looks anything like it did before September 11th... I will continue to do my PT program on my own...what this does mean is that my body is starting to rebuild muscle mass...my joints have stopped hurting (fingers crossed)...and I'm able to participate in a cardio program (your lungs and heart take a pretty big hit from the chemo). Tomorrow I will have my first transfusion since my first few days in the hospital. This is also par for the course as the meds depress red blood cell production. It will give me extra energy for the weekend. Next week I will begin my reevaluation to hopefully set a target date for me to return the other coast. Love always,
Dani

4/18 – Day 70

Dani threw up the second night in a row. We chalk it up to rich foods from my birthday celebration. At this point, it's par for the course.

This morning as Dani and I arrive on the fifth floor Triage Unit, a nurse escorts us to a small room where Dani will have her transfusion. As she prepares Dani for the transfusion, the recently inserted white Groshong line falls out. The attending triage nurse sort of panics... while Dani and I continue to remain calm. The nurse's supervisor takes over, and as she hopefully corrects the problem this time, she says to Dani, "Your gift for resiliency is a very good thing!" We laugh and say that we couldn't agree more!

As Dani and I are being moved from one room to another for the actual blood transfusion, we literally run into our Blue Team nurse, Diane, who is walking down the hallway dragging an IV pole with an intravenous solution going into her arm. She tells us that she is here for her own chemotherapy for breast cancer, and that she has recently had a mastectomy. Talk about resiliency...and strength...and courage! Dani's own nurse, continuing to care for her...while she herself is being treated for cancer. We are both stunned. Diane soon says goodbye and heads to her original destination with our best wishes and positive thoughts. At this point, Betty enters our room. After our short discussion about Diane and the Groshong Catheter crisis, we begin to speak about Dani's stomach. Betty is concerned that this is symptomatic of GvHD of the stomach. She tells us that she might prescribe Regulan to ease Dani's queasy stomach, but she wants us to take the symptom seriously, and not just attribute it to rich food. We agree to contact her if this queasiness continues.

Betty continues to prepare Dani for her transfusion. Betty thinks (as do the two of us) that Dani will be receiving A Positive blood (the blood type from her transplant donor) since Dani's blood tests now reveal that over 50% of Dani's blood type is now A Positive and we are all surprised when O Positive blood arrives. So before the transfusion begins, we ask for someone from the Transfusion Department to answer our questions (we have all learned a big lesson from the plasmapherisis snafu of February 6th). A doctor soon arrives from the Transfusion Department and explains the reason Dani is still receiving O Positive (remember that's the universal donor blood type as well as Dani's former type) blood. He says that Dani is receiving O Positive blood to be safe, as they want her to receive red blood cells from blood that she doesn't have antibodies against. He tells us not to worry, and that this O Positive red blood cell transfusion has no anti-A antibodies. He adds that, if in the future (after she leaves Seattle) Dani needs a transfusion, the blood type can be changed to that of the donor. He says that Seattle will wait until after two consecutive blood draw results show that all anti-A titers are gone, and only then will the SCCA recommend the change to A Positive blood to Dani's oncologist in Virginia. He says that this is a conservative and safe way of doing things. With this knowledge, and once more reassured that the Hutch and the Seattle Cancer Care Alliance provide the very best treatment in the world to cure Acute Myelogenous Leukemia, Dani begins her transfusion process at 10:47 a.m. It's been quite an insightful and busy morning!

4/21 – Day 73

Jay returned to the East Coast yesterday leaving Dani and me on our own for the week. Dani and I continue to "enjoy" our time together. Today, Dani has a visit scheduled with Kerry (nutritionist) this morning after her usual blood draw. Kerry is glad to see that Dani is gaining weight (Dani's not so happy about this, but understands that eating is part of the cure). Kerry is also pleased with Dani's report of normal bowel movements.

4/22 – Day 74

Yuck! Today Dani will have another bone marrow aspirate. As usual, Dani has requested pain meds. Being in a silly mood, we both sing (to the tune of the Beatles, "Here Comes the Sun") "Here Comes the Drugs…doo-dee-doo-dee…!" As Dani is sufficiently dosed, the procedure begins. Two technicians perform the task and one tells me (Dani is in La-La Land at the moment) that there appears to be a lot of growth in the bone marrow and that "it's a good thing." When the other technician tells us, "O.K., we're done," Dani (from her haze) says very softly "Good job team!"

4/24 – Day 76

Dani has a whole bunch of appointments and tests scheduled today…and she's so nervous about two of them that she actually, for the first time, forgets to fast prior to her blood draw! Dani has the dreaded pulmonary check-up as well as dental appointment this morning. Needless to say, she is a bit tense.

After she completes her blood draw at 8:15 a.m. Dani goes to the Medical Photography Department to have a base line photograph taken for any skin GvHD. Shortly after that appointment, we head to the Pulmonary Department. The technician promises Dani that the oxygen function tests will go off without any problems. The last time—pre-transplant—that Dani had these tests, the technician somehow hit a nerve, mistakenly causing Dani serious pain. Today, the testing went on without any crises.

Dani demonstrates normal functioning in all three breathing tests and her oxygen level is now at 99%. One dreaded appointment down, one to go.

Dani now visits the dentist. He speaks to Dani about mouth care to avoid peridontal disease. He tells her to floss at least once a day. In fact, he suggests that she keep floss containers all over the place and floss all the time! He suspects that Dani's dry lips and gum discoloration indicate that she has a bit of mouth GvHD. He shows her some redness and white spots in her mouth. He tells her that the side of her tongue looks patchy, there is some whiteness on the tongue surface, and her gum tissue looks delicate. He advises that once a week she should examine her mouth with a flashlight and a mirror, and that when the colors get more even, that's a good thing. For the next six to nine months, he tells her that she isn't to have any dental cleanings or invasive treatments. With that said, the appointment is over and what do you know…she survives!

The morning ends with a visit to Dani's Blue Team. As we enter the examining room, Diane asks Dani, "How's the star of the Blue Team?" After Dani confirms that she is feeling pretty good, the discussion turns technical. She tells both Diane and Betty that she is no longer using the pain patch…a pretty good sign. Diane reports that Dani's flow cytometry is clear (no blasts appeared in the bone marrow aspirate test). We all cheer. Diane runs an eye test for GvHD. Dani is able to provide Diane with tears. Dani passes the eye test with flying colors as well! Betty then advises Dani to stop taking Fluconazole and **Norvasc** (Norvasc is the brand name of Amlopidine), and to only take 12 magnesium pills a day. With that medical discussion out of the way, Dani and I invite Diane and Betty to our apartment for lunch in the near future, to thank them for all of their support. They both accept our invitation, and we agree on a date for next week. Dr. Anasetti enters the room and tells Dani that her summary conference is scheduled for May 6th, and in all probability she could leave Seattle Cancer Care by May 9th the earliest (Day 90 post-transplant).

Before we even leave the building, Dani and I are on our respective cell phones. She calls Scott with the good news as I call Jay. Jay promises to book our flight home. Through much discussion, we all agree that it will be best for us to take a "red eye" (late evening to early morning) flight home to the East Coast. By doing that, Dani will be able to sleep. We also decide that for Dani's comfort, it would be best to fly first class (boy, were we mistaken).

4/26 – Day 78

Jay arrives today (4/26) by mid-afternoon. He is so excited about our predicted departure date that, not only has he already made plane reservations for us, but as an "I love you" gift for Dani, he gives her 10 N95 face masks to wear on our flight home for added protection against flu, viruses, bacteria, mold spores, and pollen, as well as stagnant recycled airplane air. Dani is beside herself with such lovely presents! It is also Jay's and my 33rd wedding anniversary today, and we have decided to celebrate it by taking an overnight trip to Victoria, British Columbia, tomorrow.

4/27 – 4/28 – Days 79 to 80

Dani's former roommate, Elisa, arrives from San Francisco at approximately the same time that we depart for Victoria and spends some quality time with Dani. Dani is pleased that Jay and I are beginning to "let go" a bit. Although, Jay and I speak with Dani often during this 36-hour period, we all manage to have a wonderful time with our respective "good buddy!"

4/30 – Day 82

Jay, Dani, and I attend Dani's long-term follow-up meeting. We have written down a few specific questions and the team answers them and several others we neglected to ask. Dani is told that as far as sports go, she can not play golf for six months (which is okay since Dani has never played golf), and she also should not play any softball for the next year. She is given permission to observe her cousin, Heather, give birth to her second child in late June. Dani is honored to have been asked by Heather and her husband, Shawn, to be present for this miraculous occasion.

As our questions are answered, we begin to become informed about Dani's medical schedule for the next year. She will be seeing her oncologist, Dr. Christie, once a week for the first month after her homecoming, and then twice a month at least until Dani's one-year evaluation, back at the Hutch in Seattle, in February 2004. At that point, she will receive her baby booster shots. She is told, however, that before she returns to Seattle, she will need to get a flu shot. She may not, we are told, receive a smallpox vaccine, or a polio vaccine, as these vaccines include living viruses…and this is taboo for someone who is immuno-suppressed.

Additionally, Dani is directed to look for and report to her oncologist (or contact the Follow-up Care Office at the Hutch) any signs of GvHD. These signs could appear on her skin (as a rash), in her mouth (as dryness and discoloration), in her liver, in her eyes (as dryness or too much tearing), in her digestive system (as nausea, poor digestion or diahrhea), in her vagina (as tightening, dryness or irritation of the vaginal canal), in her lungs (as a persistent dry cough), or she could have any combination of these symptoms. She is also warned to be alert about joint pain, and abnormal muscle hardness. We are told that chronic GvHD occurs in about 50% of bone marrow transplant survivors, a fact that we are already aware of. The three of us understand that Dani has already experienced mild forms of GvHD in her mouth, on her skin, and in her stomach. The fact that her new white blood cells are fighting these symptoms is considered to be a good sign.

We are told that Dani will be expected to return to Seattle once a year on her new birthday (February 7th) for the next five years for a series of medical evaluations, and that she will, while living in Virginia, continue to remain under the watchful eye of Dr. Christie in Arlington. We leave the meeting even more hopeful than when we entered. We continue to take it all in stride, one day at a time. With each step we are closer to a cure! When Jay writes of Dani's progress on her website, Dani receives the following e-mail in response to this most recent update:

From Dani's high school softball catcher: *I was throwing the ball with*

*my dad yesterday and thinking and talking about you the whole time!
I am so-o-o-o-o-o-o-o-o-o happy that you're doing so tremendously
well. You are really amazing!*

5/1 – Day 83

Jay, Dani, and I head up the hill to the Hutch for her appointment with
the Blue Team. We are escorted into an examining room by our new
physician's assistant, Mark. Dani tells him that she is "excited and
nervous" as the time of her departure from Seattle nears. Mark advises
her to follow her own "common sense and good judgment" when it
comes to her becoming independent once more. He explains that, in
all probability, her shaking legs and constant chills are a result of her
hypothalamus gland (gland which regulates body temperature) "jump
starting." He is unconcerned and comments that the most recent blood
draw report shows that all her levels look good. This also means that the
Cyclosporin taper will probably begin (the taper will last approximately
three months). Kerry, Dani's nutritionist, enters the room and begins
to share with us food safety guidelines that Dani will need to follow
after she leaves Seattle. She is advised to have only pasteurized cheese;
take no herbal medications; keep hydrated; and, increase the intake of
fruits, vegetables, mono and poly-saturated fats, and foods that contain
Omega 3 (e. g., salmon). She tells Dani that currently her cholesterol
and triglycerides are high (possibly caused by the Cyclosporin and
prednisone), so that she should have this checked once she is finally off
these two medications. Kerry then reminds Dani to continue taking 2
Viactives (for calcium) as well as a multivitamin that is high in vitamin
D, even though the current bone scan was normal. Finally, Kerry suggests
that in order to maintain her body weight, Dani should consume 1,700
calories daily. Dr. Anasetti enters the room as Kerry is finishing up her
list of "Dos" and "Don'ts." He adds that right now Dani's body seems
to be accepting the transplant cells, and that she is not at high risk for
rejection. According to test results, he says that Dani's body is now
comprised of 35% donor cells. Being cautious, he wants to continue

testing for **chimerism** (Dani's own old cells versus the donor's transplanted healthy cells) for three additional months. He tells us that he has scheduled the chimerism retest for

> **Chimerism** is the simultaneous existence and function of components of both the donor's and the recipient's immune systems in the same patient, resulting in cross-regulation of immune system activities.

Monday, May 5th. Dr. Anasetti seems to think that Dani will be released from the Seattle Cancer Care Alliance on May 9th. With the appointment ended, we head down the hill back to our apartment, hopeful that within eight days we'll be back on the East Coast. Jay finalizes the purchase of our "red eye" flight home and writes an entry on Dani's website that announces the long awaited news of Dani's homecoming.

Feeling incredibly positive, the three of us decide to try once more to rise to the challenge of attempting to find the "perfect" wig for Dani to wear, until her new hair comes in. With high hopes, Jay drives us to a wig shop that has been recommended to us by another patient. Dani finally chooses a short, light, brunette-colored wig, and for about what seemed like an hour, the stylist, with her scissors in hand, shapes and reshapes the wig into what we agree almost matches Dani's old familiar "pixie" hair style. It's not quite right, but we seem to agree that because it's been so long since Dani has had hair on her head, it will take a bit for us to get used to Dani with hair! With all the snipping the stylist is doing, we feel somewhat obligated to purchase this light brunette (and now quite short) wig. With the wig on her head, Dani leads the two of us back to our rental car. Once back at the apartment, Dani and I work on adjusting the wig to get it to look "natural." Despite our best efforts, "natural" just isn't happening!

5/2 – Day 84

The plan is that tonight Dani will test out the wig, as we have planned to have a celebratory dinner with her friend, Tiffany (who is recovering from a bone marrow transplant as well, and is leaving for her home in Utah on 5/3), along with her mom, her boyfriend, our son Micah, and

David (another friend recovering from a bone marrow transplant). We will be dining at Serafina, one of our favorite Italian restaurants. We will be having a triple celebration, as all three friends have had successful bone marrow transplants.

The celebratory dinner is a bit depressing for Dani, however. Tiffany, who is not on steroids, is also wearing a wig, as she too has lost her hair…but she has no "moon face." Tiffany looks absolutely gorgeous. Our "chipmunk-cheeked" Dani manages to hold her head high and keeps a smile on her face throughout the dinner, but the wig does little to help her "Look Good, and Feel Better" (as the seminar on April 7th promised). When we return to our apartment, the wig is put away in a drawer. (To this day, none of us is sure of what ever became of that wig!)

5/3 – Day 85
Good news travels like wildfire. Dani begins to receive celebratory e-mails almost immediately after Jay posts the news of her homecoming:

A TNT coach writes: *It's great to read about your progress and the strength you are gaining daily….Your struggles and determination pulled the team through some miles of the Country Music Marathon held in Nashville. Thank you for being there for all of us as part of the BIG reason we all train so hard to fight for you and others against this battle! The total raised by the TNT family in Nashville was 1.9 MILLION dollars! May God continue to watch over your daily progress to guide you back home to the East Coast soon!*

5/4 – Day 86
Jay leaves for the airport shortly before noon for his final commute back to the East Coast. He takes with him one extra-large suitcase filled with "stuff" that neither Dani nor I will need for our remaining five days in Seattle. He has left Dani and me with 2 first-class airplane tickets for our anticipated May 9th departure from Seattle. Today, Dani and

I plan to spend a lazy day watching an MTV Real World Road Rules Challenge Marathon (the reader can well imagine that this is a brand new experience for me). As the day continues, Dani develops a migraine headache. As it becomes more severe (Dani rates the pain at an 8 out of a possible 10), we call the 24/7 clinic, and we are advised that Dani should take Tylenol for the pain. Interestingly enough, with all the drugs in our possession, Tylenol appears to be missing from our vast supply of medications. Micah, having better things to do on this lazy Sunday than hang with his mom and sister, delivers the Tylenol and heads back to his house. Dani takes 2 tablets and heads into her bedroom. With the bedroom lights turned off and lying still in her bed, Dani hopes the headache will go away. She tells me that if she lies completely flat in the darkness, she experiences no head pain. Around 8 p.m., Dani agrees to a light dinner of biscuits and tea with honey. At 11 p.m. I check on Dani, and she tells me that the headache pain has not abated. I call the clinic again and I am advised to take Dani back to the University of Washington Hospital and go to the transplant wing of the seventh floor.

I call for a taxi and for the next hour or so Dani and I enter into our own "Twilight Zone" surrealistic set of actual events. A taxi arrives, and with very little discussion the driver makes a few illegal turns and gets us to the hospital quite fast. He even goes over a restrictive curb to get us on the I-5 Interstate Highway quicker. Upon arrival to University of Washington Medical Center, I help Dani out of the cab, and we enter the hospital. We are met on the seventh floor by a doctor who takes us into an examining room, asks us a series of questions, checks Dani's vitals (BP is at 116/84), and then checks Dani's reflexes. She has Dani touch her fingers to her toes, checking her balance. Her diagnosis is somewhat vague, but, at the same time, reassuring. She thinks that maybe Dani could have twisted her neck when she was doing her physical therapy exercises, or perhaps the pain is a reaction to the Cyclosporin taper. Whatever the real cause, she tells us that we might want to stop by Triage Care at the Hutch tomorrow if the migraine continues. She assures us that the headache is nothing to worry about, and, with that said, she sends us on our way. Despite her words, we both continue to remain pretty worried. Our brief return to UW hospital is now over, so the two of us take the elevator to the lobby, walk slowly through the exit doors, hail a cab, and head back to our hotel. By 12:30 a.m. we are back in our apartment. I take care in putting my daughter (whose migraine pain is still at an "8" out of "10") to bed. Totally exhausted from this new adventure, she falls asleep immediately. As it is very late on the East Coast, I refrain from calling Jay until the morning. Sleep doesn't come to me so easily tonight.

5/5 – Day 87

Dani wakes up around 8 a.m. and reports to me that her headache pain is now at a "6." Despite this news, we agree to head up to the Hutch for her usual Monday a.m. blood draw and chimerism retest, and then head up to the Triage Unit to discuss Dani's migraines with a doctor. The friendly technicians at the first floor clinic, where Dani has had her blood drawn for the past four months, welcome Dani. They are sad to hear of Dani's lingering headache but report that she looks great and that her vitals look pretty good as well. After our short stay at the first floor clinic, we head up to Triage. Dani is escorted to a small examination room. While we wait for a doctor to appear to discuss the headache pain, Dani becomes nauseous and throws up. As if this were a miracle, Dani reports to me that her headache has now disappeared. We both agree that my mother's theory of "it is better out than in" is quite true in this instance. We meet with a doctor briefly and retell the events of the past 24 hours. This doctor also appears unconcerned about the migraines and advises Dani to rest this afternoon. We do just that. We leave Triage and head down the hill to our apartment. Once in the apartment, Dani heads to her bedroom where she "rests" all day. This prescription seems to work, as Dani reports to me in the late afternoon that her headache pain is now at a "2." Around 11 p.m. though, we call the 24/7 help line for advice on what medications Dani should take. We are advised that two Tylenol should do the trick. For the time being, it does.

5/6 – Day 88

Dani remains in bed all morning. She reports to me that, as long as she remains still, she does not have a headache. She does, however, feel a bit nauseous and has no appetite. I spend these few hours packing up my clothes, as well as our photos and other 'stuff' (that transformed our apartment into a home for the past four months).

Despite not feeling on top of her game, Dani is quite excited for today's meeting with the Blue Team, because this meeting is noted as "Summary Conference" on Dani's weekly schedule. We meet with Diane (the Blue Team nurse), Mark (Dani's new physician's assistant), and Dr. Anasetti. Dani reports to them about her loss of appetite, nausea, and continuous headache. She also mentions that she had diahrhea once today. Dr. Anasetti listens to Dani's list of concerns, reviews the results of the most recent blood draw and chimerism retest, and informs Dani that the chimerism test results look much better than they did last week. He also says that the origin of the headaches is unclear, but he too seems unconcerned about them. He is concerned about the one time diarrhea. He then tells us that he would like to remove Dani from the pill form of magnesium to check for GvHD of the stomach. He believes that since Dani is now tapering off prednisone, the GvHD symtoms would no longer be masked or hidden by the steroid. He then drops a bomb! He informs us that because of the diarrhea, he is postponing our departure for 10 days to be safe. He wants to monitor Dani's symptoms for three days, perform an endoscope on Friday, and test her stool as well then. He appears not to notice Dani's and my stunned silence, and continues his systematic commentary:

- The skin biopsy is positive for GvHD. Dr. Anasetti believes that this is a good sign as it shows that the donor's cell is keeping Dani's AML in check
- The oral dental exam also shows a mild chronic form of GvHD
- The eye exam results were very good

- Dani's pulmonary function is actually better now than it was when she first arrived in Seattle in January
- The liver function is good
- The gastro-intestinal symptoms need to be studied further. He is unsure, but this might necessitate Dani remaining on Cyclosporin for an additional month. If Dani were to have chronic GvHD of the stomach, she would also remain on prednisone for another year or more
- The donor's graft is secure. Dani's blood is now comprised of 57% donor blood type. Her marrow looks good as well, as there appears to be no abnormalities in Dani's bone marrow
- However, Dani's immunoglobulin level is a bit low, and he suggests that Dani return to Triage tomorrow to have what is called **IVIG** therapy, which he says will help her baby immune system fight infections

Dr. Anasetti concludes his comments by reiterating that the staff will need observation time of 7 to 10 days to make sure Dani is well enough to return to her home in Virginia. He then says goodbye and leaves the examination room. This would be our last time meeting with Dr. Anasetti, because Dani changes her attending physician tomorrow, May the 7th. As a result of Dani's and my shocked reaction to Dr. Anasetti's decision to extend Dani's stay, he leaves without our thanking him for his amazing contribution to Dani's successful bone marrow transplant (i.e., developing and implementing the unique cancer treatment protocol for Dani, which did not include the use of radiation). At this point, neither of us can focus on anything but that he is keeping us here, and we irrationally blame him for "bursting our bubble," which was filled with hope and joy at the prospect of our returning home to the East Coast on Saturday morning. We call Jay and Scott immediately and share our devastating news. As Dani and I walk down the hill to our apartment, the Seattle air appears as heavy as our moods.

After Dani and I have our gripe session, we both come to the realization that Dr. Anasetti's call is for the best…and what's a couple of more days of cautious study and evaluation where Dani's lifetime is at stake. That "red eye" flight home would just have to wait.

A bit calmer, I call Jay back and by reading my notes I am able to fill him in on the details of our meeting with the Blue Team. After commiserating about the recent turn of events, he tells me that he has been able to cancel our flight home and currently has two "red eye" nonstop tickets from SeaTac to Dulles Airport for use at a date to be determined. We talk about this IVIG procedure, which Dani will have to endure tomorrow, and Jay promises to find out what this IVIG infusion is all about. As a professor at George Washington University, Jay has been fortunate to gain access to all sorts of medical journals. A couple of hours later, he calls me back with the information and forwards more details to me as an e-mail attachment. He tells me that this procedure provides antibodies to patients who are immune suppressed. These antibodies are collected (screened and tested for safety) from the combined plasma of thousands of donors. The IVIG manufacturers then extract the pooled antibodies and cleanse and concentrate them into an intravenous product. When I receive the e-mail with the medical journal IVIG article attached, I can hardly believe my eyes. It seems that this procedure is incredibly expensive…it costs about $10,000 per treatment. Incredible!

5/7 – Day 89

According to the drug dosage chart provided for Dani by the SCCA pharmacy, in conjunction with the Blue Team's prescribed decisions, today is Dani's last day on the steroid prednisone…that is, unless the planned endoscope shows severe GvHD of Dani's stomach. So Dani and I have decided to hold off celebrating until we're absolutely sure that she won't have to continue taking this steroid.

In the meantime, after lunch the two of us head up to the fifth floor of the Hutch for Dani's IVIG treatment. We are greeted by the Blue Team physician's assistant, Mark, and led to the room where the procedure will take place. Dani tells Mark that she threw up this morning. Mark makes a note of this and says that he will consult with other members of the Blue Team, to see if, perhaps, Dani should be given Imitrex, an anti-migraine medication. He thinks that maybe the nausea is a result of the persistent migraine headache. Although he sympathizes with Dani's desire to go home sooner rather than later, Mark asserts that the team needs to be absolutely sure that Dani needs no further treatment for chronic GvHD. He says that we'll know better on Friday when, during Dani's scheduled Blue Team appointment, Dani's new attending physician consults with a gastroenterologist. With that said, Mark then tells us that this IVIG procedure is often used for patients who have had certain types of leukemia that result in bone marrow transplants. It's used to temporarily strengthen a patient's immune system and help it fight infections. As Dani gets comfortable in the hospital bed, Mark pre-medicates Dani with Tylenol and Benedryl . He tells us that he is dosing Dani with these two medications to help prevent her already-existing headache from getting even worse, as well as chills, which are often associated with the infusion. The IVIG infusion begins shortly after 2 p.m. When Dani begins to shake from the chills, the rate of infusion is slowed and Dani stops shaking and relaxes. Because of this, the infusion lasts over 4 hours. We head down the hill for our apartment at 6:45 p.m. Since it appears that we're not going anywhere for at least a week, the two of us spend a very quiet night together.

5/9 – Day 91

Today was to be our last day in Seattle, but instead we're heading up the hill to the Hutch for a Blue Team consult meeting with a gastroenterology specialist. Dani and I are sent by the receptionist to an examination room. But before we enter the room, Dani is weighed by the nutritionist. Mark and Diane greet us. When Dani tells Mark that she still has a headache, Mark suggests that Dani also take some Sudafed along with the Imitrex. Mark tells us that he predicts that Dani will have an endoscope and a possible biopsy of her stomach tissue performed at the hospital on

Monday morning, get the reports interpreted here at the Hutch after that, and that she'll probably be sent home, still being infused with IV magnesium. He thinks that Dani will, in all probability, be released from the Seattle Cancer Care Alliance by Thursday, May 15th. We both nod, not knowing what else to do or say.

In an instant, the examination room door opens and we meet Dr. Fero, Dani's new attending physician. He is much younger than the five other attending physicians Dani has had during her treatment here in Seattle. He reviews Dani's most current reports, and chats with Dani for a few minutes. Dani informs him that aside from the persistent headache, she feels fine. She reports that, besides her one bout with diarrhea on Monday morning, that she has had no irregular bowel movements and has a very healthy appetite. Another person enters the room. We are introduced to Dr. Steinbach, the gastroenterologist. After asking Dani a few questions, both doctors suddenly excuse themselves and leave the room for what I guess is "the consult." After about 10 minutes, Dr. Fero returns to the examination room and says to Dani, "Go home." We can hardly believe our ears…the man just told Dani to "Go Home!" He then tells us that Dr. Steinbach did not believe from all of the reports that this one episode of diarrhea warranted an endoscope or a biopsy.

Dani and I can hardly believe our ears, and we are anxious to leave the examination room before anyone changes their minds. However, Dr. Fero begins to explain to us the longterm follow-up care that the staff at the Hutch wants us to follow, beginning with weekly appointments with Dr. Christie, Dani's oncologist in Arlington. I quickly write down bits and pieces of the medical protocol. When Dani asks him about the now 6-day headache, Dr. Fero also seems unconcerned and tells Dani to continue treating it, as she has since Sunday. We thank Dr. Fero, Diane, and Mark for all their care, and ask if they don't mind if we can remain in the examination room for a few more minutes to make some phone calls. Doctor Fero says that that's fine with him as he wants to give us some medical reports to deliver to Dr. Christie. As the three leave us, Dani and I get busy on our respective cell phones. My first call is to Jay, to see what magic he can work to get us back on a flight home. While I'm waiting for his return call, I call Dani's medical supply provider and cancel the service. I also get a chance to cancel a hair cut appointment! While I'm on the phone, Dani is blubbering to her Scott…who I'm sure is as excited about Dani's homecoming as she is. Within 5 minutes, Jay calls us back, and it's another miracle…the airlines still has those 2 first-class seats on their 10:45 p.m. red eye flight on 5/9 from SeaTac to Dulles Airport! I then place a call to Micah and tell him to drop everything, pick up some boxes, and hurry up over to the Marriott, as it appears that Micah and I will have about 3 to 4 hours to pack up the kitchen and the rest of Dani's and my clothing, medicines, and toiletries before we must check out of the hotel. Before Dr. Fero re-enters the room, Dani places a call to Dr. Christie's office and makes an appointment for Monday, May 12th. As Dr. Fero finally returns to the room, we both thank him for everything…with us both agreeing that he became our very favorite Hutch doctor very quickly!

With Dani's headache taking a brief back seat to the news of our rescheduled homecoming, we both are feeling pretty good! I think we float down the hill, instead of our usual method…walking! I stop at the registration desk of the Marriott, and inform the hotel manager that it looks as if we'll be leaving later this afternoon. She tells us not to rush… that we can take as long as we want to pack. She even agrees that Micah can park his car out front for the loading of cartons and luggage. There is not enough we can say about the personnel and the services provided by the Marriott Residence Inn at Lake Union. Everyday, they made sure that Dani was receiving the best of care. From the special housecleaning services offered as a result of Dani's illness and the general hospitality — which included daily breakfasts, mail delivery, pleasant conversations, weekly dinners sponsored by a local restaurant, and the use of the gym — to the shuttle service provided that took us (on "bad days" up the hill) to the Hutch, to the hospital, to downtown, and to frequent food shopping excursions, the Marriott took great care in ensuring that our only focus would be Dani's recovery. So we thank the manager and head up to our apartment.

We arrive back in our apartment around 2 p.m. Once there, Dani attempts to pack up her stuff, but the headache returns full force…so she heads to the sofa and attempts to relax. In the meantime, my job is to empty the kitchen cabinets, refrigerator, freezer, and pack up all the extra supplies we purchased to make our four month stay feel more like our home away from home. When Micah finally arrives, he is amazed by the things that we have amassed in the last four months. Before we finish packing, Micah actually makes three trips with his Jeep, 100% filled to capacity, from the Marriott to his office near Pikes Place Market. He now has box upon box filled with spices, canned foods, and boxes of pastas, cereals, cake mixes, and varieties of rice. Then there are all the unused frozen and refrigerated foods that I had previously purchased. Of course, I also had to buy some kitchen, laundry, and cleaning supplies as well for our stay…above and beyond what the Marriott already provided us. Among these extras are plastic containers, an electric mixer, spatulas, a blender, a cheese grater, a VCR along with many videotapes, and three laundry baskets. All these items quickly become part of Micah's stash. We laugh at the fact that Micah now has enough food and supplies to completely fill not one but three apartments! It takes me over 3 hours to pack up (for Micah's use) all the things we purchased to provide a comfortable home for Dani. Then it takes another hour to pack Dani's and my clothing, books, correspondence, art supplies, and knitting, as well as shower and prepare for our flight home. By the time Micah has returned from his third trip dropping off all of the supplies, I feel like a whirling dervish. It was about 6:30 p.m. when we finally leave the apartment, say goodbye to the hotel staff, and get into Micah's car. We decide to have a farewell dinner at Brooklyn, one of our family's favorite restaurants. It's a bittersweet time for the three of us. I'm not sure whether either Dani or I taste our dinner. Our joy of finally going home is mixed with the genuine sadness of leaving Micah and the warmth and security of Seattle. Additionally, the Marriott Residence Inn at Lake Union had done such a great job providing such a safe haven for Dani since her arrival to Seattle January 13th. Also, we have anxiety about Dani's future health and well-being as well as her present general weakness and frequent migraine headaches. But the Seattle Cancer Care Alliance and the specialists at the Hutch have agreed on this very day that Dani is ready to begin a new phase of her life. And they are the experts!

By about 8:30 that evening, Micah gets us to the airport. We check in with the appropriate airline, and the three of us share a group hug prior to Micah's departure. Dani and I then go through security, and walk to our flight's departure gate. Once there, Dani attempts to get comfortable by lying down...however...the headache still remains. About a half-hour before the departure, we enter the plane. I request some blankets and pillows for Dani (remember we have first class accommodations for this flight). I am virtually ignored by one flight attendant. When I make my requests known to another attendant, I am told that there are no pillows or blankets available. I'm astounded by this bit of news, but I don't want to make the situation any worse for Dani. She urges me to calm down.... that she'll be alright. It is difficult for me to honor this request when I see how uncomfortable she is. As the plane takes off, I try to do as much for Dani as I can...since it appears that the term "red eye" for this particular airline really means minimal service from the flight attendants. I watch Dani as she attempts to sleep...but it is a long bumpy flight home... symbolic, I guess, of Dani's struggle over the past eight months.

Chapter Thirteen
A New Beginning, a New Job, and New Struggles

For the next nine months of healing, Dani will experience both pain and great joy. Her headaches, joint pain, queasy stomach, anxiety, and rashes, we are told, are all a part of the healing process. The depression sneaks up on Dani without warning. What makes it worse is that she really doesn't discuss this overwhelming sadness openly. She fights being known as "the girl with cancer." Instead she puts on a brave smile and lets all know that everything is good now. She fears what can occur if her thoughts turn negative. This anguish causes more fear and sadness…and it continues until she begins to talk about it and write about it. As the months pass, she recognizes and accepts that this is not a perfect world…that sometimes bad things happen to good people. Once she accepts this as reality, she begins to effectively deal with the "hand she has been dealt."

As she regains her ability to focus not just on today but on her future as well, Dani truly recognizes and rejoices in the friendships that helped her heal, the love of family that never left her side, the positive actions of all who surrounded her, and the excitement of new challenges. In the next few months, she and Scott will begin to share a life together, celebrating every moment they are together. They begin to make a life for themselves as Scott says, "doing what we have to," always supporting one another. Medically, Dani grows up a bit and becomes proactive, seeking out answers on her own about her queasy stomach, exercise limitations and possibilities, sleeplessness and anxiety issues, fertility concerns, rashes, and the like. She also rises to accept a new challenge when she begins her new position as a Transition Coordinator…doing a job well…a job that she was never trained for.

Each day, Dani becomes stronger and stronger. There will be setbacks, but she now takes the time to learn how to confront and deal with each problem, one at a time. Friends continue to speak to Dani about her courage, but only a few of us truly understand her passion for life. As my formal note-taking ended on Friday afternoon, May 9th, 2003, the details of the next couple of years come from our family's collective memories, Dani's journal, and Dani's website.

5/10 – Day 92

After about the worst flight, accommodations, and flight crew we have ever experienced, an exhausted Dani and I finally arrive at Dulles Airport at 6:15 a.m. East Coast time (3:15 a.m. West Coast time). Jay and Dani's housemate, Matt, meet us there. Dani and I are so grateful to be home, that we quickly put aside the horrendous last 6 hours and focus on the two men by our sides. Scott had originally planned to be with us, but Dani told him earlier in the week that our return would be delayed by almost a week. So as a result, Scott decided to join his dad in visiting his ailing grandfather in Delaware for the weekend. The new plan now was for John to return Scott to our home in Gaithersburg later this afternoon. Scott and Dani will then spend the night with us before returning to Dani's place in Falls Church, Virginia.

May 12th – May 31st

I spend as much time as I possibly can with Dani on this first week home (just to be sure everything is okay). Appointments are scheduled and I accompany Dani to them. On Monday May 12th, Dani has an appointment scheduled with Dr. Christie. He is pleased to see her in such great shape…with her blood pressure and temperature normal, her neutrophil count at 5,000, and her platelet count at 140,000. He is so pleased that he tells Dani that he won't be doing a bone marrow biopsy or an endoscope any time soon. He suggests that she schedule her visits with him every 7 to 10 days. So she schedules her next appointment for

May 20th, gives him a hug, and says goodbye.

Two days later, Dani (with me dragging along behind her) heads to the Transfusion Department of Arlington Hospital and receives two bags of O Positive blood (as was recommended by the doctors at the Hutch in Seattle). It takes what seems forever (6 hours) for this process to be over. We bide our time by chatting (because we haven't seen enough of each other), reading, and watching television. While Dani naps, I knit and continue to count my lucky stars.

Today is May 18th…and the first 100 days post-transplant are now history. Those first 100 days were about recovery; the second 100 days will be about building strength physically and making the slow but steady climb back to relative normalcy. Dani's goal is to be back at work in September. Step by step, Dani is determined to reach that goal. So the tests will continue, as will the exercises, the carefully monitored nutrition plans, the medication dosages and fluid intake, and, the staying out of harms way in terms of infection. We now know that it will take about a year post-transplant for Dani's immune system to be back to where it was before those terrible days in early September 2002. She will even need to get her baby immunization shots all over again when she returns to Seattle for her one-year post-transplant check-up. What Dani needs now is lots of rest, some exercise, positive thinking, a bit of medication, weekly check-ups with Dr. Christie, some good judgment and common sense, and continued good wishes from all of her friends and family (which she continues to receive daily).

On May 19th I reluctantly return to work. I believe that both Dani and I suffer some separation anxiety, but we both recognize that this is just one more step to recovery. Newly independent Dani heads to Dr. Christie on her own on May 20th. Although Scott, Jay, and I are in contact by telephone with her quite a bit when we're not actually in her presence, Dani's independent nature slowly returns. This second week back home has been a relatively good one…devoid of any medical crises! During this week, Dani has had some additional tests done, and it appears that all is well with her GI tract (although Seattle will check the results to be sure). The continued annoyances at this point include the lingering puffiness and skin rashes (resulting from the steroids, which are still in her body), a bit of tummy discomfort, and waiting impatiently for her hair to reappear. But in the scheme of things, none of these are major issues. The best news is that life is boring at this point. When Dani can look forward to medical tests or a doctors appointment to get her out of the house, or even to help her roommate Lori write an I.E.P. (an individualized education plan) for a special needs student, you know that life is boring. But we agree that, at this time in many ways, boring is a whole lot better than exciting. With the drug-related attention deficits disappearing as well, our girl is back to reading real books again (but they have to be humorous or they don't make the list). She is feeling so good, that she and Scott decide to head south this weekend to visit with Scott's parents at their seaside retreat down in Norfolk, Virginia. It rains for most of the weekend, but that doesn't bother Dani in the least, as she can neither be in the sun nor go swimming at this point in her recovery. But the view is spectacular, and the company is even better…so the weekend is just perfect!

A well-rested and relaxed Dani receives her first IVIG since returning home on May 27th. I join her at Arlington Hospital for the procedure (just to keep her company). About 2 hours into the procedure, a very pleasant doctor stops by. He asks Dani how she is doing, and Dani says that she is doing quite well, thank you. He then hands her a Hershey's milk chocolate bar and departs. We both agree that this doctor has the bedside manner thing down pat!

As the rainy month of May (a record 24 out of 31 days of rain) finally comes to an end, Dani receives an e-mail on her web-site from a friend and work colleague that seems to sum up all of our feelings. He says, *"So, so, so happy to hear that things are slowly but surely getting better for you, Dani. You are truly a masterpiece and an inspiration!"*

June 2003

Dani announces to anyone who will listen today (June 1st) that she can see signs of wispy blond hair coming in on top of her head. She is quite relieved by this occurrence, as she was beginning to think that it would never reappear. Besides her weekly visits with Dr. Christie, Dani begins to pack up her things from her group house on Hillman St., in Falls Church, Virginia, for the move to an apartment about 1 mile away that both she and Scott will share. This is a huge step for the two of them. Their excitement can hardly be contained. July 1st is the date that they will make this move. However, the amount of packing that Dani can do is extremely limited, by an oddity. Dani's sweat glands don't seem to be working properly yet. For that reason, Dani cannot tell when she is overheated, and needs to drink a lot of water lest she become dehydrated. This problem keeps Dani not only from her exercise plans, which were designed for Dani by her SCCA physical therapist in Seattle, but also limits her "packing-up for the big move."

This strange and unexpected (by us) reaction to the transplant is quickly overshadowed by a major milestone. On Thursday, June 19th, Dani finally has her Groshong Catheter removed from her chest. Dani is now totally on oral medications, and hopefully these drugs will continue to be tapered throughout the summer. This is a major step in Dani's return to normalcy.

A few days later on June 22nd, just like normal times, we celebrate Dani's 27th birthday with a tea party at our home. Jay and I provide two very special surprise gifts for Dani, as Micah comes in from Seattle and Dani's Grandmom, Geri, visits from Del Ray Beach, Florida, to help celebrate Dani's big day. The day is perfect!

At the end of the month, Dani receives an e-mail from my former boss who herself is a cancer survivor. She passes on some wisdom as she says, *"Dani, I'm so glad to hear that things continue to go well for you. Progress seems slow at times, but if you glance backward, I'm sure you will see how very far you have come. Hang in there and keep moving toward your goals. With love and best wishes...."* It's like we've been saying to Dani all along...slow but steady wins the race.

July 2003

Today (July 1) Scott, Dani, and Phoebe (their Labrador Retriever) move into their new apartment in Falls Church. Their very cute one-bedroom apartment is on the first floor with a sliding door in the living room that opens to lovely common parkland. This will make it easier for both Dani and Scott to exercise Phoebe. They spend a lot of their spare time over the next two months getting their "first home" into shape. Getting into shape seems to be the vogue this summer, as Dani herself is doing the same thing!

At her appointment with Dr. Christie on July 9th, Dani receives great news. The doctor tells Dani that her hematocrit went up this week on its own (Yippee!), which generally means that Dani is producing red blood cells faster than they are being depleted. The medication that Dani is on tends to slow the development of new blood cells, so her hematocrit is normally supposed to slowly drop until it reaches the point where Dani would need a transfusion (which was tentatively scheduled for this week). So this is excellent news, as Dani would certainly like to avoid additional transfusions if she can. Dr. Christie cancels the planned transfusion. It is one more sign that Dani continues to stay on course. Dani reports to Dr. Christie that she is having good days along with some bad days, but she reports that the general trend is certainly on the positive side!

The very next day (July 10), Dani heads to Arlington Hospital Center for another IVIG. It lasts about 4-½ hours. Again, the same very pleasant doctor stops by and hands Dani another chocolate bar. Once more, we are so "impressed" with this doctor's kindness not to mention his treats. It's only when we receive the hospital bill for the services performed on IVIG infusion days that we realize just how "impressive"—not to mention costly—this brief visit and sweet gift actually was. Despite this dose of reality, this infusion of concentrated immunoglobulin invigorates Dani, which is the desired result of such a procedure.

Dani feels so good that she and Scott decide to go to the pool later on in the week. They have an easy walk to the pool. Scott places Dani under a large umbrella, as he goes into the pool for a dip. He is away from Dani no longer than 5 minutes. When he returns to Dani, he finds her with flushed skin and completely dehydrated and drained of energy. Scott thinks quickly and just about carries Dani back to their air-conditioned apartment, where he sits her down and gives Dani cool water to get her rehydrated. This appears to be another one of those bumps on the road to recovery. It seems the heat of the day, combined with Dani's inability to produce sweat that would cool her body, just about caused Dani some serious heat stroke. This condition lasts a few more months. Dani finds out later in the summer that one benefit of not sweating is that biting insects are not attracted to her, as she lacks any kind of scent! This is just another example of Dani's way of viewing life. We continue to be amazed by her talent for "making lemonade out of lemons!"

As each day passes, we see our Dani physically getting stronger and stronger. However, she never pretends that this recovery is a snap. We all can see our Dani struggling with her recovery…but she still chooses to live each day with a smile on her face. On rare occasions, she shares with us her anxieties and concerns. Mostly, she maintains a positive front…or so we think. In actuality, our Dani is experiencing mental, as well as the obvious physical, discomforts. She decides on her own (and without telling a soul) to keep a journal, in hope of purging these anxieties. For as Grandmom always says, "It's better out than in." (Dani doesn't share these entries with us until several months later, when she is feeling like her old self again.) Here is Dani's first journal entry, which she writes on July 26th:

I can go a whole week without a negative thought running through my head. Even through stomach aches, headaches, nausea and discomfort, I can stay positive. But when the depression hits, it hits hard! I think that this stuff must only happen to strong people. I don't know how a weak person could handle being sick for 10 months. My illness is no longer in my blood stream, and no one has to assist me out of bed or walk me to the bathroom. My sickness is sometimes in my belly, sometimes my head, and even sometimes my emotions. I don't want any of this to bother me. I want to put on my best face and walk out into the world, and say, "Look at me! I beat this thing!" But...I don't. I still...even with hair...don't feel beautiful. I still...even with most of the swelling gone...don't feel confident. I sometimes want all the attention and affection of the world, and at other times want everyone to just leave me alone. I want people to stop giving me pep talks. I'm allowed to be sad. My world has turned upside down. I was a special education teacher with a masters degree. I had parents of my students requesting me as their child's teacher a year before their children even entered the school system. I was so proud of myself. I was an athlete. I have pitched dozens of no-hitters. I made 1st Team Patriot League in my freshman year at Lafayette. I was so proud of myself. I used to walk into rooms and honestly believe that I was one of the most beautiful people there. I know that in the long term that means nothing...but...I've never ever lacked confidence. I never cried on a weekly basis. I never felt so needy, weak, and distanced from the world all at once.

I know there are people to talk to about all of this. In fact, I have spoken with quite a few. I am open to my doctors, my boyfriend, my parents, my friends...but the truth is...no one wants to hear that you are feeling down. The easiest and most accepted comment is... "I'm fine."

I'm sad and lost. I feel like my days are filled with mindless errands: packing, unpacking, e-mailing, working out, cooking, cleaning, meeting for lunch, playing with the dog, shopping, etc., etc., etc. I want to work. I want to feel like I make a difference. I want to come home and have a story about my day, whether good or bad. I know that all of this is coming in my future...but...I am losing patience, and becoming more and more frustrated all of the time.

I want the hair to stop growing on my back, my neck, my shoulders, my arms, my face, and my legs. I want to feel pretty and thin. I want people to approach Scott and tell him how pretty his girlfriend is. I know this is stupid...but...it's what I want! I don't want to feel like people know me before they meet me as "the girl with cancer."

I'm worried that I am pushing away one of the best things that ever happened to me (Scott) because my personality is currently hit or miss. I feel crazy sometimes. I feel out of my head.

I know that good things came out of this past year. I am closer to my brother than I have been in years. I re-established old and neglected friendships. In just one year, Scott and I know each other better than I have ever known anyone.

People call me "heroic." It's weird. I'm thankful for the lessons learned this year...but...I'm not thankful for the possibility of infertility in the future; and, I'm not thankful for the increased chances of getting another form of cancer. I know that my body can handle all of it. It has already been put to the challenge...but...that doesn't mean that I want to repeat this experience all over again! I want a baby! Not now...but I want one. I was meant to have a child. I will adopt and maybe even carry Scott's baby with some donor's eggs...but...I will never be able to look at my child and say, "he has my eyes," or "she has my lips," or even "he has my ugly feet!" It is not fair! I can't beat myself up for it, because that won't change anything...but...it is not fair. It is not fair. It is not fair. I want someone to wake me and tell me that this was all just a bad dream. I'm starting to lose faith in that as a possibility. This is my current reality, situation, and life. It is such a cliché...but...boy was I dealt a shitty hand.

And so...September is coming and so...yea...I get to go back to work. I'm trying to stay positive about it. I keep telling myself and others that it will be a good learning year for me. It'll be a lot of paper work... but...it will still be a good learning year for me. Bull shit! I went into teaching because I love children, and I knew that I could make learning fun, and because I knew that I did not want to sit in front of a computer and do paper work.

Maybe I should just be thankful for being alive. Maybe this all happened for a reason. But...I can't think of one good reason for this to happen to anyone. I still, to this day, look at people with cancer with sympathy until I remember that I myself have had it. I have survived it. I never thought while I was having heart palpitations, running high fevers, or vomiting that I wouldn't make it. I knew that I had to make it for my dad, my mom, Scott, my family, and my friends. I have already lost friends to disease. For those lost...I believe that I didn't do enough for them. I hope that all of my friends believe that they did enough for me. I hope that I will be able to pay them all back for a long time to come.

I wish someone could tell me on what days I would feel fine, and on what days I would feel like shit! I wish someone could tell me the exact day that all of this nonsense will leave my head, and I will go back to fun, sweet, sensitive Dani. I'm tired of being this other person. I don't recognize her, and she doesn't physically or spiritually fit my body.

Dani's second journal entry is written the day after we attend my father's Unveiling on July 27th (an Unveiling is a Jewish tradition when the family of a departed person gathers around his or her gravesite, uncovers the gravestone, and celebrates the memory through words and prayer). My dad had passed away during Dani's first week in Seattle over six months ago, and as a result of that, Dani was unable to attend his funeral. She never had a chance to say goodbye to her "Poppy." So this ceremony took on an even deeper meaning for Dani.

I went to Poppy's Unveiling yesterday. I guess it gave me closure to a certain extent. I imagine that he now knows that I'm okay. It is not fair that he passed on so worried about me. I just want to see him one more time to tell him that the engraftment took, that my donor had strong marrow, and that I will return to normalcy. I wish that I could communicate with him.

My Uncle Bruce opened up to me today. He told me that he distanced himself from me upon my return from Seattle because my physical features (i.e., swollen face) made him feel horrible. He thought that I was in a great deal of pain and he couldn't bear to see me suffer. He said it was "Too hard." Finally, somebody was honest with me. Everybody has been so busy telling me how strong I am, how great I look, and how much I have impressed them...that they haven't taken the time to be *honest. He then went on to tell me that now I look beautiful…*I believed him. *It took so much courage for him to tell me the negative, that now the positive comment must be true. Right? He also said, "Scott is some guy. He must be made of pure gold." I'm not sure that I've ever heard such an amazing compliment. Uncle Bruce surprised me with his words and actions today. It made me look forward to speaking to others, which hasn't been my thought for an awfully long time.*

Somehow journal writing has not had the positive impact that Dani was hoping for. She decides to share with Dr. Christie these concerns about her continuing migraines, anxiety, insomnia, anger, poor appetite, and general depression. He prescribes a mild anti-depressant for her. He says that these reactions are "par for the course," especially as she has recently been tapered off of prednisone and is currently being tapered off of Cyclosporin. He continues to be very optimistic about Dani's recovery. Although he says that she is certainly not ready to pitch a complete game on the softball diamond, things continue to go well, and the target is still to be back to work by September. He then adds that if the medication doesn't have the desired effect of easing these symptoms, then maybe she would want to see a psychiatrist. At this point, Dani declines, but recognizes that such a physician may need to be added to her long list of medical support in the future. Instead…after much searching, Dani finds a cancer survivor support group and begins to attend their monthly meetings.

August 2003

If it wasn't for some migraine headaches that haven't been pinned down as to the cause, Dani says that she would be feeling superb. She looks great (thick curly hair), is settled into her new place, and is looking forward to a new set of work experiences this coming year. In September, Dani will return to Arlington County Public Schools, not as a pre-school special education teacher, but as a Special Education Transition Coordinator. Dani will serve for the year as one of five Transition Coordinators for graduating special education students who need support transitioning to the (as Dani puts it) 'real world'. She will assist these students in the areas of further schooling, housing, and job procurement and training. Through attending meetings with these students, their parents, and other specialists, it will be Dani's responsibility to develop a transition plan in the student's Individualized Educational Plan. Dani will be working in the Arlington Education Center, so she will not be in daily contact with the "little ones" or their germs. Although she's sad about not being with her kids for another year, she is excited about the opportunity to rise to a new challenge (as if she hasn't been challenged enough in the past year). She's already had some ideas in her head about developing special programs for these transitioning students and their parents. Finally, she can get back into the "real world" as opposed to watching it on MTV! Jay puts out an all-points bulletin to his colleagues for special education resources that can help our early childhood special education-trained daughter with the transition services she will now provide to adolescent students with disabilities.

Dani is now six months post-transplant and everything continues on course. Medications continue to be slowly tapered, with an early October target for reaching the end of the Cyclosporin taper. Blood work is checked every two weeks, and she now sees Dr. Christie every three weeks. Dani will be getting her first round of immunizations ("baby shots") in February 2004, to continue on the road to building back her immunity to illness. She will go back to Seattle for her first annual checkup in early February. All things considered…a very good place to be compared to where she was 11 months ago.

Scott is also in a good place! Right now, he is planning for another gathering of the "Friends of Dani" to participate in the Washington D.C. Light the Night Walk for the benefit of the Leukemia and Lymphoma Society. He passes along an email he hopes will reach all those whose positive spirit surrounded Dani during the past year. His hope is that the "Friends of Dani" group will be one of the largest walking together on October second.

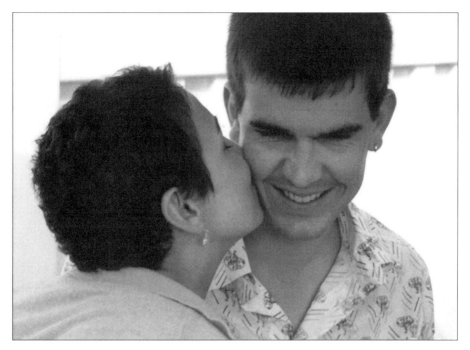

Check out the curly dark hair!

Looking at Dani, with that thick dark curly hair, the cute little pixie face returning to normal size, and the continuous smile on her face, you would think that this world is a pretty sunny place. Unfortunately at this time, she is hiding some dark thoughts. Dani's third journal entry on August 20th focuses on death.

I think I forget sometimes that people can die from cancer. I don't ever remember feeling close to death during the past year. Even though Rob [longtime camp friend] and Mona [Dani's friend Ally's mom] both passed away from the disease recently, I never really thought much about death or dying. However, this month one of the women in my cancer support group died. I attended two sessions with Patricia. She told us that she had an understanding with God and was prepared for death. She had suffered twice from breast cancer and in her last days developed brain tumors. I'm really not sad for her as I'm sure she's finally at peace. But the mere thought of death as a result of a cancer is completely terrifying to me.

September 11, 2003 (Day 216)

Still completely unaware of the depth of Dani's depression, we mutually agree to have a rather odd celebration. Dani has decided that this September 11th and every subsequent September 11th (the date of Dani's Acute Mylogenous Leukemia diagnosis one year ago), she will demonstrate to everyone that she is really BACK! She has decided to co-host (along with her partner Scott) a special dinner party. She invites John and Gayle and Jay and myself. Unfortunately John is unable to join us…so it becomes just the five of us for dinner. Dani prepares a delicious dinner, sets a beautiful table, and adorns their apartment with lovely floral arrangements to add to the celebration.

In the meantime, I've been in contact with a few of Dani's friends…and they have come to the conclusion (along with my input) that a quiet little dinner party just won't do. They want to be part of the celebration. So we secretly plan for them to drop by Dani and Scott's place after Dani's planned dinner party. I decide not to tell Scott (I came to regret this decision very quickly), as I really don't want to take any chances that Dani would suspect anything out of the ordinary occurring tonight.

So after the five of us finish a lovely dinner, we head into the living room where we chat and listen to some music. All of a sudden, there is a banging at Dani and Scott's front door. Phoebe is barking wildly as Scott opens the door. Into the room burst six very important "Friends of Dani!" Sandy D, Liz, Ryan and Ally, Marissa, and Yvonne surprise Dani with balloons, confetti, silly gifts, and lots of laughter. Dani has a grin from ear to ear and, after a few moments of stunned silence, runs to embrace the group. Scott remains standing at the door as if in a state of shock. Tonight I learn that my daughter's boyfriend Scott really, really, really doesn't like surprises! Scott eventually closes the door and joins the party that is already taking place in the living room. The celebration continues for about an hour…and then we all hug, say, goodbye to one another, and plan to have many, many more celebrations.

Sept. 12 – 30, 2003

Today the *Potomac Almanac* runs a follow-up article to the one that was published about one year ago, regarding Dani's illness and the subsequent bone marrow drives. Both Dani and Scott are interviewed for this article. Their love, devotion to each other, and positive outlook for Dani's future is quite apparent in this excerpt:

DANI'S TEAM CELEBRATES – *(Potomac Almanac)* - *9/17/03*
By Ari Cetron

Dani Shotel has two birthdays. The 1994 graduate of Wootton High School was born in June, 27 years ago. But her bone marrow transplant took place in February. "Next birthday I'll be one year old," Shotel said... Her donor was found in Germany... "My only match," Shotel said. Donor regulations prohibit Shotel from contacting the donor for two years after the procedure...but Shotel plans to contact him as soon as possible. "I want to thank him," she said. Shotel needed to take some time off in order to have the transplant and received help from her colleagues in Arlington Public Schools. "I had over 100 days of sick leave donated to me," Shotel said. Once the match was found, Shotel went to the Fred Hutchinson Cancer Research Center in Seattle to undergo the transplant, because they have experience with Shotel's specific condition. "We weren't a perfect match," she said. One major problem was that she had a different blood type than her donor so special precautions had to be taken to ensure that her body did not reject the stem cells from the marrow of the donor. "I was O positive, now I'm A positive," Shotel said. After the procedure, Shotel experienced minor complications from graft-versus-host-disease, sometimes called GvHD. "Your body needs to accept the donor cells, but it's fighting the donor cells," Shotel said. In her case, the GvHD manifested as a rash. While there are no longer visible symptoms, Shotel still tests positive for the illness. "It's actually good to have a little," Shotel said. A mild case of GvHD is actually considered a good sign, since it means that the patient's immune system is functioning.

"I think she's the epitome of how they want you to be," said Scott Greene, Shotel's boyfriend. Motivated by his girlfriend's illness, Greene is managing the Friends of Dani team in the annual Light the Night Walk, sponsored by the Leukemia and Lymphoma Society. Last year, Dani's team raised approximately $800. For this year Greene hoped to exceed that mark. (Dani's team actually has so far raised over $3,000 for this year's Light the Night Fundraiser.) Last year, Shotel had been diagnosed just before the walk and couldn't take part, but this year she looked forward to walking with her team and easily completed the three mile course. Dani has returned to work, although in a different capacity than before her transplant. "[The school system] really made it so I could come to work every day," Shotel said. Shotel's immune system is compromised as a result of the heavy chemotherapy she had prior to the transplant, and is unable to have the vaccinations necessary to work with children. As a result, Shotel has been working as a transition coordinator, assisting young adults with disabilities as they integrate into the community.

Next February, one year after the transplant, she will be able to get the necessary shots and resume working with children, which she plans to do at the start of the 2004-05 school year. Shotel believes that her experience working with young adults with disabilities can help her when she deals with parents whose children who have recently been diagnosed with a disability. "I think it will help me a lot in my discussions with parents," Shotel said. "I can tell them there is hope."

October 2003

On a beautiful, clear-skied, warm, just perfect Thursday, October 2nd evening, about 40 "Friends of Dani" gathered on Wilson Plaza to participate in the Leukemia and Lymphoma Society's Washington D.C. Light the Night Walk. These good people…Dani's friends as well as ours…represent a small cross-section of those who supported us during this last year. A few of us remember the very same walk held one year ago in the same location. Scott, Micah, and Matt Levine walked that evening in the icy cold rain. The three later returned to Dani's hospital room totally drenched, holding a couple of limp balloons and a very damp "Friends of Dani" banner. Jay, Dani, and I were so very proud of the commitment and love they showed to Dani that night. They walked that evening...despite the weather conditions. They walked for Dani. Tonight we will not only walk for Dani, we'll walk for everyone afflicted with these dreaded diseases. We'll walk for them...and we'll hope for a cure. We'll walk with thousands of people tonight....we're walking with the millions who complete this walk every year in support of this cause.

We were able to find that very same banner, and each of us took turns walking in front of our group holding the banner. I can't remember an evening where I felt prouder of my daughter, her boyfriend, and all of her friends. And the truth is...I can't remember an evening when my daughter looked happier.

That Sunday night (October 5th) was the eve of the Jewish High Holy Day, Yom Kippur. Yom Kippur is known as the Day of Atonement for Jewish people all over the world. On the evening before the holy day begins, families get together and go to synagogue to pray for forgiveness for acts committed during the past year, and also pray for a peaceful new year. Scott and Dani join us that evening and together the four of us go to our synagogue, Temple Beth Ami. The service is beautiful, and Dani is even more so! After the service is completed, Rabbi Luxemburg rushes over to Dani and embraces her. What he says to her at that moment is unforgettable. We all smile with his words, and agree with him completely. In fact, I come home that evening and copy down his words in a little notebook that I keep on the book shelf by my bed.

It is actually the first and probably the last time that I will write in this small notebook. The very next morning Dani uses her journal one final time to transcribe the very same blessed message of our rabbi. She writes:

Last night (October 5th) at the conclusion of Erev Yom Kippur [the eve of Yom Kippur] *services, Rabbi Jack greeted me by hugging me and saying, "It's good to know a miracle!"*

It is my belief that Dani's journal has finally served its' purpose!

Christmas Day 2003 – Day 321
On Christmas Eve, Dani becomes ill with severe stomach pains, diarrhea, and vomiting. These pains have continued throughout the night and into Christmas morning. After speaking with Dr. Christie, an alarmed Scott follows the doctor's advice and brings Dani to the hospital. So early on this special morning, instead of celebrating their first Christmas together in their own home, Scott brings Dani to the Emergency Room at Arlington Hospital where she is immediately attended to. The staff in the Emergency Room hook Dani up to an IV solution that will aid in hydrating her. For the next few hours the attendants monitor her vitals, and make sure that Dani is able to eat without the previous night's symptoms continuing. Jay and I arrive at the hospital and sit with Dani for a couple of hours, until the staff is satisfied that Dani's condition has improved and that she does not need to be admitted to the hospital. At this point, Dani is wished a Merry Christmas and released from the ER. Later on in the day, the four of us agree that Dani and I will return to Dani and Scott's apartment so that Dani can rest, while Jay will accompany Scott and go to John and Gayle's home to join the Greene family for Christmas supper. We're sad that we can't all be together for this Christmas, but we all also know that the greatest gift any of us can receive is Dani's complete recovery. So, as a group, we practice patience.

January 31, 2004 – Day 359
Since Dani won't be home for her one-year post-transplant anniversary (which Dani now calls her new "birthday"), she decides to organize a celebration a week early. She chooses the Clarendon Ballroom for her pre-birthday celebration, as it is a smoke-free environment. Approximately 25

"Friends of Dani" join Dani and Scott for this special celebration. I don't think any of us will ever get tired of celebrating Dani's good health. At last count, we have three Dani special celebrations a year: her real birthday on June 22nd, her September 11th celebration of no longer having leukemia, and her February 7th celebration of being given a new life!

February 2004

Scott, Dani, Jay, and I arrive in Seattle on February 1st. We have decided to join Dani for her one-year post-transplant check-up. Micah has offered us the use of his apartment, as it is located conveniently in downtown Seattle (near Pike's Place Market and his business office, the home of the graphic design company he and two college roommates started several years prior: {Nsurgents}), as well as pretty close to the Hutch. The apartment is pretty tiny…hardly enough space for our son and his cat, Teka…so Jay and I stay nearby in the new Marriott right on Elliott Bay while Dani and Scott stay at the Ace Hotel, a European style boutique hotel that Micah has recommended. At 7:45 a.m. on the second of February, Jay and I pick up Dani and Scott and head to the Hutch, where Dani will undergo her first series of appointments that are all part of her one-year check-up. I actually get back into the swing of things, and for the first time in months take notes today, although they will be the last notes of medical exams that I'll take for Dani. She and Scott have become pretty self-sufficient and are managing her care quite well.

We arrive at the Hutch at 8 a.m. February 2nd and Dani heads to the first floor clinic for her blood draw. There, as usual, she is warmly greeted by the same nurses and technicians who saw her so frequently nine months ago. Once the blood draw is completed, Dani heads upstairs to the Pulmonary Department to get her chest X-rayed. Then, she is off to another cubby for the dreaded bone marrow biopsy. What a day!

We then go to the sixth floor for Dani's meeting and physical exam with Dr. Mary Flowers, who heads the Transplant Follow-up Program of the SCCA. Dr. Flowers briefly reviews Dani's medical history and then it is Dani's turn to talk. She openly speaks to Dr. Flowers about her depression, fatigue, lack of perspiration, shortness of breath at times, decreased appetite, and difficulty sleeping. Dr. Flowers nods in understanding, saying, "You look great. The first year is so hard as you are redefining who you are." She also comments that all of these symptoms are very common to survivors of Acute Mylogenous Leukemia. She then asks Jay and Scott to leave the room so that she can physically exam Dani. On the spot, Dani performs a miracle by undressing and donning a hospital gown without baring any skin! The three of us share a laugh at such a feat.

During the exam, Dani informs Dr. Flowers that there is no history of breast or colon cancer in our family. Dr. Flowers suggests that Dani have a mammogram when she returns to Virginia. The two of them then discuss gynecological matters. Dr. Flowers informs Dani that she will need to decide what form of hormone replacement to use, as she believes that all forms of hormone replacement carry risks; but she suggests that Dani discuss this matter directly with her gynecologist in Virginia (who works with cancer survivors). She is pleased that Dani continues to maintain her menstrual cycle…but she believes that Dani should go off of the birth control patch completely for two months to see if her menstrual cycle returns naturally. She is quite direct with Dani regarding her ability to naturally conceive a child, telling Dani that the Busulfan chemotherapy protocol, which Dani underwent to save her life, is quite sterilizing. This "no-holds barred" conversation about Dani's predicted inability to conceive continues to be quite painful to both of us. Although I know that Dani is hearing what Dr. Flowers is saying and respects her breadth of knowledge…I also know that she will still want to consult further with fertility specialists back in Virginia…because Dani continues to believe in miracles.

The exam continues. Dr. Flowers recommends that Dani see a psychiatrist for her symptoms of depression. She also prescribes some ointment for skin GvHD; reminds Dani to take her daily multi-vitamin, calcium, and Vitamin D; and suggests that Dani eat little meals often each day. Dr. Flowers again repeats to Dani that she is so happy to see that

Dani has made such progress in her recovery. The doctor then proceeds to list the reasons for her positive outlook. The first reason is that Dani is now off of all medications except for calcium and a multivitamin. The second reason is that Dani's new blood system seems to be working really well. Although Dani still has some mild symptoms of graft vs. host disease (GvHD), her doctors on both coasts have agreed to "wait it out" and see if her own immune system can work out the continuing process of her new blood system getting to know her original equipment body. We are once again told that a little bit of GvHD is a good thing because it shows that Dani's new immune system is functioning well. Our German donor's bone marrow and Dani's body seem to have gotten along famously. The third reason is that Dani's bone marrow is perfect; her blood counts are perfect, her bone density is normal, and it seems that our German friend even transferred a certain amount of his immunity to disease to her, so she will more than likely not need a second round of immunizations. With the exam over, Dani thanks Dr. Flowers for her care and tells her that she'll see her again next year!

Today, February 3rd is the day that Dani has dreaded for over one year. For today, she is scheduled to receive her "baby shots." Just like other 1-year-olds, Dani has to get a set of immunizations. In total, she receives six immunization shots in various parts of her body and, along with the bone marrow biopsy on Monday, Dani is quite ready for Tylenol and some well-deserved rest by Tuesday night. Dani seems to be having a reaction to the anti-pneumonia shot she received earlier in the day, as her right thigh (place where she received the needle) is quite sore. Despite this new pain, Dani sleeps through the night and some of the following day. The miracle of Tylenol! Dani is two days away from her first birthday after transplant, and today (February 5th) she finished her one-year check-up at the Hutch. All of the medical tests have proven to be normal, and although she has lost a few pounds since her upset stomach episode over Christmas, the doctors are confident that lots of smaller meals and regular exercise will bring the appetite back and gradually increase Dani's overall stamina.

For the past three-and-a-half days Dani has been poked and prodded. What we have all learned is that Dani's life after the bone marrow transplant is very different from the life and day-to-day routines experienced prior to her illness. In many ways Dani, in this first year post-transplant, has experiences just like that of a newborn baby, who needs lots of rest, nutrition, and nurturing to grow and maintain its health. Every day Dani is a step closer to resuming her daily routines, doing the things she used to take for granted. Today her appreciation of these ordinary experiences has changed significantly. There is no question that the events of the past year have had their impact on Dani, but fortunately for all of us she hasn't lost the sweet "Dani-isms" we love so much.

On the evening of February 6th, just a few hours before Dani, Scott, Jay, and I leave Seattle, we have a celebration of sorts at Micah's office (we have decided that his apartment is way too small to contain the festivities). Dani, Scott, Micah, Jay, and I are joined by a couple of Micah's friends, as well as Tiffany and her mom (who are also in town for Tiffany's one-year post-transplant check-up). Together we celebrate Dani and Tiffany's "birthdays." The evening ends early, as tomorrow is a travel day for at least six of us.

February 7th finally arrives, the one-year anniversary of Dani's successful bone marrow transplant. Dani and Scott arrive home from Seattle today. Exhausted, Dani rests up. Some birthday! Dani will return to work on Monday. Her continuing goal is to be back in a direct instructional role next fall with the kids she loves, and as of right now that goal appears to be a reasonable one. With a little luck, lots of love, lots of prayers, and the best of care, every day seems a bit brighter. Happy Birthday, Dani. Here's to many, many more!

Chapter Fourteen
Life Goes On: February 2004 to June 2005

Winter 2004

The reader might remember that way back on December 6th, 2002, we were informed by Colleen Duffy, the Search Coordinator for Unrelated Transplants at the Seattle Cancer Care Alliance, that an acceptable match had been found for Dani. A 30-year-old German male matched on 9 of 10 characteristics, with the mismatched characteristics not sufficient to eliminate the donor. Although we didn't know it at that time, Dani's one match in the entire world was Thomas Heimhuber from Munich, Germany. The rules with regard to protecting both the donor and the patient's identity are very specific. When the donor is from another country, the rules of that country apply. For instance, in the United States, if both parties agree, direct contact between the donor and the recipient can be made after one year. But in Germany there is a two-year waiting period. We are told by the Transplant Center not to get our hopes up too high, because approximately one-third of all donors prefer to remain anonymous. It takes Dani approximately one year to find the words to thank her donor.

Today, February 23rd, 2004, a few days past the one-year post-transplant anniversary, and with a lot of nagging by her parents (okay... by me), Dani finally completes her letter of thanks to her donor. Her letter is sent through the Seattle Cancer Care Alliance Transplant Center, where it is screened to ensure that there is no identifying information included in it. Responses are dealt with in the same manner. So Dani's donor is known as Donor URD, DEAKB 117626 and Dani is Recipient # 42319. She sends it to the attention of the Search Coordinator (Colleen Duffy). This is the only communication allowed at this time. Both parties are to remain anonymous to one another for at least another year. Dani knows, that under German regulations, she cannot communicate as Dani Rebecca Shotel with her donor until two years post-transplant...and then only if the donor wishes to be known. So at this time, she writes:

February 23, 2004

Dear? [She did not know her donor's name]

Location: Somewhere in Germany!
It has been a little over a year since the day that I received your bone marrow. It has also been a little over a year for me to be able to even try to write this letter. I have no idea what to say, how to thank you, explain to you what a miracle gift you gave me, or even try to explain my fears of the transplant combined with my total respect of you. You saved my life. You gave me a gift that is nearly impossible to give. A day doesn't go by where I don't thank god for your existence. I don't even know who you are, but my blood sure does.

I have done so well since the transplant. Your marrow was some of the strongest that my transplant team has ever seen! I'm currently back at work. I have begun to get back into an exercise routine. I just got a new dog with my boyfriend. I have started painting again. You have started a new life for me. Thank you.

I hope that one day I will be able to meet you. I will travel to Germany if you will allow for that to happen. Until then I will continue to appreciate my mystery superhero from Germany. You gave a gift that is neither forgettable nor duplicable.

Respectfully yours,
Dani

After sending this note to Colleen Duffy at the SCCA Transplant Center, Dani will now have to wait at least a year for a response, if her donor decides to correspond with her. It's a good thing that Dani has inherited her father's patience!

In March 2004, as a result of Dr. Flowers' suggestion, Dani reluctantly makes an appointment to see a psychiatrist; but when she finally has her appointment, and after she tells the doctor her story, she decides that this is not for her, so she leaves before her hour is even up. At that moment, she decides to find another support group instead.

Dani feels so much better at this time, that she decides that maybe she can offer her fast pitch softball pitching prowess to assist the coach of the local high school fast-pitch softball team. As her place of employment, Arlington Education Center is right next door to Washington and Lee High School, Dani contacts the softball coach and offers this expertise. For a couple of hours a week during the spring of 2004, Dani works with the junior varsity and varsity pitchers. Slowly but surely the love of the game returns. She enjoys herself so much that she agrees that during the spring and summer she will join the coed slow pitch team that Scott plays on. She continues to be very careful as she actively participates in the games, since she is not in her prime physical shape. Besides that, Dani is still not sweating. But by just having the opportunity to participate in a team sport her spirits are lifted.

As the summer of 2004 begins, Dani's sweat glands start working again. Although the good news is that she is returning to her normal pre-leukemia self, the bad news is that, despite using "acceptable" insect repellents, Dani does get mosquito bites. And every time she gets a mosquito bite, the bite gets infected. So at this point in her recovery, Dani needs to go to her primary care physician to get a cortisone shot every time she gets a bug bite.

After a pretty uneventful summer, Dani returns to teaching in the fall. Because the developmentally disabled 2-year-olds are medically considered a bit dangerous for Dani's developing immune system (because of live virus vaccinations they receive at this stage of their young lives), she "graduates" to teaching a pre-kindergarten special needs program at a different school, Jamestown Elementary. Dani thrives on the trials and tribulations of her new charges. The parents of her students are provided with some information about Dani's illness and her continuing recovery. Despite this news, Dani's new students and their parents can't help but fall in love with Dani's enthusiastic, positive approach to teaching.

Unfortunately the quote "into each life, a little rain must fall" is fulfilled, as Jay's mom and Dani and Micah's beloved Philly Mom-Mom passes away in October. Our family and friends are all deeply saddened to lose this wonderful, enthusiastic, joyous, and loving little lady. Yet, at her funeral, and even today with every mention of her, a smile comes to our faces. There is no question that Dani often demonstrates traits similar to those of her Philly Mom-Mom. Dani's positive attitude, work ethic, and general disposition, not to mention her somewhat quirky taste in clothing, have all been influenced by this special lady.

Medically, Dani develops a mystery bronchial cough this fall. Originally we think maybe it's an allergy like hay fever or something. But this dry cough doesn't go away despite the allergy medications. It appears as if no one is able to figure out just what is causing this cough. Visits to all kinds of doctors and subsequent testing follow but nothing seems to work very well. Besides seeing her primary care physician, Dani also visits with a pulmonary specialist, a gastroenterologist, and an ear, nose and throat specialist, but the coughing continues day and night. This cough causes Dani some difficulty sleeping as well as producing a sore throat. All of these conditions two years ago would have been considered a minor nuisance, but today they only serve to makes us all quite nervous.

Despite the cough, we all manage to get through the holiday season. Jay and I even get to join the Greenes and Dani and Scott for Christmas Eve dinner. We're all breathing a bit easier this year. It looks as if we all will get our wish...good health and lots of love for the new year.

Winter 05

On Valentines Day of 2005 Dani and Scott become engaged...finally!

The special guy Dani started dating three months before she was diagnosed, and who thereafter worked tirelessly to support her, commuted to Seattle to be with her, and stuck with her through this long, tough road, is joining the family, and we are all very excited.

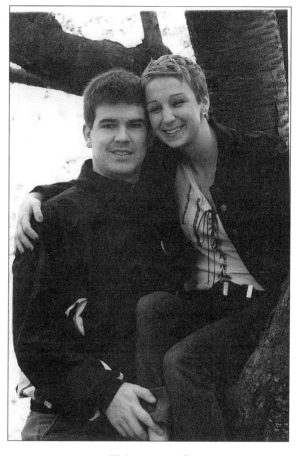

Spring 2005

It is March 2005, a little over two years post-transplant, and Dani schedules her visit to Seattle during her school spring break. Scott and Dani head

We're engaged!

west to the Seattle Cancer Care Alliance one more time, while Jay and I stay at home in Maryland this time, and look forward to continuing good news. For some reason, Dani's cough disappears during the Seattle two-year check-up. The news is, indeed, good, and Dani is told that her next visit will be at the five-year mark, when The Hutch will consider Dani completely cured.

Upon her return from Seattle, the cough returns. One highlight that comes to mind is the Passover Seder that Carol and Bruce have at their home with their kids and grandkids and Dani, Scott, Jay, and me. Throughout the entire Seder, during the reciting of the Passover story, the songs, the traditional multi-course Seder meal, as well as the "family time" post dinner, Dani's cough is non-stop. Although our worrying about this condition never really stops, we come to accept the cough as part of what happens to a person's body after he or she has a bone marrow transplant. Some days, there is no cough, and then there are other days when it seems continuous. Dani, in the meantime, continues to visit with various doctors to determine the cause of this nemesis and find a way to stop the cough.

As the weather warms and the flowers begin to bloom, Dani receives an incredible gift in the mail. We didn't know how long it would take for Dani's "thank you" note (which she sent in February 2004) to get to her donor. But once the two-year time limit has passed (February 2005), Dani is finally able to find out who her donor is only if the donor agrees to be identified. Days and then months pass…we hear no word from the Hutch's Transplant Center in regard to the donor. We have almost all given up hope of ever communicating with him when, in early May 2005, Dani receives a legal-sized manila envelop from the Hutch.

Chapter Fifteen
Tom

May 2005

On May 2, 2005, Dani receives a very large envelope from the Search Coordinator at the Hutch. It contains two letters. The first letter is correspondence from Colleen Duffy of the Transplant Center, and it contains both congratulations and a well-deserved apology. The congratulatory part of the letter states that her donor has given permission for Dani to contact him directly. The apology stems from the fact that her donor had actually written a letter to Dani in December 2004, but the letter was never forwarded to Dani. This following letter is also enclosed in that very large envelope from the Hutch.

December 2004
Germany

Dear ? [Tom had not been given Dani's name yet either]

When getting mail from the hospital with your letter inside, I was really nervous. I didn't know anything about the transplantation...if it was good for you or not. And after I had read your letter — wow — I was so happy to know that you are fine. All the time I kept my fingers crossed for you, and it worked... Yippee!

But please, I'm no hero or something else, just another guy, that's it (I hope, that this is not disappointing for you now). And it wasn't me that started a new life for you, that was and still is your job and you hopefully made it. There was just a little push from me, nothing more. The hero is you. I wish you all the best. And if you want to come to

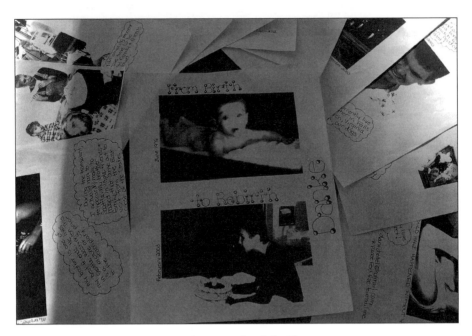

Dani's picture book for Tom

Germany, feel free to do this whenever you want to — next year, in two years, in five years... I don't mind. It's your decision, take your time. But it would be an honor for me to meet you.

I wish you, the people you love and your dog a happy new year, much time and many, many days still to come and to enjoy.
Best regards from a German guy

Dani follows up quickly with a second letter, her contact information, a booklet made up of pictures, and a brief summary of her young life. Dani does not hear back from him right away, so Jay attempts to call the phone number in the contact information but is not successful in reaching the donor.

After what seems to be an eternity, on Monday August 8, 2005, Dani receives her first e-mail from Donor URD, DEAKB 117626 (or as we've come to call him...Tom).

From: Thomas
To: Dani Shotel
Date: Mon, 08 Aug 2005 17:54:54 +0200

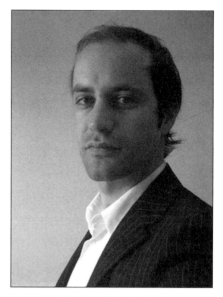

Thomas Heimhuber

Hi Dani!

First of all, I'm sorry that I did not reply to your dad's phone call. The problem is: I can't find the number any more that he gave me... and as it was a very busy time for me during the last two months, I didn't put much effort in getting it again. But last week, I received your wonderful picture book and I am so happy to see that you are feeling fine. I was wondering quite often how you are and if everything is ok with you, and of course, whenever possible, I would like to accept your invitation (if you did not marry already). You just have to tell me in advance about the date and the location where I shall come.

...Well, the reason, why I really had a lot to do the last months, was because I moved from Munich to London and to manage all the stuff (looking for a flat, handle all the furniture and the things that I accrued the last few years in my old Munich flat, talk to the insurance companies, talk to the government, write to the health services, organize a good-bye-party... blah, blah, blah...) took me a lot of time. Now I have done the major tasks and I am able to relax a little bit; and if you have a look at my website, you can find my address and phone number that I use currently (and also a few pictures of me ;-) and in terms of university and companies that I have worked for you also can find information there. But I think, that is only the official part of my life and therefore maybe a little bit boring. On the other hand, I cannot tell you about hobbies or something like that, because I do not have specific ones. I *like everything (almost!).*

For example things that I have never done before, or things that simply allow me to enjoy the moment...like drinking a cappuccino in a cafe and having a look at people, talking to people (especially to those I like), making a breakfast; a heavy beer drinking afternoon (as happened last weekend); traveling (to Asia or just to the next village), driving, skiing, open water diving, reading, listening to music (music is the best invention man has made), watching TV.... So everything I just would like to do that specific moment. Often I don't know what I would like to do next. I rarely have plans...so sometimes I just do nothing (or wash the dishes and clean up my flat, but that does not happen too often).

Maybe that's it...why I became a donor...it was around 1997 or 1998 when my sister and her boyfriend had an accident with his motorcycle; fortunately both recovered completely but particularly for my sister's boyfriend the situation was quite serious. During the time he was in the hospital, my mother and I read an article in the newspaper about a little girl that needed bone marrow... and so we decided spontaneously to offer ours (unfortunately it didn't match hers). My blood or the data about my blood was recorded into a database. I forgot all about this.... My sister married another man and someday in November or December 2002 my mother gave me a phone call "Hello Tom," she said, "Your bone marrow is needed, you have a matching person! There's a letter." At first I didn't really know what she was talking about, but then I remembered... Well, then I gave the doctor a call, the doctor came to my flat, got some blood out of me (a lot of blood and that before I had my first coffee of the day)...phew!

Weeks later, they told me, that you are able to handle my kind of blood or marrow if I am still willing to donate. "Yes, of course," I said. So I had to go to the hospital for a detailed checkup of my health constitution. It appeared that I was ok. They chose me as donator and that's it! I spent the donation act under general anesthesia, so I cannot tell you anything about this. The only thing is that they took the marrow from my pelvis with thick needles. I was just able to walk with some difficulties ;-). After three days, I was allowed to leave the hospital (in the meantime I could walk almost normally) and to continue my life. That was the day I started to wonder: Did this reach you (it was a really snowy day. The night before the operation, there had been a heavy snow fall so the anesthetist was late. The doctor was getting really nervous. Could you need this? Does this work? .... So for me this was not nearly as difficult as for you. I cannot imagine what you had to stand, what your feelings have been, of what you were thinking all the time

...So, please, I am not the hero. You are the hero (but you know this already). I even received a gift from the hospital: a watch (not really nice), and a certificate. They also paid for one dinner with my girl friend I had during this time.

I really hope to hear or read from you and I wish you all the best....

Have a nice day ;-)

Tom

Dani shares her e-mail with us, and makes Jay and I promise that we won't contact Tom until she writes him back (which she does quite quickly...for Dani)!

Dear Tom,

It was so great to receive your email. I had been slightly worried that you never received my booklet. Fortunately, the postal service seems reliable enough to even track you down in London, England. How exciting for you! That seems like a pretty big move. I assume that the rest of your family is still in Germany. I actually spent some time in London a couple of summers ago. I taught in a program called Intern Exchange International. The program basically took 17-year-olds from America and placed them into Internship Programs in London. I worked with a group of 17- year-olds that were interested in Special Education. They interned in the schools there, and then attended a seminar that I had to teach. It was an amazing experience. Although I haven't traveled nearly as much as you have, London was one of my favorite places to visit. There was a bar in Soho, called "Lab" that I made nightly visits to.

Lately, my traveling has pretty much been between here and Seattle (where I had my transplant). Scott and I are actually on holiday right now on the beach in Virginia. His parents have a home here.

We've had some pretty exciting times within the last couple of months. Besides planning a wedding, we have recently bought a home (a "flat" in your terms). We actually will move in to it in about a week. Scott recently was called upon to be a bone marrow donor as well. Fortunately for him, this patient was able to use stem cells rather than bone marrow, which appeared to be a less intense process. It only took about 6 hours, and he was able to leave the hospital that same day. However, he did not receive a watch from the hospital!

It seems as though everything happens for a reason. If it weren't for your sister's accident (which I was so sorry to hear about), you may never have been on the registry. Then I would have never had a match to save my life. If it weren't for me getting sick, Scott would have never been on the registry, and this other woman who matched him would have never been given the opportunity to continue her life. It's truly amazing how strangers can save strangers and not think twice about it.

This may seem like a slightly bizarre question, but do you have any Jewish lineage? I am Jewish and I know that most of these "bone marrow matches" occur based upon your heritage. I'm just curious....

Our wedding is scheduled for Sunday, 9 October 2005. I know that you enjoy traveling, so if you wanted to make a trip here, we would love to have you. However, if it is not possible we are extremely excited about you living in London and would love to make it there at some point. But, if your schedule is free and this interests you, I know that my parents would love to pick up the expenses of your flight and hotel for the weekend. Also, if you would like to come a couple of days prior to the wedding, you would certainly have a place to stay with Scott and me. No pressure...but we wanted to extend the invitation. One last thing...I greatly enjoyed perusing your website. It sounds as though you are a very determined individual. I greatly enjoyed looking at your photographs as well. It looks as though you have quite an artistic interest as well.

Love always,
Dani

PS. My parents will be sending you a wedding invitation by mail, and I'm sure they'll also contact you by email regarding wedding plans. Again, please feel no pressure in attending the wedding. I know that in starting a new job, it may be difficult to find time to get away. Of course we would love to have you!

At this point, Jay and I can no longer contain ourselves. We begin corresponding with Tom as well. I thought that Tom needed to know a bit more about Dani. Below is an excerpt:

Subject: thank you and more
Date: 8/11/2005 2:26:45 PM Eastern Daylight Time
From: Sue Shotel
To: Thomas Heimhuber

Hi! I'm Dani's mom...and have been looking forward for over 2 years to have the opportunity to thank you for saving my daughter Dani's life. I hear that I might have that opportunity to hug you in person in October...but for now this e-mail will have to do. Your kindness exceeds you being 'one in a million' because you actually were one in eight million!!!!

I thought that maybe this e-mail could tell you a bit more about Dani, her family, and what brought you two together. As you already know, Dani is a delight! She is beautiful both inside and out. All through school, her teachers recognized this and always sat her next to the 'new' student or even the incorrigible ones...as her kindness would always put a positive light on events. As a result, she developed friendships with many... including teachers, coaches, other parents, etc. She is truly our sunshine. During her middle school years, she expressed an interest in girls' softball... and began to work at being the best at it. Dani is a little thing (not the image of a muscular fast pitch pitcher)... but with her dad's help, patience, practice and perseverance...she developed into a star athlete. Because of her size, the coaches recommended that she use her whole body for each throw. Consequently, she employed the 'Monica Seles' grunt with each pitch. She became an all-star in her high school years. I'm telling you this, because these same skills came in to play as she tackled her illness.

Dani's dad is a college professor, the department chair of teacher preparation at George Washington University, and I'm a retired social studies (World and U.S. History, Government, Psychology, etc.) teacher (23 years) and administrator (11 years)...so it was no surprise that Dani decided early in her college career to become a teacher...but not just any kind of teacher...a teacher of children with disabilities.

The summer of 2002 was wonderful for her...she had fallen in love with Scott, her teaching job was great (working with 2-3 year old special needs children)...she was on top of the world. During Labor Day weekend (the first weekend in September) she began feeling poorly. She visited the doctor...they tested her for strep and gave her some medicine. Still the symptoms continued (sore throat and a fever), she took herself to the emergency room of a hospital...they said she had strep. All in all she visited her doctor 6 or so times in the next 2 weeks. They told her...not to worry...she was in great shape...she just needed to be patient and let the medicine take effect. They even prescribed some steroids to help mask the pain of the sore throat. She was so sad...she felt awful... she missed work...she had no energy. On September the 9th, she called me on the phone and told me that she was developing bruises all over her body. I didn't know what to say (not being very medically astute)... but for some reason I told her to march into her doctor's office the next day and demand a blood test. She did this on September the 10th...even though the doctor told her that she had nothing to worry about. The next day was September 11th; the first anniversary of 9/11...and the 3 of us (Jay, myself and Dani) had discussed the possibility of another terrorist attack...and planned our possible meeting if such a thing occurred. Because Jay's office is 1 block away from the Department of State building in Washington D.C. he decided not to go to work on that day but to go to Dani's home to make her breakfast...to cheer her up instead. He was with her when she got a frantic call from the doctor's office telling her that she needed to see a hematologist immediately (she had no idea what a hematologist or an oncologist was at the time, having had a pretty boring previous medical history). Dani and her dad met with Doctor Christie, the hematologist, who took some bone marrow from Dani's hip as well as a couple of other tests to confirm the diagnosis that he was 99% sure that Dani had acute myelogenous leukemia and that she needed to go to the hospital and begin treatment immediately. Dani's take on this was positive because there was that 1% possibility that they were wrong even though at that time her white blood cell count was 140,000 (normal is from 6,000 to 10,000). Without waiting, Dani was admitted into the hospital. Within 11 hours her chemotherapy began. We only began to realize how 'lucky' we were. The doctor said we dodged the bullet...by about 12 hours. AML advances that quickly! For the next month Dani remained in the hospital. It was a pretty awful time for her. The hospital couldn't keep all of her friends, or family from visiting her. Her room was filled with student drawings, and cards, stuffed animals, laughter and love. Her nurses and medical residents became close friends. This love and affection was pretty good medicine! My husband began his research to learn all he could about this disease... we learned about treatments and were put in touch with hospitals that specialized in AML and bone marrow/stem cell transplants. We also began fund-raising activities to pay for the bone marrow match search and transplant costs, and began blood drives to test for a possible match. Over 1000 people were tested in local drives that our friends and Dani's friends had organized. As an addendum to all of this...about 8 people in those drives have been identified as matches for other people in need... but no match for Dani came from these drives. Her brother, Micah, was devastated that he could not help his beloved big sister with his bone marrow, but he began to research where the best transplant centers were located. Soon, our decision was made...we would go to the Hutch in Seattle...which was where our son Micah lived (only 3700 miles away from our home!) All we needed was a donor...and finally...on Micah's birthday, we received a call that there was a donor from Germany. There were no matches in our family, or in the US registry of 5 million...but in searching in the International Registry, you were found!!!!

We began our preparations for departure to Seattle. The plan was that I would take leave from my job and I would stay with Dani as her primary care giver. Scott and Jay would commute to Seattle on a regular basis.

By early January 2003, we took up residence in Seattle, Washington and Dani began the pre-transplant regimen. Soon after our arrival, Dani entered the hospital and began the final 2 phases of the strongest chemotherapy. When we found out that her donor (you) were a 30 year old German male...the doctors were ecstatic (it seems that there's always the chance that a potential donor will back out or the transplant center won't react quickly enough, but this rarely happens with Germany). In preparation for your bone marrow, they needed to change Dani's blood type (pretty amazing when you think of it). On February 6th, your marrow was in route from Germany. We learned that bone marrow has a 72 hour shelf life...your marrow somehow flew to San Francisco first... and then was routed to Seattle. It arrived around midnight. The head of the infusion team extracted the stem cells from your bone marrow in its purest form in a pretty risky procedure. Apparently, they were able to extract twice as many stem cells from this process as were needed...and on the morning of February 7th, Dani was transfused with 2,000,000 or so of your stem cells. After less than 2 weeks of post-chemo and transplant reactions (like rashes, an inability to eat, high liver counts, depression, and pain) Dani's white cell, red cell and platelet count began to rise. The graft had taken!!!!!!!!! Your stems cells took over! Dani left the hospital at the beginning of March. We traveled daily to the Fred Hutchinson clinic for tests, appointments, daily blood draws, etc. Dani began her healing. We were given the o.k. to go home on May 9th. Over the summer, she continued treatments to build her immunities. Did you know that the chemo wiped out all of her immunizations? She actually inherited some of yours believe it or not...even some of your allergies! As she was taken off of some immunosuppressant drugs she developed severe migraine headaches... her summer was dismal. She could not return to the classroom in 2003 because she still needed to get her immunization (baby) shots. She received some of these shots and got great reports when she returned to Seattle for her 1st year check-up. She was allowed to return to the classroom in 2004, and began working with 5 and 6 year old special needs children.

So here we are...with a wedding just 58 days away. It's been an amazing journey. I've learned a lot about hope, love, and faith...and the goodness of people. You did a good thing...a great thing...you saved a life and gave hope to many, many others. We don't know you yet...but we now consider you a member of our family. We are hopeful that you will add to our joy when you join our family as our guest on October 9th for Dani and Scott's wedding. The formal invitation as well as Jay's information about flights, etc. will be forthcoming. Thank you for being you! I look forward to hearing from you soon...and meeting you in person. Please give your mom, dad, and your sister our best, and take care.

Sue

Within a week, Dani hears from Tom again. She shares this e-mail with Scott, Jay, Micah, and me. She says, "He is quite funny and endearing!"

From: Thomas

To: Dani Shotel

Date: Mon, 15Aug 2005 16:01:57 +0200

Hi Dani.... I just asked my chief for holiday and he told me that's fine. So I would like to join your wedding and if this is ok for you I'd arrive at the 7th of October in the evening (Friday) or Saturday in the morning and leave on the 10th back to London. Are you sure that your parents want to pay for the expenses for the flight? I'm used to traveling first class... ;- (Ok, that was a joke...) to be serious and to let you know, your parents do not have to pay for this. But, of course, I will not reject the offer, if they want to.

Generally, please do not think that you are bound to anything because of me as donator (I do not know how to express this correctly in English, but what I want to say is...) You do not have to give me anything, neither flights nor anything else you think you have to... I appreciate everything I receive from you. I am very happy to see your photographs and to read your stories or maybe to receive gifts from you or your parents. But only if you really want to do so and not because you think you have to do so - you owe me nothing, Ok!? I very much hope that you do not misunderstand this....Nevertheless, Dani, thank you very, very much for the invitation. I am quite excited about this! I would be happy to meet you, Scott and your family. By the way, the very best regards and wishes from my family: my mum (Marianne), my dad (Johann), my sister (Melanie) and from Tobias (my sister's son, two years old).
and no, I am not Jewish...hope, this is no bad news for you ;-)

In her next e-mail to Tom, Dani explains why she asked the question abut Tom's religious heritage. It appears that through these few e-mails, the two of them have struck up a real friendship! Dani writes:

16.08.05 19:33:55:

Tom:
The reason I asked you about being Jewish is that during all of our searches our doctors as well as the bone marrow registry made us believe that our most likely match would be from someone from a similar

background, including being Eastern European and Jewish. I'll make sure to let my doctors know that their assumptions are not always true.

Great to hear back from you! I'm so excited about getting to know you and meeting you in person for the first time. My family and friends are so happy to hear that you will be coming to the wedding. Have you ever been to Washington, DC?

It's a pretty wonderful place. There is a lot to do. All of the museums are free (and they are amazing). There are also many, many coffee shops! :)

Now, don't worry yourself about my family feeling that they owe you anything. I don't think anyone feels that way. However, they do feel that you saved my life...you were my only match in the entire world. Without you, my cancer would have certainly taken over my body and I would not be here typing this email today. I understand your degree of modesty, and completely respect that. I will certainly thank you again in person for your act of kindness, but then I will just be content to say I have a new friend from London. I guess I'll just have to return that Movado watch, and those diamond encrusted cuff links that I got for you!!!! :) ha ha!

Enjoy your new home in London. I can't wait to meet you in October. I hope to keep up our correspondence as well.

Love always,
Dan

Tom responds promptly:

To: Dani Shotel
Date: Wed, 17Aug 200511:26:04 .0200

No, it's the first time for me being in Washington! But, wow, I am very interested in seeing this city, and I am much more interested in meeting you and Scott, so actually I do not mind where we meet. Washington is absolutely ok. In Germany, we would say, this is the cream on top of the cake... (Sahnehaeubchen ;-)

But what I am wondering is, do you not need to take preparations for the wedding? Do you have time to take care of me or will I have to make cakes, salads, prepare soups and the lobster...?

Yippee..., I am looking forward to meet you all, take care, and have a nice day.
See you,
Tom

Tom also takes time to respond to my voluminous email!

Hi Sue

Wow, thank you for this wonderful email. As you maybe can imagine I have nearly no idea what hard times Dani had to pass. Of course, I was informed very well from the transplant team during several meetings before the transplant, but this has been theoretical. They told me, what you wrote in the email: that the patient's (Dani's) blood type has to be changed, that the patient will inherit my immunization (however, I did not know about any allergies I have, could you please keep me updated? ;-). They told me about all the procedures necessary for preparation, during the transplant and those afterwards. For me, this meant just three days in hospital, a break from my 'normal' life. After that, everything was as it had been before. Well, almost everything, as I was thinking very often on the person that received my cells and wondering if everything went fine. I had, of course, this good feeling that you have after helping other people (quite egotistical, I know) - and I became always nervous when I received letters from the transplant center at Munich: Anything new? Did it work or not? But I would like to tell you all this personally: I wrote just before to Dani that I will be able to visit you from the 7th to the 10th of October. I am very happy to accept this wonderful invitation and quite excited, looking forward to this weekend. My mom and sister and dad also wish you all the best (especially my mom who is very curious in what you and Dani are writing. I really had to fight for the photo book Dani sent me, as she wanted to see it for herself... she did so, of course, but she cannot speak or read in English, that was her handicap)!

Thank you very much for the invitation. I am happy to accept this.
See you soon,
Tom

On the Friday before the wedding, we get a few frantic calls from Tom, who is fogged in at Heathrow Airport with all flights cancelled for the day. Jay urges Tom to let the airline personnel know about the importance of getting to Washington quickly. They do their best, and Tom makes it to Washington D.C. with a brief stopover in Paris, France, 24 hours later than originally expected. Dani, Scott, and Micah pick Tom up at Dulles Airport in time for the rehearsal dinner Saturday evening, October 8th.

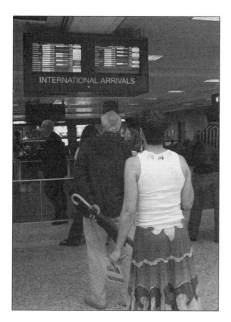

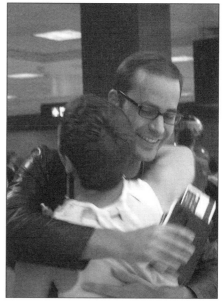

Dani awaiting Tom's arrival at Washington Dulles International Airport

Dani and Tom's first meeting

At the dinner, Tom is an instant celebrity! He is a delightful young man, instantly at ease with strangers. He is especially happy to make the acquaintance of Dani's girlfriends!

We venture to guess that in the scheme of things, this bright, personable, warm, and fun young man named Tom gave us the absolute best present any one of the Shotels ever received. What first appeared to be a casual blood test, taken to pass the time in a hospital, turned into a gift of life for our Dani. Throughout the past couple of years, we have personally observed the miracles of modern medicine and those incredibly talented professionals who dedicate their lives to the health and welfare of others. We continue to also be in awe of the heroes, like Tom,

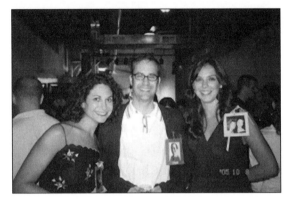

Two of Dani's best friends and bridesmaids (Ally and Marissa) with Tom at the rehearsal dinner

who take a few minutes out of their busy days to perform a simple act… having their blood drawn. But this one single act of human kindness becomes a great gift…and this gift winds up making the world a better place for all of us.

Chapter Sixteen
It's Gonna Be a Lovely Day

It is a busy and exciting time. RSVPs are coming back and almost all them say "yes." We are getting a bit nervous that the room won't be big enough, but we can't say we're surprised. Dani and Scott are a very special couple and this day is a celebration in more than the traditional way. Dani is still coughing—but the cough miraculously disappears during the wedding weekend. The rain however does not. Torrential rains hit the East Coast on Friday, October 7th. It rains non-stop for two-and-a-half days. We have heard that rain on your wedding day is good luck—but enough is enough! Two hours before the wedding, the skies clear…It's a lovely day!

Over time we all are beginning to move from thinking about the present to looking toward the future. On October 9, 2005, Scott and Dani Greene take their marriage vows. We look for a ballroom large enough to hold all those "Friends of Dani" and Scott. In the end we decided that this would be a time for all of the special friends, who were more supportive than one could ever imagine, and the place would have to be a special one…one that could only complement this wonderful love story. After looking at many places both in Washington, D.C. and the Eastern Shore of Maryland, there was a perfect setting in the Fairmont Hotel in downtown Washington that was like none we had ever seen. Weddings are always special…but this place would make the fairy tale come true. This wedding would be extraordinary, for this celebration will mark the union of a most loved and special couple. This couple had the faith, the courage, the strength, and the love to do everything in their power to make the dream of matrimony into a reality despite the

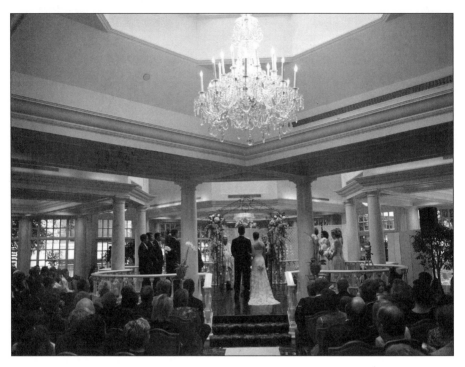

Dani and Scott exchange vows in The Colonnade Room at the Fairmont Hotel

adversity they had faced.

The wedding proves to be a double celebration. Not only do our guests witness and celebrate the marriage of two beautiful young people, Scott and Dani, they also get to rejoice in the undeniable permanent union of Tom and Dani.

Dani and Scott are surrounded that afternoon by their devoted friends and family, who had prayed for Dani's recovery, even forming prayer circles with their particular religious communities; organizing blood drives and special fundraising events; volunteering at the various bone marrow drives (with a few actually becoming bone marrow donors themselves, having the opportunity to save a life); donating generously to a worthwhile cause; participating in marathons to raise money for the Leukemia and Lymphoma Society and other life-saving causes; sending uplifting cards and e-mails to Dani that would bring a smile to her beautiful face; visiting Dani in the hospital in Arlington or in

Seattle; never losing faith in Dani's ability to heal; contributing to Dani's sick leave; donating air mileage so that Scott and Jay would be able to maximize their time with Dani in Seattle; ensuring that Dani, Scott, Jay, and myself have the professional support when we were unable to perform our jobs; and always surrounding us with sunshine, even though dark clouds threatened our days.

The moment had finally come. Dani and Scott Greene arrive on the dance floor to share their first of many dances as a married couple to Bill Withers' "Lovely Day."* The sweet words seem to be written with Dani and Scott in mind.

> *When I wake up in the morning, love*
> *And the sunlight hurts my eyes*
> *And something without warning, love*
> *Bears heavy on my mind*
>
> *Then I look at you*
> *And the world's alright with me*
> *Just one look at you*
> *And I know it's gonna be*
> *A lovely day*
>
> *When the day that lies ahead of me*
> *Seems impossible to face*
> *When someone else instead of me*
> *Always seems to know the way*
>
> *Then I look at you*
> *And the world's alright with me*
> *Just one look at you*
> *And I know it's gonna be*
> *A lovely day.....*

The honeymoon is perfect. It does much better weather-wise than the wedding weekend in Washington, and the cough that has followed Dani around for a year continues to lay low. But when the newlyweds return from their honeymoon…the cough returns as well with a vengeance.

In the past year-and-a-half (since October 2004), Dani has made countless calls to the Hutch, consulted often with Dr. Christie, and had many medical referrals in regard to her incessant

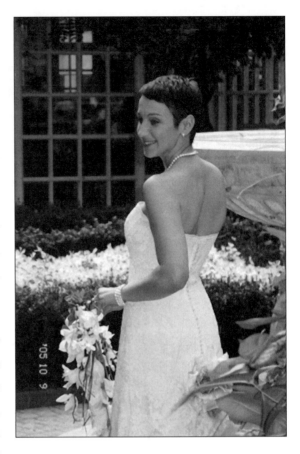

Mrs. Dani Greene

cough. She visited with a pulmonary specialist, had several chest X-rays (that never showed any fluid in her lungs or chronic bronchial condition), and continued her visits with her gastroenterologist, who insisted that Dani's stomach was just fine. Dani was not too crazy about her first ENT (Ear, Nose, and Throat Specialist) doctor, who suggested that this cough was caused by acid reflux. It really was a puzzle to all of us. In my head I thought, and I suspect others also thought, this may be some GvHD-related condition or something maybe even worse. Finally in January 2006, I believe Dr. Christie suggested to Dani that maybe she should just see another ENT (Ear, Nose, and Throat) doctor for a second opinion. This one specialized in allergies, and perhaps he would test Dani for various allergic reactions. Collectively, we sarcastically thought

"SURE…like it's an allergy!!" Well guess what? It was! Remember Dani had an immune system similar to that of an infant, and it turns out that, like an infant, she was lactose intolerant! Dani, who by the way, adores dairy products of any variety, shape or size, immediately does as the doctor advises and cuts all milk products out of her daily diet. The coughing stops within 24 hours. Gradually (after going cold turkey on the dairy products for about three months) Dani reintroduces these favorites back into her diet…and to our utter amazement…the cough is gone! An interesting sidelight I feel I should mention here is that, as we were writing the book, I relied heavily on my notes. And in February 2007 as I was writing Chapter 11 of this book…right there in front of my eyes… right there in our second notebook…right there on the February 20th entry was the answer. Because, on February 20th, 2003, Dani was visited by the SCCA Nutritionist who said to Dani, "Be cautious when trying dairy products, as you might become lactose intolerant post-transplant."

As Dani and Scott settle into married life, their thoughts turn more seriously to having their own children become a part of their lives. They have begun the adoption process. The extended family can hardly contain themselves with the joy that a child will bring to all of our lives. In the meantime, Dani continues to work with her class of pre-kindergarten special needs children in Arlington County, where her popularity gives the system headaches, as it seems that many want their children in Dani's class. Scott continues his career counseling work with army civilian personnel, while pursuing his master's of science degree in management, and has just recently been selected to participate in a leadership training program for civilians working for the military. Our Micah, still in Seattle, is working hard and enjoying every minute. I retired after 30 years as a teacher and administrator and spend my time consulting for Montgomery County Maryland Public Schools, reading, cooking, knitting…and taking some time to "smell the roses." Jay is actually beginning to think about retirement, and together Jay and I are beginning to truly enjoy thinking about our future, including a bit more relaxation, travel, and grandkids.

We have learned many lessons in the past four-and-a-half years. We have (as Scott has said many times) done what we've had to do. We have learned a great deal. And through all of this time, we have remained positive. We now have "the present of a future," as Dr. Flowers once promised Dani. What's more…we can all agree…

It's *good* to know a miracle!

Appendix: Resources on the Road to Recovery

A: Lessons We Have Learned

B: Transplants are Expensive

C: Fundraising

D: Bone Marrow Drives

E: Publicity

F: The Website – Purpose and Design

G: Medical and Disability Insurance, Social Security, Retirement Benefits, and Other Stuff that Nobody Wants to Think About

H. Organizations that support patients and their families

I: Glossary

J: The Cast of Characters

A: Lessons We Have Learned

Have good medical coverage!

Insurance is only important when you need it! Young people view themselves as invincible until a life-altering experience like this one occurs. How does one convince a twenty something that medical coverage is critically important? Perhaps one can use our experience to help in that regard. Dani's friends and acquaintances now know how important it is. We all were fortunate that our daughter listened to our advice. Because of advice that was heeded, we were fortunate enough to be able to make medical decisions for medically relevant reasons other than cost.

Ask questions!

In our society the medical profession is held in high esteem as well they should be. In our parents' generation it was considered inappropriate to ask a doctor a question. In the time in which we live, self-advocacy is part of our recognition of equality, whether it is race, gender, or age. There was a point in our story where we stopped asking questions. Perhaps we relaxed a bit because we were in good hands…because everyone told us that the care we would receive would be the best, or that there was no greater expertise in the world, but mistakes can still be made. Do not take anything for granted. Well-meaning, very smart people who are the best in their field can still make mistakes. Never stop being a self-advocate and never let your guard down.

Keep notes!

I'm not sure who told us this, but from the moment Dani was admitted to the hospital we took notes on everything that was said and done. No detail was too small. No information was insignificant. Perhaps it was because we didn't know what was or would be significant; but whatever the reason, we never stopped. Whenever I left Dani's side, someone else was then charged with that responsibility. As we reviewed the three loose-leaf binders of notes, the additional binders of medical reports, bills and informational documents we found that there were things that we didn't understand at the time that explained something later on, e.g., an allergy-related cough that we would be warned about by a nutritionist, or migraine headaches caused by sinus issues that are common with transplant patients. In retrospect, we probably should have gone back through the notes more frequently after the transplant. If we would have done that we would have been able to solve some problems that surfaced later in Dani's recovery more quickly. Perhaps this paragraph should be titled, *"Keep notes and keep reading them!"*

Your friends truly want to help – Use that energy!
Our family was fortunate to have many good friends…more than we could ever imagine. How to use the overwhelming level of energy and support was almost a fulltime job but a critical one. True friends really want to help, but they need direction and focus. Some provided comfort to Dani and the family…some became actively involved in supporting our various fund-raising activities or in securing potential donors. Others gathered information for us or used their professional contacts to give us information. The old adage that "you find out who your real friends are in times of need" rings true. Although our family tends to be a fairly self-reliant group, the support of friends became more critical as time went on. Moving across the country was no easy task, but friends stayed in contact, visited when they could, and continued to send little reminders of how important we were to them. It is something that we will never forget, or be able to repay, but it has changed our priorities and our way of looking at the world.

Educate yourself!
Information is critically important. You can't ask questions if you don't know the options that are available. The web is critical to gathering relevant information that the layman can understand. To know that there are options and to discuss the options with the medical professionals

requires them to justify their recommendations. In the end this information becomes the facilitator of a *conversation* rather than a *lecture.*

The patient's job is to focus on getting well!

We know that not everyone is as fortunate as we were…to have the support system that we had; but it seems to us that the most critical focus for patients is getting well. They can't spend their time worrying about paying the bills, or taking care of the dog, or meeting the requirements of their job. If at all possible, one must depend on others to pick up those responsibilities and do them as well as can be expected. There is no substitute for the patient being singly focused on recovery. The resources are out there to assist the patient…you just need to utilize the systems that are in place to help you find them.

The show must go on!

Appearances are critical. As Dani's Philly Mom-Mom always said, "The show must go on." That show, on its face, is for others, but in the end it is for us. Dani vowed never to walk with her head down. We can hear Philly-Mom-Mom sing, "Just let a smile be your umbrella on a rainy, rainy day…." We need to continue to keep up appearances despite the "rain." Dani made a pledge to herself to do this. We truly believe that if we can continue to push ourselves…to look the best that we can…to fight the good fight…it will help us win the battle in the end. Cancer will not get us…we will beat it!

Fluffy towels and nice P.J.s are really important

Soft P.J.s, fluffy towels, the scent of lavender, get-well cards, photos, stuffed animals, etc. All serve an important purpose in a patient's recovery…for they communicate warmth, love, and comfort.

"Multi-Taskers" may have to change their style!

For the patient the focus must be on getting well. For the primary caregiver that focus must be to ensure that this will occur. Each of us had a job to do. Whatever our job was, we needed to be single-minded in that focus. In our society, we seem to have all become multi-taskers. At least it appears that that is what is needed to succeed. Looking back on the experience, we believe that multi-tasking is not a good strategy for the life- changing event that we experienced as a family. We reverted back to a strategy of a single- minded focus and it appeared to serve us well.

You must be your own advocate!

There are no secrets to be kept for the bone marrow transplant patient. If one doesn't feel "quite right," that feeling needs to be expressed — and quickly. If there are things that the patient or the caregiver doesn't understand, then they have to ask questions. This is not to say that we should be less than cordial to those whom we entrust with our care, but no one will stand up for us better than we can for ourselves.

Show appreciation!

None are more committed to their patients than oncology doctors and nurses!

This is probably said too infrequently, but we have come to realize that most medical professionals do not develop relationships with their patients like oncology doctors and nurses. Oftentimes the care is longterm. Dani developed substantial friendships with the primary care staff that will never be forgotten. We are sure that the patient–professional relationships that develop in longterm care settings can take their toll on medical professionals. We are only stating here that we recognize the power of these relationships, and the energy that it must take for these professionals to do their work—and we salute them for it! It was the kindness, the sincere concern for the individual, the support, and the expertise that we all valued. Let them know how much you appreciate all of their efforts.

B: *Transplants are Expensive!*

One thing that became abundantly clear to us was that the expenses associated with a bone marrow transplant would far exceed what was covered by Dani's health insurance plan. When Dani started in the world of work we suggested that she get the best health insurance plan available, and in this particular instance, somewhat surprisingly we might add, she had listened to her parents' sage advice! Her plan, administered by Blue Cross and Blue Shield of the National Capital Area, was the best that Arlington County Schools had to offer. They assigned a case manger to Dani's case, and we were told that a million dollar reserve would be set aside to handle the covered expenses that would relate to the disease. Although we didn't quite understand this at first, we were informed that the Arlington County Public School System is self-insured, which means that the money is set aside in the budget to fund the health insurance costs of their employees. Blue Cross and Blue Shield administers the plan, and essentially determines what costs are allowable and what should and should not be paid. As the shock and initial treatment associated with the diagnosis began to settle in, the work began in earnest to seek the best treatment option disregarding cost, but fully realizing that a great deal of time, effort, and energy would need to be spent on making sure that Dani was reimbursed for anything the coverage would allow, and that appeals of denied expenses would more than likely be a part of that process. The biggest kink in the armor was a clause in Dani's insurance coverage documents that included the actual cost of a transplant but excluded the cost of finding a donor. That cost for the donor search was estimated to be approximately $50,000!

Cost should never be a factor when one is trying to save the life of a child and, we knew that we would not shy away from whatever needed to be done to allow our child to be saved; but the reality is that transplants are expensive. We learned throughout this experience that one should always have a "safety net." Our "safety net" in this case was a birthday present that I gave Jay on his 50th birthday. It was called the Boat Fund and I had $50 deducted from each of my paychecks to support that plan for the future. Now, five years later, our Boat Fund was looking pretty good. This account now became known as the "Donor Search" Fund, unless we got real lucky and could convince the insurance company that it was a bit absurd to approve the expenses of a transplant if they didn't approve the expenses of a search for a donor.

It was clear that, short of declaring bankruptcy, Dani would need significant resources to support her fight, and most importantly, allow her to focus be on her job, which was to fight the disease and not worry about the associated costs. Her co-workers in Arlington had now come through with 120 days of sick leave that would allow her to continue to receive a regular pay check through March of 2003. At a minimum, the pressure of her continuing expenses (rent, phone, food, etc.) would be covered. As mentioned earlier, on October 12, 2002, approximately 30 of Dani's and our closest and dearest friends, as well as co-workers, met at Dani's house to discuss a set of strategies to mobilize a series of fundraisers, etc., to support Dani's need for assistance in this area.

Prior to the meeting, we had discussed with our close friend Steve, an attorney, the possibility of forming a 501C3 foundation, as a vehicle to support Dani's medically related expenses. After some significant research by Steve and several legal associates, it was determined that the establishment of a 501C3 might not be in Dani's best interest. Some of our own research allowed us to connect with an established 501C3 that was focused on the specific needs of transplant recipients of all kinds. The National Transplant Assistance Fund (NTAF) appeared to be a good match for our needs. Steve turned his research efforts in that direction, and concurred that this seemed to be the way to go. We submitted an application to NTAF on September 26, 2003.

NTAF also gave us an additional rationale to feel good about our decision to fundraise, and allowed people to feel secure in their contributing. Fundraising empowers family, friends, neighbors, and community, by allowing them to help in a concrete way. Obviously, these supporters cannot change your medical condition, but they are able to make your healing easier. People want to help. Fundraising with NTAF provides a mechanism for your supporters that can be trusted, that donors and supporters alike can be fully confident that the support will be utilized appropriately.

The organizing meeting on October 12 gave us the opportunity to channel the energy of friends, relatives, and co-workers into the many tasks that needed to be accomplished in a relatively short period of time. Those tasks included the design and implementation of various fund-raising strategies, the organizing of bone marrow drives, and suggestions for the development and use of a website. An important consideration in our discussion, and something Dani felt strongly about, was that everything that we did should both help Dani and other persons fighting blood-related cancers; and so this was a consideration in our discussions. We functioned under the assumption that our application would be accepted to the NTAF, so that a vehicle would be in place for reimbursement of transplant-related expenses not covered by insurance.

On October 21, 2002, we were informed that the National Transplant Assistance Fund had accepted our application to establish a fund in honor of Dani Shotel. "The NTAF Bone Marrow Transplant Fund in Honor of Dani Shotel" was a regional restricted fund, established under the auspices of the National Transplant Assistance Fund (NTAF), in accordance with IRS requirements. NTAF qualifies as a 501C3 nonprofit organization and all monetary contributions or gifts-in–kind are tax deductible to the extent allowed by the law. NTAF serves as administrator for the fund, to assure the contributors that the money raised will be used for its intended purpose, that is, to assist with any expenses directly related to the treatment of organ/tissue transplantation (including stem cell/bone marrow), of transplant patients meeting this restriction. NTAF sends acknowledgements to all contributors of $250 and above; otherwise, the donor's canceled check serves as a tax receipt. All financial records for the management and administration of the fund are maintained by NTAF. With the vehicle for receiving the fruits of our efforts in place, we began to proceed with the initial set of ideas first discussed at that early October meeting.

Those ideas were bolstered by the materials that were sent to us by NTAF. They included a variety of fundraising ideas, many of which were utilized from November through the beginning of May. Some of the ideas were picked up by Dani's friends and some by people we didn't even know. Whatever the source, we appreciated everything that was done on Dani's behalf...and some of the ideas were rather unique.

C: *Fundraising*

Fundraising had not been an area of expertise for any of us when all of this began, but it became something in which we developed a fair degree of knowledge. The National Transplant Assistance Fund was tremendously helpful in this regard, by providing helpful hints, ideas, and sample materials to facilitate our activities. From our meeting in early October, we knew that we had a cadre of friends who were willing to help. What we did not realize was that there were many others who would come to Dani's assistance, by not only making donations but also by volunteering to help our initiatives and organizing activities on their own. The following is a partial list of those activities that supported our efforts in this area.

Direct Solicitation

The National Transplant Assistance provided us with a sample fundraising

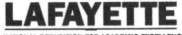

A NATIONAL REPUTATION FOR ACADEMIC EXCELLENCE

Classmates help Shotel '98 with leukemia battle

Friends organize fund drive to cover costs of transplant

EASTON, Pa.(www.lafayette.edu), November 7, 2002 — On September 11, 2002 alumna **Dani Shotel '98** was diagnosed with an acute form of leukemia. She is 26 years old, and is currently a teacher of preschool children with developmental disabilities in Arlington, Virginia. She has been told that her only chance for her survival is a bone marrow transplant that has been scheduled for mid-January. Dani will travel to the Fred Hutchinson Cancer Research Center in Seattle, Washington for this procedure and will be in Seattle with a required caregiver for a minimum of three months.

Friends from the classes of '96, '97, '98, and '99 are organizing a fund drive to help cover the estimated $80,000 in costs not covered by insurance. Alumni leading the fund drive are: **Kelly Butterfield '97, Melissa Carnahan '98, Amy Hessels '99, Marisa De Zego Khachaturian '98, Adam Khachaturian '98, Liz Lichtman '98, Kat Palotta '98, Harry Psilopoulos '98, Topher Patterson '98,** and **Matt Schapiro '96.**

The National Transplant Assistance Fund is accepting donations for Dani Shotel and will administer the fund. To contribute, make your check payable to NTAF Bone Marrow Transplant Fund for Dani Shotel, and mail to: NTAF Bone Marrow Transplant Fund, Suite 230, 347 West Chester Pike, Newtown Square, PA 19073. Credit card donations are accepted at 1-800-642-8399; for online contributions go to www.transplantfund.org.

If you wish to send Dani your best wishes, get more details, or find out how you might be able to help, you can reach her at www.nsurgents.com/dani/.

This article can be found at
http://www.lafayette.edu/news.php/view/1198/

letter, which we posted on our website. Jay worked with several groups to create letters on their own. Ten of Dani's friends from Lafayette put together a solicitation to Dani's friends and acquaintances from her undergraduate days. With the help of the Lafayette Alumni Association a version of this letter was direct-mailed to the over 400 alumni whom she knew personally. In addition, the notice on the previous page was posted on the Lafayette alumni website.

We received several copies of letters individualized by Dani's friends and colleagues, which helped in the fundraising activities. The following is a sample letter that was adjusted to meet the needs of the individual audience:

Send a Letter to Friends Requesting a Donation

(Today's Date)

Dear Friends:

On September 11, 2002 my friend Dani Shotel was diagnosed with an acute form of leukemia. She is 26 years old, a graduate of Lafayette, and is currently a teacher of preschool children with developmental disabilities in Arlington, Virginia. We have been told that Dani's best chance for a cure is a bone marrow transplant that has been scheduled for mid-January. Dani will travel to the Fred Hutchinson Cancer Research Center in Seattle, Washington for this procedure and will be in Seattle with a required caregiver for a minimum of three months. Besides the risks associated with the bone marrow transplant procedure, it is extremely costly and insurance will not cover all of her expenses. The Hutch has estimated that the expenses related to transplant and not covered by insurance will be in excess of $80,000 barring any complications.

I am writing this letter to ask you to help my friend financially. On October 21, 2002, we were informed that the National Transplant Assistance Fund had accepted her application to establish a fund in honor of Dani Shotel. The NTAF Bone Marrow Transplant Fund in Honor of Dani Shotel is a regional restricted fund established under the auspices of the National Transplant Assistance Fund (NTAF) in accordance with IRS requirements. NTAF serves as administrator for the fund to assure the contributors that the money raised will be used for its intended purpose: that is to assist with any expenses directly related to the treatment of organ/tissue transplantation (including stem cell/bone marrow), of transplant patients meeting this restriction. If you are able and would like to contribute to this fund please make your check payable to:

NTAF Bone Marrow Transplant Fund - Dani Shotel

Mail your donations to:
NTAF Bone Marrow Transplant Fund
Suite 230, 3475 West Chester Pike
Newtown Square, PA 19073

The NTAF is able to accept credit card contributions for your convenience by calling them at 1-800-642-8399 or for secure on-line contributions, log onto www.transplantfund.org . Be sure to note your donation is for the Dani Shotel fund. If you would like to make a donation of stocks, please call the number above for assistance. NTAF qualifies as a 501(c)3 nonprofit organization and all monetary contributions or gifts-in-kind are tax deductible to the extent allowed by the law. NTAF sends acknowledgements to all contributors of $250 and above, otherwise the donor's canceled check will serve as a tax receipt.

Thank you for your generosity and desire to help.

Concerts
Another fund-raising opportunity that didn't work out for Dani, but can work for others, involves concerts. The band OAR had graduated from

the same high school as our son and daughter. They were enthusiastic about doing a benefit concert for Dani, but as it turned out, they were already booked for a date in Washington, D.C., and were contractually excluded from performing at another venue. The band made a substantial contribution to Dani's fund, but it was an enlightening experience for those of us who are not typically involved in these kinds of activities. Nevertheless, smaller bands did donate their services as a part of several club nights scheduled in and around D.C., and we are convinced they can work for other persons in need of support. We were amazed by the fund-raising potential of events of this kind.

Athletic Events

As mentioned earlier, arrangements were made to sell reduced-price tickets to two Washington Wizards basketball games. Tickets were set aside at reduced cost so that we could charge half-price for the tickets, and Dani's fund received the differential between the cost of the ticket and the price we paid. Scott took the lead in organizing and marketing the event. Flyers were distributed throughout our network of friends, places of employment, and Dani's website. The first fundraiser was so successful for the game on December 7th (all 500 tickets were sold) that Scott had to mail checks back to people who got their checks in too late. It turned out that Dani was in-between rounds of consolidation chemotherapy and was able to attend the game as well. A request was made and approved for tickets for a second game. This game occurred on March 1, while Dani was in Seattle, and 200 additional tickets were made available, which also sold out. On the following page is a sample flyer that was produced for the second game.

Other Events Looking for a Cause

We found out that many fund-raising events actually pick a cause each year. These range from golf tournaments to religious institution-sponsored events. Several of these events decided that Dani was worthy of support. Some examples include a local golf tourney that looks for a cause each year and a fundraiser at our synagogue, with the proceeds going to a person or persons in need within the community. Both of these events picked Dani as a recipient during the spring of 2003.

Restaurants and Clubs

Ray's the Steaks in Arlington, Virginia, became our home-away-from-home for dinner, when we spent those first few months at Arlington Hospital Center; and Mike Landrum, the owner, became a personal friend of Dani and Scott's. He agreed to have a special fund-raising evening at the restaurant, where the profits went to Dani's fund. Scott's parents, Gayle and John Greene, organized a similar fundraiser at the Austin Grille in Springfield, Virginia, and some of Dani's Lafayette friends, led by Topher Patterson, did the same at Garrett's, which is both a watering hole in Georgetown and a local Lafayette alumni hangout. Topher also utilized *On Tap* magazine, which focuses on entertainment in Washington, to support the fund-raising activities. Two of Dani's camp buddies, Yvonne Townsley and Jason Zymkoviak, did the same at Mrs. O'Leary's in Gaithersburg, which turned into a reunion for Camp Seneca Creek, where Dani spent many summers as a camper, counselor, and, finally, director. Brother Micah organized a similar fund-raising event at a club in Seattle.

The Austin Grille fund-raising flyer has been included as an example. It is particularly interesting because it was part of a community support project that the restaurant had participated in for a number of years. Scott's parents were able to reserve a "First Monday" community support night

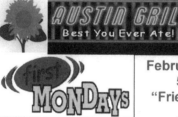

AUSTIN GRILL
Best You Ever Ate!

February 3rd, 2003
5-10 P.M.
"Friends of Dani"

If you know Austin Grills you know about First Mondays. They're the restaurant's way of giving back to the communities they call home, by donating a portion of dinner sales the first Monday of every month to a local non-profit organization. The first Monday of every month, one or more of Austin Grill's restaurants sponsors a community organization for the evening. The organization invites their friends and supporters to dine at Austin Grill. They donate a portion of the restaurant's sales after 5pm to the organization.

They held their first First Monday in November of 1995. In 1999, Austin Grill was a finalist for the Restaurant Neighbor Award, an initiative by the National Restaurant Association to recognize "exceptionally innovative and effective community service projects."

Help Dani Shotel as she wins her fight against Acute Myeloid Leukemia. 50% of your check will be donated to her assistance fund simply by signing your name and "Friends of Dani" on the back of the dinner bill.

It is perhaps only in times of sadness that we realize the importance of those around us. These times inspire us to give of our resources, whatever they might be to help those in need. Take this opportunity to help our beloved friend and sister Dani Shotel. Dani has spent a great deal of her time reaching out to those around her...now it is our turn to give back. It is impossible to put a value on someone's life, the means necessary to save one, however it can be devastatingly expensive.

Dani is busy preparing for the next phase of her journey at the Fred Hutchinson Cancer Research Center in Seattle, where she eagerly awaits her bone marrow transplant. Join us in celebration of Dani's continuing success on February 3rd at Austin Grill.

Simply by attending, having dinner, and signing your name and "Friends of Dani" on the back of the dinner bill, 50% of your check will be donated to the NTAF Bone Marrow Transplant Fund in honor of Dani Shotel. Dani, her friends, and loved ones offer their sincerest gratitude for your generosity.

to benefit Dani. This is another example of an "event looking for a worthy cause."

Pledges for Activities

Several other events were planned to benefit both leukemia victims and transplant recipients generally, and included: several "Light the Night" leukemia fund-raising teams in D.C., Philadelphia, and New York (the Lafayette alums); four bone marrow registration drives that added more than 1,000 potential donors to NMDP and related registries; and support for Team in Training Marathons, the Leukemia and Lymphoma Society's signature national fund-raising initiative. Marathons were run in New York, Boston, and D.C. on behalf of Dani. The largest of these was in Washington, where Dani's former roommate, Alyssa Walstein, organized a team in honor of Dani. Alyssa and 87 other participants trained rigorously through many adversities to participate in the Washington D.C. Marathon, on March 23rd, 2003. They were part of a team that raised over $151,000 for the fight against blood-related cancers. Scott even participated in one of the Lance Armstrong Bicycle fundraisers for cancer research.

The organizers of several fund-raising events scheduled in our area initiated a call to us on Dani's behalf. An annual charity golf tournament, a synagogue fundraiser, and several other yearly events made a determination that Dani would be the benefactor of their fund-raising efforts.

The most unique event on Dani's behalf, was an activity at Wootton High School in Montgomery County. Her high school newspaper published an article about Dani's plight, and followed up with several fund-raising activities by both alumni and current students. One of those fundraisers, led by a science teacher, Sanford Herzon, and the DNA Club at Wootton High School, titled "DNA for Dani," raised more than $1,500. It involved students purchasing a paper ring for one dollar on a DNA "chain" that went up and down the hallways of the entire building.

A group of Dani's college buddies from Lafayette even held a fundraiser in New York, while watching the Leopards beat Lehigh at football for the first time since 1994, and raised more than $1,000 for Dani. (The Lafayette/Lehigh football rivalry is one of the oldest in college football.)

Miles for Smiles – Another Benefit of the Drives

At our first Bone Marrow Drive, a gentlemen by the name of Ted Moon, a senior manager at NEXTEL, walked up to Jay, introduced himself, and asked if we had begun to solicit frequent-flyer miles for people who would like to support our trips back and forth to the West Coast for Dani's transplant. Ted was a resident of Arlington and didn't know any of us. He came to be tested. This good samaritan's suggestion led to 150,000 miles being donated for trips back and forth from Seattle, for both Jay and Scott, during Dani's treatment at the Hutch. The donation of miles for trips is a fabulous way to keep spirits up in addition to being a tremendous financial benefit. Marriott points were donated as well, which covered the first week of our stay in Seattle.

Continuing Fundraising to Support Patients and Families

Light the Night Walks

Dani continues to support fund-raising activities for cancer patients and their families. The first event that Dani participated in directly, upon her return from Seattle, was the Leukemia and Lymphoma Society's Light the Night Walk in the District of Columbia. Dani felt it was critically important to walk with the team that walked for her in 2003. She has participated every year since, and in 2006 her team raised more than $5,000 for cancer- related programs.

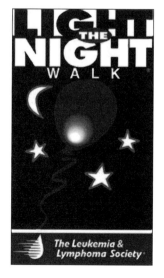

Virginia Turkey Trot

The next event Dani and her friends participated in on Thanksgiving Day, 2003, was the Virginia Turkey Trot to raise funds for local programs. Specifically, support is directed to "Life With Cancer," an Inova Health System nonprofit program for cancer patients and their families.

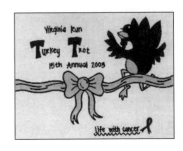

Relay for Life

Dani also organized a "Relay for Life" team for the American Cancer Society in 2004. Her team was called "Team Bald Days" and she did a painting for the team T-Shirt (which is the cover of this book).

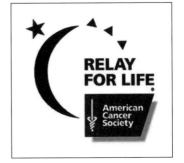

Pennies for Patients

In 2004 Dani was named the spokesperson for the "Pennies for Patients" portion of the School and Youth Programs for the Leukemia and Lymphoma Society. The Leukemia and Lymphoma Society's School & Youth℠ Programs offer children hands-on experiences, which cultivate caring, respect, and sharing with others. School & Youth Programs also give schools the opportunity to extend fund-raising to the larger community, involving faculty and administration, school service organizations, community businesses, and the students' extended families. Since 1994, millions of dollars have been raised in pennies and other spare change by more than 10 million elementary, middle, and high school students throughout the country. The funds, collected during a three-week period, benefit The Leukemia and Lymphoma Society. The goal here is a simple one: "One of life's most valuable lessons — best learned at a young age — is that we're all made better when we help others." Dani's letter to children and teachers across the country follows:

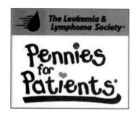

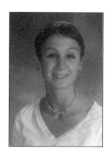

Dear Educators and Friends,

I have been fortunate to learn many important lessons thus far in my life. In pre-school, Mrs. Santee introduced me to the wonders and simplicity of Flavor-ice. Mrs. Kuhn began my mathematical education in first grade by using apples as props. In fourth grade, Mr. Smith helped me realize that I could be funny and should also be more self-confident. In my freshman year of college, Dr. Leibel handed me my first failing grade on a test, which helped me learn from my mistakes. Collectively these teachers helped me to learn my own potential as a teacher.

After finishing school I pursued my dream and became a teacher. I taught special education in both Arlington and Montgomery County for the next three years. Just when I thought that my learning was over, and teaching had begun, I learned I had cancer. Dr. Christi and his team made me realize that learning is constant and ever expanding.

On September 11, 2002, I was diagnosed with Acute Myelogenous Leukemia (AML). I learned that AML is an extremely fast-acting form of cancer. I was extremely sick and had been so for about 10 days prior to my diagnosis. The doctors later told us that had I not received treatment on that very day, I would have surely died.

We quickly learned about donor banks, treatments, percentages of survival rates. I underwent three rounds of chemotherapy at Virginia Hospital Center in Arlington and was in the hospital off and on for over two months. I then traveled to the Fred Hutchinson Cancer Research Center in Seattle, Washington for a bone marrow transplant. The treatment was not easy, nor was being away from all those who supported me since my diagnosis. However, I was blessed with superb care and extremely nurturing nurses and doctors.

Today, I am a survivor! I am thankful to The Leukemia & Lymphoma Society, which continues to support me and so many others. Supporting The Leukemia & Lymphoma Society gives many patients a chance when they would otherwise not have one.

I personally want to thank you for supporting the Society through participating in Pennies for Patients. Because of the work your school is doing you are helping researchers move closer to finding a cure. Most importantly you are helping individuals like me get through the toughest battle of their lives.

Thank you! Dani

Bone Marrow Transplant Newsletter Calendar Fundraiser

Dani had been informed that she would be one of a group of survivors who had been selected to be a part of the 2008 Calendar Fundraiser for BMT InfoNet.

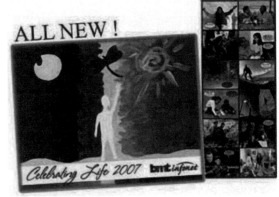

Since 1990, BMT InfoNet has provided quality information and emotional support to more that 100,000 transplant patients, survivors, and their loved ones. The BMT InfoNet is a resource for patients who need help with the following:

Patients: who are interested in being matched with survivors and are willing to provide emotional support.

Survivors: who are willing to provide emotional support to patients undergoing similar treatment.

Insurance Difficulties: For patients covered by US insurance plans who are having difficulty securing insurance reimbursement for a bone marrow, peripheral blood stem cell, or cord blood transplant.

D: *Bone Marrow Drives*

By early October, contact had already been made by Liz with the Red Cross of Washington, which was linked with the National Marrow Donor Program (NMDP) and its local branch office, located at the National Institutes of Health in Bethesda. They would provide the materials and the personnel necessary to do the actual testing of people interested in becoming bone marrow donors. The cost of the testing was approximately $50 to $100 per person, but the Red Cross could cover a portion of the cost.

In addition, the "Fair Lakes League," a community-based organization in Virginia, and the Friends of Allison, a nonprofit corporation providing funding for the recruitment of potential marrow donors, were also contacted and agreed to support our efforts. The Foundation was established in honor of Allison Atlas, who was diagnosed in August 1989 at age 20 with a rare form of leukemia. Doctors informed Allison and her family that her only chance for survival was a bone marrow transplant. No one in Allison's family had the perfect tissue type that matched hers, so she was forced to appeal to the community for help. The Atlas family also turned to the NMDP. Family and friends also formed the Friends of Allison in October of 1989. The purpose was to recruit more potential bone marrow donors. A campaign was launched to find a life-saving donor for Allison and the thousands of other patients who needed a matching donor. Unfortunately, a donor was not found in time for Allison. Allison's search sadly failed but, thankfully, her effort was not to be in vain. The Friends of Allison continues to fund marrow testing for other cancer victims because Allison believed "No one should die because they do not have a donor." Mr. and Mrs. Atlas both advised us on the bone marrow drives, and members of the family were present at both the Wood and the Beth Ami drives. The Atlas family and the continuing support of other groups and organizations, such as the Gift of Life Foundation, the Red Cross, NIH, and the National Marrow Donor Program, have been key to developing a worldwide registry, which now totals over 13 million potential donors.

Although we knew that there would be a slim possibility of Dani finding a match from local bone marrow drives that were sponsored on her behalf, we, as a family, became very involved in this activity, and several of our friends devoted their time, effort, and energy to these events. Enough support was gathered for the four drives supported by the "Friends of Dani" that no person who wanted to be tested was asked to pay anything. To date, we are aware of eight people who were tested during the drives for Dani who were selected as potential donors for other persons needing transplants, including Scott, now Dani's husband. These four drives would not just be supported financially by these organizations but, also, with voluntary professional personnel.

With Liz, Laurie, Bonnie, Steve, Sandy, Wendy, Burton, and Susan ready to set up the respective drives, they had their work cut out for them. In addition we would need both publicity for the drives and volunteers to man the various activities not associated with the actual blood draw necessary for typing (i.e., the welcome station, sign-in and form completion, screeners to review eligibility, the babysitting area, and a station to take voluntary contributions to defray the cost of the testing). We all agreed that no monetary donations would be taken for Dani specifically at the Bone Marrow Drives.

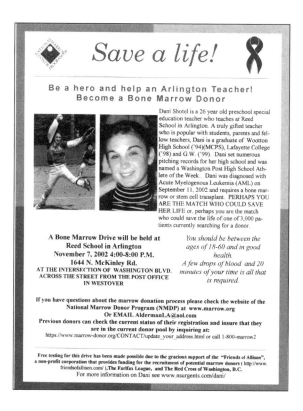

Save a life!

**Be a hero and help an Arlington Teacher!
Become a Bone Marrow Donor**

Dani Shotel is a 26 year old preschool special education teacher who teaches at Reed School in Arlington. A truly gifted teacher who is popular with students, parents and fellow teachers, Dani is a graduate of Wootton High School ('94)(MCPS), Lafayette College ('98) and G.W. ('99). Dani set numerous pitching records for her high school and was named a Washington Post High School Athlete of the Week. Dani was diagnosed with Acute Myelogenous Leukemia (AML) on September 11, 2002 and requires a bone marrow or stem cell transplant. PERHAPS YOU ARE THE MATCH WHO COULD SAVE HER LIFE or, perhaps you are the match who could save the life of one of 3,000 patients currently searching for a donor.

**A Bone Marrow Drive will be held at
Reed School in Arlington**
November 7, 2002 4:00-8:00 P.M.
1644 N. McKinley Rd.
AT THE INTERSECTION OF WASHINGTON BLVD.
ACROSS THE STREET FROM THE POST OFFICE
IN WESTOVER

You should be between the ages of 18-60 and in good health.

A few drops of blood and 20 minutes of your time is all that is required.

If you have questions about the marrow donation process please check the website of the National Marrow Donor Program (NMDP) at www.marrow.org Or EMAIL AldermanLA@aol.com
Previous donors can check the current status of their registration and insure that they are in the current donor pool by inquiring at:
https://www.marrow-donor.org/CONTACT/update_your_address.html or call 1-800-marrow2

Free testing for this drive has been made possible due to the gracious support of the "Friends of Allison", a non-profit corporation that provides funding for the recruitment of potential marrow donors (http://www.friendsofallison.com/),The Farifax League, and The Red Cross of Washington, D.C.
For more information on Dani see www.nsurgents.com/dani/

Contributions would be directed to the groups that made the drives possible. In the four drives scheduled on behalf of Dani, close to 1.000 people were tested.

E: Publicity

We found that publicity was tremendously important in supporting our fund-raising events. Our friend, Sandy Davis, and Jay put together a "press release" about Dani. Sandy made the rounds to various local newspapers in the area. Five local papers in both Northern Virginia and Maryland carried an article publicizing the bone marrow drives and included Dani's "story" in various forms. Two local television networks picked up the story as well.

WUSA, the CBS affiliate in Washington, showed up at a bone marrow drive at Temple Beth Ami in Rockville, Md., and later at Dani's hospital room to do an interview; and the drive at Wood Middle School was attended by a reporter and photographer from the local cable news channel, News Channel 8, a subsidiary of the ABC affiliate in Washington, D.C. All of these activities both raised leukemia awareness and were helpful in direct support to Dani.

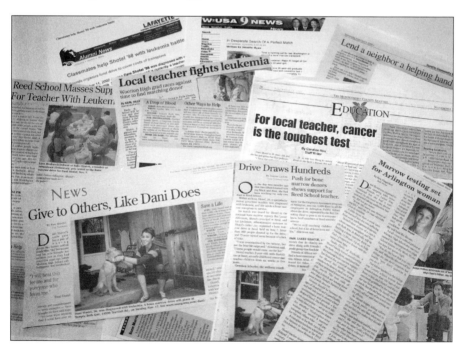

A press release and personal follow-up generated lots of publicity in the difficult D.C. area media market

The Gazette Papers in Maryland, *The Arlington Connection, The Potomac Almanac, The Montgomery County Sentinel*, the *Montgomery Journal*, and the *Washington Jewish Week,* all carried stories about the drives. They carried Dani's story as the illustrative "poster person" for the importance of registering to be a donor. Several even carried information about the website and the fund, and two actually did follow-up articles when she returned from Seattle.

F: The Website — *Purpose and Design*

With regard to the website we felt it was important to have a vehicle to communicate with the hundreds of friends and acquaintances that Dani had touched over time, without the burden of having to make individual contacts. The website had to be interactive, updatable, and user-friendly. The expertise to do this was no further away than Dani's brother, who had recently started a graphic design and web development company, Nsurgents, during his junior year of college with two classmates. The website would be a primary vehicle for communication about Dani's progress, as well other information (e.g. fund-raising activities, becoming a potential donor, donating to her fund, etc.).

There was probably no single item that helped us more than the website that Micah created! As we discussed the idea of a mechanism for communicating on a regular basis with Dani's friends, a website seemed to meet every objective that we had, while at the same time reducing the time, effort, and energy necessary to provide effective communication. The website accomplished the following:

- It provided a vehicle to update Dani's friends and relatives about her condition. Updates on Dani's condition and other information were uploaded to the site by Dani's Dad on a weekly basis, or more frequently as needed. Jay put together a list serve to keep close friends and family informed of Dani's progress, and these "postings" were then archived so that people who became aware of Dani's fight after the first few skirmishes could "catch up."

- It gave us the opportunity to link people with information about Dani's illness, the transplant process, and the medical resources that were supporting her fight. For people who didn't live in the Washington D.C. area, Dani's website acted as a resource for people who wanted to find out how to be tested. Links were set up to facilitate access to the National Transplant Assistance Fund, the Gift of Life Foundation, the National Marrow Donor Program, and the Seattle Cancer Alliance, among others. A parent of one of Dani's students even helped us out by putting together a list of out-of-state bone marrow drives for the website. This list of out-of-state bone marrow testing drives was updated as new information became available.

- It gave people information about the various fundraisers that were being sponsored on her behalf, and also served as an information-sharing mechanism for people who wanted to make donations to her fund directly or develop a fund-raising mechanism of their own.

- It gave people the opportunity to communicate with Dani both publicly and privately, as the website had an interactive capability that allowed people to post general greetings and best wishes, comment about specific updates, or send Dani private messages that were password-protected. After each posting, readers also had the ability to click on the word "comment" as another way of communicating with Dani. As Dani's condition improved, she was able to answer the messages that were posted on the site.

- It gave us the opportunity to post pictures and news articles written about Dani, so that people could truly stay current and also provide content to make it easier to write to Dani.

Micah's love and devotion to his sister was never in question. His visits, his encouragement, and his reality-based points of view all were so vital to Dani. But his amazing ability to visualize—and then implement—this interactive website proved invaluable to so many… and for so many reasons. For Dani, this website, taken in daily doses, proved to be as beneficial as the life-saving medications she was given each day. Although a bit out of date, the website is still available for viewing at: www.nsurgents.com/dani.

G: Medical and Disability Insurance, Social Security, Retirement Benefits, and Other Stuff That Nobody Wants to Think About!

The Health Insurance Maze

As mentioned earlier, upon reviewing Dani's health insurance policy, and after our visit to Seattle, it was unclear that Dani's medical insurance would cover the search process to locate a donor. In a letter dated October 21, 2002, Colleen Duffy, Dani's search coordinator, wrote us with the following information:

The Seattle Cancer Care Alliance (SCCA) identifies most of their donors through the National Marrow Donor Program, a Minneapolis-based registry of over 5 million donors worldwide. In addition, they access every registry worldwide, utilizing an on-line search program managed by the Europdonor Foundation in The Netherlands, to obtain a summary of potential donors in most foreign registries. When contact was first made with Seattle and Dani's records were forwarded, a preliminary review of the NMDP and BMDW found two U.S. donors and four non-U.S. donors who were potential, based upon broad antigen matching (6 of 6 "broad antigen matches" rather than the 10 of 10 that Seattle prefers for a matched unrelated donor transplant.).

Seattle was in contact with Blue Cross/Blue Shield, in order to determine whether the insurer would cover donor search costs. If it was determined that search costs were *not* a covered benefit, then pre-payment of costs is required in order that the search progress.

Dani had to have her blood retyped at the Hutch to assure that no errors had been made. (This had already been done when we visited Seattle on October 18th.)

Dani had to sign and return the consent form, so that further testing of potential donors could begin. (This was signed and faxed back to Seattle on October 25th.)

After a review of the language in Dani's health insurance policy, the financial representative at the Hutch was certain that the administrator of

Dani's Health Plan (Care First Blue Choice) would not cover the search process, and was not optimistic that an appeal would be successful. She went ahead and contacted Care First and informed us that the cost of the transplant was covered under Dani's policy, but that the cost of an unrelated donor search was not covered under Dani's plan, despite what we considered to be language to the contrary. At any rate, it was agreed that we would fund the search process as needed, and wage the good fight, to show the plan administrator and the school system, if necessary, that approving a transplant without approving the search for a donor made little sense. We made three payments directly to the Hutch as requested, to ensure that the search would proceed as expeditiously as possible. (The payments were $2,440 on 10/25, $2,075 on 11/1, and $2,305 on 12/03/02.)

The language of the policy was quite clear, and was specific in its coverage of an allogeneic bone marrow transplant for acute leukemia. The language of the policy was less clear with regard to the search. The only specific language in the policy stated the following:

"If you are the recipient of a covered organ/tissue transplant, we will cover the Donor Services (as defined below)...Donor services consist of services covered under your contract which are related to the surgery, including evaluating and preparing a possible or actual donor (emphasis ours) and recovery services after the operation which are directly related to donating the organ or tissue."

Appeal Writing

While Seattle was not optimistic that an appeal would be successful, Denise Lim, of the Office of Patient Advocacy at the National Marrow Donor Program, was. In addition to sending us materials to apply for support from the Donor Foundation administered by NMDP, to specifically fund a portion of the search, she wrote a letter of support for our appeal. In her letter supporting Dani's appeal of November 18th she included the following:

"Most payers acknowledge that the donor search is a medically necessary and reimbursable part of the matched unrelated donor (MUD) stem cell transplantation process. As previously indicated, it is impossible for Ms. Shotel to have the transplant you approved, without completion of the donor search process. We appreciate your documented support of the medical necessity of MUD transplantation for Ms. Shotel and trust that you will incorporate and reimburse all aspects of care needed to affect the desired outcome."

In the letter denying our appeal received on December 21st, and dated December 18, 2002, the appeals nurse analyst reiterated the language on Page 28 of the contract (stated above), and then stated, "A donor search is not an evaluation." It should be noted the Arlington County Schools is self-insured and Carefirst Blue Choice is the plan administrator for the system. This fact was critical in our continuing quest for coverage.

In a document received from the Maryland Insurance Administration, CareFirst's role is clearly defined in the following language:
The employer provides to their employees a self-insured, self-funded plan. CareFirst is not acting as an insurer for any services subject to the inquiry. Care First Blue Cross/Blue Shield is a provider of administrative and claims processing services only.

On December 23rd, 2002, we appealed the decision of CareFirst to the Associate Superintendent for Personnel of the Arlington County Public Schools. As advised by Ms. Lim, we could file an appeal directly with the school system. That letter follows.

December 23, 2002

Dr. ------- -------------
Arlington Public Schools
1426 N. Quincy St.
Arlington, Va. 22207

Dear Dr. ---------:

Re: Dani Shotel

I am writing this letter on my own behalf as a teacher in the Arlington Schools and a policy holder within Care First Blue Cross Blue Shield to request a recommendation for coverage or an exception to the existing policy interpretation to allow coverage for the search process for potential donors related to a transplant that is required for my catastrophic illness. On September 11, 2002 I was diagnosed with Acute Myelogenous Leukemia (AML) and my doctors have informed me that an allogeneic unrelated stem cell transplant is required in my case. During the week of October 15, 2002 my family and I made consultation visits with Dr. Douglas Smith at Johns Hopkins University and Dr. Ranier Storb of the Seattle Cancer Care Alliance and both gentlemen agreed with Dr. Robert Christie, my hematologist at Arlington Hospital, that a matched unrelated donor transplant protocol is medically necessary in my case due to the high risk nature of my illness. When we met with the financial representative at Seattle she informed us that she would contact Blue Cross Blue Shield to confirm my coverage and about a week later informed me that the cost of the transplant is covered under my policy but the cost of an unrelated donor search is not covered under my plan despite words to the contrary in my insurance booklet supplied by Arlington County Schools.

It is difficult for me to understand how the policy can approve an unrelated donor stem cell transplant without approving the evaluation of possible donors for the transplant (these are the words in the policy I was provided that says that in fact this activity is covered under the Point of Service Plan). In the denial that I received on December 21ˢᵗ (dated December 18, 2002) the Appeals Nurse Analyst reiterated the language on Page 28 of the contract which states the following:

"Donor services consist of services covered under your contract which are related to the surgery, including the evaluating and preparing a possible or actual donor and recovery services after the operation

which are directly related to donating the organ or tissue." She then adds "A donor search is not an evaluation." The statement in the policy is ambiguous at best. It is both unclear and undefined in the policy the services that are part of a search and the services that are part of the evaluation but it would seem to me that a process that costs thousands of dollars for each identified donor is much more than a "search." Further, it is quite clear that the policy covers both possible and actual *donors. The bone marrow registry analysis performed by the National Marrow Donor Program determines a list of* potential *donors. In my case the "search" yielded six potential donors. Once* potential *donors have been found through registry analysis, HLA typing of the patient and* potential *donors is performed and* possible *donors are identified. This typing is essential in order to identify the most appropriate unrelated donor for stem cell procurement. Of the six potential donors that were the result of the search process on my behalf further testing/evaluation had to be done on those donors. The cost of this evaluation is significant and I was required to pay for this evaluation for each* possible *donor that passed the initial screening and whose blood products were shipped to Seattle. A donor from England was rejected and two potential U.S. donors were unavailable. It would seem to me that the early rejection or screening out of these potential donors might be considered to be part of the search process. The donors who remained potential candidates for donation by passing the initial screening had blood products shipped to the Seattle Cancer Care Alliance for further* evaluation. *The cost of this* evaluation *is significant. The overall cost of these* evaluative *procedures has been approximately $10,000 and it was suggested to me that this cost is significantly lower than average because I had so few potential matches. It is these costs that have been rejected by Blue Cross Blue Shield. In my case a German donor has been identified through this process as a potential match for me. In order to have the evaluation process continue on these potential donors I have wiped out my savings and have had to borrow money to cover this process. I am not sure that* this is what you had in mind when the system prepared a quality health insurance plan with Blue Cross Blue Shield. The language in the policy and, I believe, any reasonable person would agree that the level of detail required in the process I have described would be far beyond what one would suggest is a search and more in line with the cost associated with the evaluation of potential *donors which is the language in the policy. It is my understanding that as a self-insured plan you can intervene on my behalf and recommend coverage for the services I have described or make an exception on my behalf to cover the described services.

I have been informed by D_____ L___ of the Office of Patient Advocacy of the National Marrow Donor Program that most payers acknowledge that the donor search is a medically necessary and reimbursable part of the matched unrelated donor (MUD) stem cell transplantation process. It is my understanding that it is impossible for me to have the transplant that is approved under my policy without completion of the donor search process. It should also be noted that although some costs (such as housing and transportation) are excluded from our policy the search process is not. It is my hope that you will review this matter and find it appropriate to recommend reimbursement for all aspects of medically required care needed to effect a positive outcome in my case including the coverage of the unrelated donor search.

In closing let me say that my supervisors and the school based personnel in Arlington County as well as the parents of my students have been exceptional during this time. These various communities have supported me beyond what I ever could have expected and has reassured me that when I left Montgomery County Public Schools to join the Arlington Schools in the Summer of 2001 I made the right decision. I hope that your support in this matter will be consistent with the tremendous affirmation I have received from both the school system and the Arlington community. I have enclosed an article that documents the support that I have received thus far. I look forward to your response.

Sincerely,

Dani Shotel
1935 Hillman Rd.
Falls Church, Va. 22043

cc: Ms. _____Case Manager, National Marrow Donor Program

In the end, the combination of Donor Foundation support for Dani's search and a positive response regarding payment by the public schools to cover a portion of the search procedures allowed us to recoup the majority of funding directed at the search process. This support allowed us to redirect the money that was initially paid for the search to cover the patient responsibility portion of the out-of-area expenses not covered by the plan.

The Will to Persevere

Over 400 separate payment requests were generated during the period from diagnosis in September of 2002 until Dani was released back to the East Coast in May of 2003. Several notebooks were filled with copies of bills, payments by the plan administrator, and the application of those payments by the various doctors, hospitals, and treatment centers. It was amazing to us that as efficient and effective as the primary medical care was at each of the treatment facilities, the billing for services was not nearly as consistent or as accurate. At times, the only way one could determine whether a bill was paid was by the exact amount, to the penny, that was charged for a specific service. In the end, approximately 10% of the bills were never fully accounted for, until approximately one year after the services were delivered. Fortunately, the difference in amounts for the majority of those bills was several dollars, but one credit for $750 was never fully accounted for. Vigilance and perseverance are once again the watchwords in this area. Reconciling payments and reimbursements, as well as coordinating benefits from the Social Security Administration, the Virginia State Retirement System, and the private disability insurer contracted by the county became Jay's other full-time job during this period. While Dani was concentrating on recovery, and I was the fulltime caregiver, Jay picked up this responsibility along with meeting his obligations at the office, making sure we had the information to ask the appropriate questions, and coordinating the travel schedule of a weekly commuter. There is no question that it takes a bit of luck and a whole lot of resources to have a successful outcome from this process.

Blending Compatible Sources of Support

Although each person's situation is different, Dani had several sources of financial support during the time when she could not work. The first of these came from the generosity of her fellow teachers in Arlington, Virginia. Teachers in Arlington were allowed to donate sick leave to a colleague in need, and despite Dani's short tenure in the county, 120 days of leave were donated to support her during this time. In addition to her continuing to be paid, it allowed her to focus her attention on fighting the disease. During this time, we were able to gather information on the "gap" disability insurance coverage that the school system provided and the benefits that were available to her from the Virginia State Retirement System, and concentrate some of our energy on a careful navigation of the Social Security Disability system. Social Security cannot be applied for right away, so the support of her colleagues through the donation of sick leave and the gap insurance coverage become critically important. In the end, the sources of support cannot exceed an existing salary, but the combination of sources allowed Dani to continue to make her payments to Blue Cross/Blue Shield and receive the same net salary that she was making while she was working. Careful monitoring of the combination of sources is critical, as "gap" insurance coverage is designed to fill the gap between other sources of income from retirement benefits, social security, etc. The insurance company must be kept informed of those sources, and in Dani's case social security approval allowed us to refund a portion of the gap coverage to the insurance company. The Human Resources personnel in the Arlington County Public Schools were excellent in helping us negotiate the maze of insurance and coverage possibilities. In addition it is strongly recommended that a source book such as Tomkiel's *Social Security Benefits Handbook* be obtained. With the Social Security Code taking up over 700 pages, some additional source of information is critical in negotiating the maze. Negotiating the maze is time-consuming and frustrating at times, and if some of those excess energy people that we spoke about earlier are up to the challenge, it is a marvelous assignment for them.

H: Organizations that Support Patients and Their Families

The following is a list of resources that is available to leukemia patients and their families. We have put an asterisk next to those organizations with which we have had personal contact during our experience. Much of this information was updated from the BMT InfoNet website listed below.

*Angel Flight America
Phone: 877-621-7177
Website: www.angelflightamerica.org
Description: Free air transportation for patients in financial need who must travel to receive medical treatment. They also work with several travel agencies that can assist in getting reduced fares for emergency flights. Regional information is available by accessing the website.

*BMT InfoNet
2310 Skokie Valley Road – Suite 104
Highland Park, Il 60035
Phone: 847-433-3313
888-597-7674
Website: www.bmtinfonet.org
Description: The Blood & Marrow Transplant Information Network is a not-for-profit organization dedicated exclusively to serving the needs of persons facing a bone marrow, blood stem cell or umbilical cord blood transplant. Founded in 1990, BMT InfoNet strives to provide high quality medical information in easy-to-understand language, so that patients can be active, knowledgeable participants in their health care planning and treatment

*Bone Marrow Foundation
337 E 88th Street - Suite 1B

New York, NY 10128

Phone:212-838-3029 800-365-1336

Fax: 212-223-0081

email:theBMF@bonemarrow.org

website: www.bonemarrow.org

Description: Financial aid for some transplant-related expenses. Request for aid must be initiated by hospital affiliated with this organization.

Children's Leukemia Foundation of Michigan

29777 Telegraph Road - Suite 1651

Southfield, MI 48034

Phone: 800-825-2536 (Michigan only) 248-353-8222

Fax: 248-353-0157

email: info@leukemiamichican.org

website: www. leukemiamichican.org

Description: Information, financial assistance and emotional support for patients and their families (Michigan residents only).

Children's Organ Transplant Association (COTA)

2501 Cota Drive

Bloomington, IN 47403

Phone: 800-366-2682

 Fax: 812-336-8885

Email: cota@cota.org

website: www. cota.org

Description: The Children's Organ Transplant Association helps children and young adults who need a life-saving transplant by providing fundraising assistance and family support.

Immune Deficiency Foundation

40 W Chesapeake Avenue - Suite 308

Towson, MD 21204

Phone: 800-296-4433   410-321-6647

Fax: 410-321-9165

email: idf@primaryimmune.org

website: primaryimmune.org

Description: To improve the diagnosis and treatment of patients with primary immune deficiency diseases through research, education and advocacy. They provide publications, referrals to support groups as well as scholarships for seniors graduating from high school.

Jeffrey Katz Bone Marrow Transplant Fund for Children

Los Angeles Ronald McDonald House

4560 Fountain Avenue

Los Angeles, CA 90029

Phone: 323-666-6400

Fax: 323-669-0552

Description: Financial aid for children transplanted at UCLA.

*Leukemia and Lymphoma Society

1311 Mamaroneck Ave 3rd Floor

New York, NY 10605

Phone: 800-955-4572   914-949-5213

 Fax: 914-949-6691

email: infocenter@lls.org

website: www. lls.org

Description: The Leukemia & Lymphoma Society is the world's largest voluntary health organization dedicated to funding blood cancer research, education and patient services. They provide publications, support groups, and financial aid.

Leukemia Research Foundation

2700 Patriot Blvd. Ste 100

Glenview, IL 60026

phone: 847-424-0600

fax: 847-424-0606

email: info@lrfmail.org

website: www.leukemiaresearch.org

Description: The Leukemia Research Foundation (LRF) is dedicated to conquering leukemia, lymphoma and myelodysplastic syndromes by funding research into their causes and cures, and to enriching the quality of life of those touched by these diseases. Programs at LRF include over $2 million in annual funding for young, investigative researchers in leukemia and related blood cancers; patient services including counseling and support, and direct patient financial assistance.

*The Marrow Foundation

400 Seventh St. NW #206

Washington DC 20004

Phone: 202-638-6601   202-638-0641

email: tmf@nmdp.org

website:www.themarrowfoundation.org

Description: Provides financial assistance for unrelated donor search and procurement expenses not covered by insurance. Patients must apply through a medical center affiliated with the National Marrow Donor Program.

My Friends Care Bone Marrow Transplant Fund

148 S Main Street - Suite 101

Mount Clemens, MI 48043

Phone: 586-783-7390

Fax: 586-783-7404

email: MFC@MICH.com

website: www.myfriendscare.org

Description: Help for Michigan residents needing a stem cell transplant in the areas of; fundraising, assessing financial need, assist in bulk mailings, provide materials, talk with donors, work with hospital staff, assist with travel and living arrangements, and set up bone marrow drives

National Association of Hospital Hospitality Houses (NAHHH)
PO Box 18087
Asheville, NC 28814
Phone: 800-542-9730   828-253-1188
Fax: 828-253-8082
email: helpinghomes@nahhh.org
website: nahhh.org Description: Referrals to free or low cost lodging near medical facilities.

National Children's Cancer Society
1015 Locust - Suite 600
St Louis, MO 63101
Phone: 800-532-6459 314-241-1600
Fax: 314-241-6949
email: PFS@children-cancer.org
website: www.nationalchildrenscancersociety.org
Description: The mission of The National Children's Cancer Society is to improve the quality of life for children with cancer and their families by providing financial and in-kind assistance, advocacy, support services and education

.
National Foundation for Transplants
1102 Brookfield - Suite 200
Memphis, TN 38119
Phone: 800-489-3863 901-684-1697
Fax: 901-684-1128
email: jhill@transplants.org
website: www. transplants.org
Description: provides advocacy, support and financial assistance to transplant candidates and recipients when they face major transplant-related costs not covered by insurance

National Leukemia Research Association
585 Stewart Avenue - Suite 18
Garden City, NY 11530
Phone: 516-222-1944
Fax: 516-222-0457
email: info@childrensleukemia.org
website: www.childrensleukemia.org
Description: provides financial aid to leukemia patients (children and adults) and their families who show financial need to offset the costs of outpatient chemotherapy, radiation, and other leukemia-fighting medications

*National Marrow Donor Program (NMDP)
3001 Broadway Street NE - Suite 500
Minneapolis, MN 55413
Phone: 800-627-7692
Office of Patient Advocacy: 888-999-6743
fax: 612-627-5877
website: www.marrow.org
Description: The NMDP maintains the largest, most diverse Registry of potential volunteer stem cell donors, provides resources for patients and physicians, and conducts research to improve outcomes of stem cell transplants. The NMDP's Office of Patient Advocacy (OPA) works with patients to remove barriers to obtaining an unrelated donor transplant. The OPA connects patients to transplant-related resources, helps patients find a transplant center, or assists them with financial and insurance matters.

National Patient Travel Center
Mercy Medical Air Lift
4620 Haygood Road - Suite 1
Virginia Beach, VA 23455
Phone: 800-296-1217 757-318-9145

Fax: 757-318-9107
email: mercymedical@erols.com
website: www.PatiemtTravel.org
Description: Referrals to charitable medical air transportation programs.

National Transplant Assistance Fund (NTAF)
150 N. Radnor Chester Road Suite F120
Radnor, PA 19087
Phone: 800-642-8399 610-535-6100
Fax: 610-535-6106
email: NTAF@transplantfund.org
website: www.transplantfund.org
Description: Fundraising assistance: See Appendix C

Needy Meds
email: info@needymeds.com
Website: www. needymeds
Description: Lists pharmaceutical manufacturers who provide drugs free of charge to patients with limited financial resources.

Nielsen Organ Transplant Foundation
580 W Eighth Street
Jacksonville, FL 32209
Phone: 904-244-9823
Fax: 904-244-9821
email: nielsenfoundation@yahoo.com
website:www.geocities.com/nielsonfoundation
Description: Financial aid and fundraising assistance for North East Florida residents who need a transplant

I: *Glossary*

Abelcet is used to treat a variety of serious fungal infections. It is often used in patients who cannot tolerate or who do not respond to the regular amphotericin treatment. It works by stopping the growth of fungi.

Acyclovir, or Valcyclovir or Valtrex prevents and treats herpes virus infections.

Acute Leukemia is a rapidly progressive malignant disease of the bone marrow, which results in the accumulation of immature, functionless cells, called blast cells in the blood.

Afebrile means without a fever.

Albumen is a simple water-soluble protein found in many animal tissues and liquids.

ALL (acute lymphocytic leukemia), a rapidly progressive cancer that starts by the malignant transformation of a marrow lymphocyte, is the most common form of leukemia.

Allogeneic transplant is a marrow or stem cell transplant using blood products from another person who is not the person's identical twin but could be a sibling, relative, or a matched unrelated donor (MUD).

Alpurinol is a drug used to treat gout.

Ambien or Zolpidem is a mediation to control insomnia

Amlodipine or Norvasc is a calcium channel blocker used to treat angina (chest pain) and high blood pressure. Amlodipine affects the movement of calcium into the cells of the heart and blood vessels. As a result,

Amlodipine relaxes blood vessels and increases the supply of blood and oxygen to the heart while reducing its workload.

AML (acute myelogenous leukemia) is a rapidly progressive cancer that starts by the malignant transformation of an immature cell in the bone marrow. AML will be diagnosed in more than 13,000 people in the United States in 2007, and close to 9,000 are expected to die of the disease (American Cancer Society Website).

Apheresis means to take away. There are several different types of apheresis but the procedure is essentially the same. It is used to remove specific cells or plasma from your blood. One can be a plasma donor through the Red Cross where they would hook up two lines (one in each arm) and draw blood out of your body with one line, send it through a centrifuge-like machine to separate the blood into its various components (plasma, red blood cells, and white blood cells), and return it through the second line. If one is a plasma donor, then the plasma is retained. This process is then called a plasmapheresis.

Ara-C (Cytarabine) is one of the older chemotherapy drugs which has been in use for many years. Ara-C is a clear, colorless liquid given by intravenous route. It is most commonly used in treatment of several forms of leukemia and lymphoma. Ara-C is normally given on a daily basis for five to seven days.

Ativan, or Lorazepam is a medication used to relieve anxiety.

Autologous transplant is a marrow or stem cell transplant using the patient's own blood products.

Aztreonam is an antibiotic that is used to treat infections caused by bacteria by either killing bacteria or preventing their growth.

Bactrim, or Trimethoprim/sulfa, is used as a preventive (prophylactic) medication for certain types of infections while leukemia patients are immune suppressed…most typically pneumonia.

Betadine is an antibacterial solution.

Bilirubin is a pigment that is produced from the breakdown of red blood cells.

Blasts are immature white blood cells.

Bone Marrow Aspirate and Biopsy is a medical procedure in which a small volume of bone and or marrow is removed under local anesthesia from the hipbone; cells from the sample are then examined to identify any abnormality.

Busulfan (byoo-SUL-fan) belongs to the group of medicines known as alkylating agents. It is used to treat some kinds of cancer of the blood. It may also be used as a conditioning regimen prior to a bone marrow or stem cell transplant.

Butterfly is a children's size needle utilized to draw blood.

Cephalosporin is a drug which is used in the treatment of infections caused by bacteria.

Chemo-mucositis is a raw throat caused by the shedding of fast growing cells in the throat caused by chemotherapy.

Chimerism is the presence in an individual of cells of different origin, as of blood cells derived from a transplant donor. It is the simultaneous existence and function of components of both the donor's and the recipient's immune systems in the same patient, resulting in cross-regulation of immune system activities.

Colace is a stool softener.

Clostridium difficile, or **C. dif** is a bacterium that causes diarrhea and more serious intestinal conditions such as colitis. It is the most common cause of infectious diarrhea in hospitalized patients in the industrialized world. It is also one of the most common infections in hospitals and long-term care facilities. The use of antibiotics increases the chances of developing C. difficile diarrhea. Treatment with antibiotics alters the normal levels of good bacteria found in the intestines and colon. When there are fewer of these good bacteria, C. difficile can thrive and produce toxins that can cause an infection. The combination of the presence of C. difficile in hospitals and health care settings and the number of people receiving antibiotics in these settings can lead to frequent outbreaks. In these settings, C- difficile infections can be limited through careful use of antibiotics and the use of routine infection control measures.

Consolidation Chemotherapy is a course of treatment with anti-cancer drugs given while in remission, with the aim of killing as many of the remaining leukemic cells as possible.

Creatinin level is a measure of kidney function.

Cyclosporin is a member of a family of drugs that possess immunosuppressive activity. These chemicals are very useful in helping the body to overcome the body's natural tendency to reject transplanted organs and prevent GvHD.

Cytogenetics is the study of chromosomes and the diseases caused by numerical and structural chromosome abnormalities.

Cytoxin, or Cyclophosphamide is in a class of drugs known as alkylating agents; it slows or stops the growth of cancer cells in your body. It may also be used as a conditioning regimen prior to a bone marrow or stem cell transplant.

Decadron, or Dexamethasone, a corticosteroid, is similar to a natural hormone produced by your adrenal glands. It relieves inflammation (swelling, heat, redness, and pain) and is used to treat certain forms of arthritis; skin, blood, kidney, eye, thyroid, and intestinal disorders (e.g., colitis); severe allergies; and asthma. Dexamethasone is also used to treat certain types of cancer.

Dexascan, or DXA scan of the spine and hip, is considered the gold standard for diagnosing osteoporosis. DXA stands for dual energy x-ray absorptiometry. It is a low dose x-ray that can be performed with the person lying on a flat table in street clothes. The amount of x-ray is similar to what one would get on a trans-Atlantic flight. It is painless and can be completed in approximately 15-20 minutes.

Diflucan or **Fluconazole** is an anti-fungal medication.

Dilantin (Phenytoin) is the most common drug prescribed to prevent or stop seizures.

Endoscope is an instrument for examining visually the interior of a bodily canal or a hollow organ such as the colon, bladder, or stomach.

Dilaudid, or Hydromorphone is used to relieve moderate to severe pain.

Fentanyl acts in the central nervous system (CNS) to relieve pain.

Fluconazole is used to prevent yeast infections in patients who are likely to become infected because they are being treated with chemotherapy or radiation therapy before a bone marrow transplant. Fluconazole is in a class of antifungals called triazoles. It works by slowing the growth of fungi that cause infection.

Flow Cytometry refers to analysis of biological material by detection of the light-absorbing or fluorescing properties of cells or subcellular fractions such as chromosomes passing in a narrow stream through a laser beam.

Fortaz, or Ceftazidime, eliminates bacteria that cause many kinds of infections, including lung, skin, bone, joint, stomach, blood, gynecological, and urinary tract infections.

Gastroenterologist is a medical doctor who specializes in diagnosing and treating people with diseases of the gastrointestinal tract, the stomach, and the intestines.

Groshong Catheter is a long, thin tube made of flexible silicone rubber. It is surgically inserted into one of the main blood vessels leading to the heart (this is basically done to dilute potentially damaging medications by having them flow into a main artery so they can be diluted quickly inside the body). They can be used for drawing blood samples and for giving intravenous fluids, blood, medication or nutrition. It basically reduces the number of needle sticks you need to have while you are being treated.

GvHD (Graft vs. Host Disease) occurs when infection-fighting cells from the donor recognize the patient's body as being different or foreign. These infection-fighting cells then attack tissues in the patient's body just as if they were attacking an infection. Tissues typically involved include the liver, gastrointestinal tract and skin.

Hematocrit is the percent of whole blood that is composed of red blood cells.

Heparin is (Lock Flush) a solution used to prevent clots from forming in a venous catheter, allowing continuing access to veins in the body when multiple injections or blood samples are required.

HLA typing, also known as the human leukocyte antigen (HLA) test, or tissue typing, identifies antigens on the white blood cells that determine tissue compatibility for organ transplantation. There are six loci on chromosome 6, where the genes that produce HLA antigens are inherited: HLA-A, HLA-B, HLA-C, HLA-DR, HLA-DQ, and HLA-DP.

Hydrea, or Hydroxyurea is in a class of medications known as antineoplastic agents. Hydroxyurea treats cancer by slowing or stopping the growth of cancer cells.

Idarubicin treats acute myelocytic leukemia (AML) in adults. Recent research suggests that using Idarubicin results in higher rates of complete remission (CR) and longer survival for patients. CR is the total elimination of all diseased cells detectable following therapy.

Imipenem (Primaxin) is a drug which is used to prevent and treat bacterial infections.

Induction Chemotherapy is the initial course of treatment given to a patient upon admission to a hospital, which is intended to remove all evidence of leukemia or lymphoma.

Immunocompromised is the inability to fight disease caused by the lack of white blood cells or neutrophils.

Immuno-suppression is suppression of the immune response, as by drugs or radiation, in order to prevent the rejection of grafts or transplants or to control autoimmune diseases. It is also called immunodepression.

Intraconazole (Sporanox) is an anti-fungal medication.

IVIG, Intravenous Immune Globulin (IVIg), is also know as IGG, IGIV, globulin, immunoglobulin and immune globulin intravenous (human) (systemic). It is an intravenous solution of highly purified immunoglobulin G, derived from large pools of human plasma. IVIg contains antibodies against a broad spectrum of bacterial and viral agents. IVIg also confers passive immunity in the treatment of immunological disorders.

Lasix, given to help reduce the amount of water in the body, works by acting on the kidneys to increase the flow of urine.

Leukoreduced red blood cell units contain leukocytes in a specifically reduced amount. The blood is filtered to make leukoreduced red blood cell units. Leukoreduced red cells are usually effective in preventing certain types of transfusion reactions for most patients.

Levaquin, or Levofloxacin (lee-voe-FLOX-a-sin), is an antibiotic used to treat bacterial infections in many different parts of the body.

Lorazepam, or Ativan is a medication that controls nausea and vomiting.

Lung Scan is a nuclear scanning test that is most commonly used to detect a blood clot that is preventing normal blood flow to part of a lung.

Magnesium is used as a dietary supplement for individuals who are deficient in magnesium. Magnesium supplements may be needed by patients who have lost magnesium because of illness or treatment with certain medications. A lack of magnesium may lead to irritability, muscle weakness, and irregular heartbeat.

Mesna is a medication used to protect the bladder wall from the harmful effects of some cancer-fighting drugs.

Methatrexate is classified as an antimetabolite drug, which means it is capable of blocking the metabolism of cells. As a result of this effect, it has been found helpful in treating certain diseases associated with abnormally rapid cell growth, such as cancer; it also lowers the likelihood of developing acute GvHD, so that patients typically receive a combination of Cyclosporine and Methatrexate.

Mugascan is a test designed to measure how efficiently your heart is pumping blood.

Mycelex troche is a lozenge used to ease the throat pain.

Myoclonic Jerks or **Myoclonus** refers to sudden, involuntary jerking of a muscle or group of muscles. Myoclonic twitches or jerks usually are caused by sudden muscle contractions, or by muscle relaxation. Myoclonic jerks may occur alone or in sequence, in a pattern or without pattern. They may occur infrequently or many times each minute.. A hiccup is an example of this type of myoclonus. Other familiar examples of myoclonus are the jerks or "sleep starts" that some people experience while drifting off to sleep. These simple forms of myoclonus occur in normal, healthy persons and cause no difficulties.

Nadir is the term given to the lowest point in white blood cell count following chemotherapy.

Nebulizer is a machine that changes liquid medicine into fine droplets (in aerosol or mist form) that are inhaled through a mouthpiece or mask inhaler (MDI). It is powered by a compressed air machine and plugs into an electrical outlet.

Neutrophil is a particular type of white blood cell that is made in bone marrow, whose absence would put a patient such as Dani at continuing risk for disease. Its job is to find and kill any germs (bacteria) in your body. Neutrophils seek and destroy bacteria and keep you healthy.

Norelgestromin and ethinyl estradiol transdermal system (patch) are, respectively, a progestin and an estrogen which help control menstrual bleeding.

Norvasc®, Amlodipine besylate, is the most prescribed brand name high blood pressure medicine.

Neupogen, or Filgrastim is a protein that stimulates the production of white blood cells.

Neutropenia is an abnormal decrease in a type of white blood cells. The body needs white blood cells to fight disease and infection.

Nubain is a potent analgesic. Its analgesic potency is essentially equivalent to that of morphine on a milligram basis.

Oxycodone is a medication to control severe pain.

PCA, or patient controlled analgesic, is a method by which patients control the amount of pain medicine they receive.

Petechiae are small red or purple spots on the body, caused by a minor hemorrhage (broken capillary blood vessels). Petechiae are a sign of thrombocytopenia (low platelet counts.)

PICC line, a peripherally inserted central catheter, is a form of intravenous access that can be used for a prolonged period of time, e.g., for long chemotherapy regimens, extended antibiotic therapy or total nutrition.

Phenergan is a medication utilized to ameliorate allergic reactions to blood or plasma; it is also used to prevent and control nausea and vomiting.

Plasma Exchange involves removing blood from the person, mechanically separating the blood cells from the fluid plasma, mixing the blood cells with replacement plasma, and returning the blood mixture to the body. The rationale for plasma exchange is that the plasma contains immune factors that may stimulate disease activity. Substituting replacement plasma may dilute the strength of these potentially destructive immune factors.

Platelets are one of the main components of the blood that form clots sealing up injured areas and preventing hemorrhage.

Prednisone is used to treat or reduce the severity of Graft vs. Host Disease (GvHD) after a bone marrow transplant. For both acute and chronic GvHD, the main treatment is to give steroids that weaken the immune system. The most common is prednisone along with Cyclosporine.

Premarin, or estrogen, is in a class of medications called hormones. It works by replacing estrogen that is normally produced by the body.

Protonix is an antacid used for acid reflux.

Sitz Bath is a warm-water bath taken in the sitting position that covers only the hips and buttocks. It may be used for either healing or hygiene purposes.

Solumedrol (methylprednisolone) is the intravenous version of prednisone. It is used at the time of transplant to help prevent an immune response.

Taper refers to a very slow and gradual decrease in medication.

Thrombocytopenia refers to low platelet counts.

Thrush is an infection of yeast fungus, Candida Albicans, in the mucous membranes of the mouth. Candida is present in the oral cavity of almost half of the population. These changes can occur as a side effect of taking antibiotics or drug treatment such as chemotherapy.

TPN, total parenteral nutrition, is used for patients who cannot or should not get their nutrition through eating. TPN may include a combination of sugar and carbohydrates (for energy), proteins (for muscle strength), lipids (fat), electrolytes, and trace elements.

Titer is a measurement of the amount or concentration of a substance in a solution. It usually refers to the amount of medicine or antibodies found in a patient's blood.

Tumor lysis syndrome is caused by the sudden, rapid death of cells, particularly cancer cells in patients with leukemia or lymphoma, in response to cancer therapies.

Ursodiol is used in the treatment of gallstone disease. It is taken by mouth to dissolve the gallstones or to break down sludge in the gall bladder caused by chemotherapeutic breakdown of fast growing cells.

Vancomycin-Resistant Enterococci (VRE) are bacteria that are normally present in the human intestines and in the female genital tract and are often found in the environment. These bacteria can sometimes cause infections. Vancomycin is an antibiotic that is often used to treat infections caused by enterococci. In some instances, enterococci have become resistant to this drug and thus are called Vancomycin-resistant enterococci (VRE). Most VRE infections occur in hospitals and can be best treated with "designer" antibiotics other than Vancomycin.

VOD, venal occlusive disease, is a complication of transplantation in which the liver's ability to remove waste products from the body is impaired. It is most likely to occur during the first month after a transplant.

Zofran is a medication used to prevent nausea caused by chemotherapy.

J: The Cast of Characters in Order of Their Appearance

(Mentioned more than once in the story)

Personal Friends

Dani – the star

Scott – the boyfriend

Jay – the dad

Sue – the narrator and the mom

Micah – Dani's brother who lives in Seattle

Jeff and Joann – Sue and Jay's cousins

David Laskin – Jay and Sue's cousin and a medical doctor

Aunt Carol – Sue's sister (Dani's aunt)

Uncle Bruce - Aunt Carol's husband, and a pharmacist

Ari – Dani's cousin and Carol and Bruce's son

Liz Lichtman – Dani's good friend and Jay's administrative assistant at G.W.U.

Laurie Alderman – Dani's principal in Arlington County Public Schools

Ben Busey – one of Dani's former students

Philly Mom-Mom – Jay's mom and Dani's Grandmom

Poppy – Sue's dad and Dani's grandfather

Grandmom – Sue's mom and Dani's Grandmom

Gayle and John Greene – Scott's mom and dad

Matt & Estelene Boratenski – Dani's high school coach and family friends

Bonnie and Steve Spivack – life time family friends

Rabbi Jack (Luxemburg) – the rabbi of our synagogue in Maryland

Kat and Fitz Fitzpatrick– Dani's college roommate and husband

Don Dillingham – one of Dani's first pitching coaches

Matt Levine – Dani's high school friend and housemate

Topher Patterson – Dani's college friend

Sandy Davis– a longtime family friend

Wendy and Burton Katzen– longtime family friends

Susan Hoopes – the PTA president of Earle B. Wood Middle School

Rochelle Sislen – a volunteer for the Gift of Life Bone Marrow Foundation

Ally (Samuel) and Ryan Frank – A life long friend of Dani's and her husband

Heather – Carol and Bruce's daughter and Dani's cousin

Jason – Carol and Bruce's son and Dani's cousin

Phoebe – Dani's Chocolate Labrador Retriever

Dave Brubaker – the principal of Earle B. Wood Middle School

Abby and Justin Botts– Scott's sister and brother-in-law

Yvonne Townesly – A longtime friend of Dani's

Susan Kaufman – the owner of *Serafina*, a restaurant in Seattle

Kat, Cameron and Beth – Micah's Seattle friends

Medical Personnel (D.C. Metropolitan Area)

Sharon Gallop – Red Cross/NIH representative at blood drives

Dr. David Schreiner – Dani's primary care physician

Dr. Deluca – Dr. Schreiner's partner in the family care practice

Medical Personnel (Virginia Hospital Center – Arlington)

Dani's nurses at the Virginia Hospital Center (VHC) Oncology Wing in Arlington: Katrina, Joanne, Dot, Dina, Erica and Lisa

Dr. Thomas Butler – the senior partner in the oncology practice

Dr. Robert Christie – a partner in the oncology practice and Dani's lead doctor

Dr. Robert Meister – a partner in the oncology practice

Dr. John Feigert – a partner in the oncology practice

Dr. Patricia Rodriguez – a partner in the oncology practice

Dr. John Schnable – the resident assigned to Dani's case at VHC Arlington

Dr. Pamela Herbert – a fourth-year Georgetown medical student assigned to Dani's case

Jack – (known as medical student Jack) a third-year Georgetown medical student
Caroline – a fourth-year medical student who replaced Pamela
Dr. William Furlong – the Infectious Disease Specialist at VHC
Dr. Frederick Schwab – Radiologist at VHC
Dr. Leonardo Mendez – Gastroenterologist at VHC
Dr. Anthony Casolaro – Pulmonary Medicine Specialist at VHC

Medical Personnel (Seattle Cancer Care Alliance)
Dr. Rainier Storb – an oncologist at the Seattle Cancer Care Alliance
Colleen Duffy – Unrelated Donor Search Coordinator SCCA
Dr. Mary Flowers – Director of Long Term Follow-up Care, SCCA
Christy Aplin – social worker
Shoshana Devorah – rabbi/chaplain
Diane Stayboldt – head nurse of the "Blue Team" at the Hutch
Corrine – nurse at University of Washington Medical Center Transplant Wing
Dr. Paul Martin – Oncologist in residence, Dani's first attending physician, SCCA
Betty Stewart – Physician's Assistant, SCCA
Dr. Michael Linenberger – Director of Blood and Blood Component Services SCCA
Dr. Terry Gernsheimer – Director of Transfusion Services SCCA
Dr. F. Mark Stewart – Medical Director/Vice President at SCCA; Dani's attending physician post-transplant at University of Washington Medical Center
Dr. Fred Appelbaum – Director, Clinical Research Division, SCCA and Dani's third attending physician
Dr. George McDonald – Head of the Gastroenterology at the Fred Hutchinson Cancer Research Center
Kerry McMillen - Nutritionist, SCCA
Andréa Leiserowitz - Physical Therapist, SCCA
Dr. Mark Khan – Fertility Specialist, University of Washington